Essentials of Visceral Surgery

Franck Billmann • Tobias Keck
Editors

Essentials of Visceral Surgery

For Residents and Fellows

Springer

Editors
Franck Billmann
Department of General, Visceral and Transplant Surgery
University Hospital Heidelberg
Heidelberg, Germany

Tobias Keck
Department of Surgery
University Hospital Schleswig-Holstein
Lübeck, Germany

1st edition under the title "Specialist knowledge in visceral and general surgery"

This book is a translation of the original German edition „Facharztwissen Viszeralchirurgie" by Billmann, Franck, published by Springer-Verlag GmbH, DE in 2021. The translation was done with the help of artificial intelligence (machine translation by the service DeepL.com). A subsequent human revision was done primarily in terms of content, so that the book will read stylistically differently from a conventional translation. Springer Nature works continuously to further the development of tools for the production of books and on the related technologies to support the authors.

ISBN 978-3-662-66734-7 ISBN 978-3-662-66735-4 (eBook)
https://doi.org/10.1007/978-3-662-66735-4

Planung/Lektorat: Fritz Kraemer

This Springer imprint is published by the registered company Springer-Verlag GmbH, DE, part of Springer Nature.
The registered company address is: Heidelberger Platz 3, 14197 Berlin, Germany

Preface

"First comes the word, second comes the medicine, and last comes the knife"[1]—solid knowledge and a structured knowledge of general and visceral surgery are obligatory prerequisites, especially for doctors in advanced training, fellows and future specialists in general and visceral surgery.

Medical expertise in visceral surgery and bystanding subjects has seen a continuous and rapid increase in knowledge in recent years. The increasing specialization in surgery has led the editors to the present concept of a short compendium, which allows the reader to access the current up-to-date knowledge summarized by specialists in a condensed and clear manner.

Our book aims to provide the readers with a clear understanding of the main aspects of general and visceral surgery. In a condensed, bullet point form, the current and actual knowledge of visceral and general surgery is summarized in this book, to which numerous renowned specialists have contributed in its 16 chapters.

For learning residents and fellows, special emphasis is placed on detailed and precise recommendations concerning the diagnostic procedure and the indication for therapy. The surgical procedure is described step by step in a compact and comprehensive form. New technologies and evidence-based treatment strategies are taken into account and brief overviews facilitate the targeted memorization of the most important facts. This new, completely revised second edition takes into account the rapid development of our field on the one hand and the high response to the book on the other.

For the preparation of the specialist examination in general surgery or visceral surgery, the book is therefore an ideal companion as well as a reference in everyday clinical practice.

Tobias Keck
Lübeck, Germany

Franck Billmann
Heidelberg, Germany
March 2021

1 Christian Albert Theodor Billroth (1829–1894).

Contents

Contributors

Holger Bannasch Department of Plastic, Hand and Aesthetic Surgery, Schwarzwald-Baar-Hospital Villingen-Schwenningen, Villingen-Schwenningen, Germany

Franck Billmann Department of General, Visceral and Transplant Surgery, University Hospital Heidelberg, Heidelberg, Germany

Therezia Bokor-Billmann Department of Dermatology, University Hospital Heidelberg, Heidelberg, Germany

Raoul A. Droeser Clarunis—Universitäres Bauchzentrum Basel, University Hospital Basel, Basel, Switzerland

Michel Gagner Sacré Coeur Hospital, Clinique Michel Gagner, QC, Canada

Courtney Elizabeth Gibson Department of Endocrine Surgery, Smilow Cancer Hospital at Yale, New Haven, CT, USA

Torben Glatz Department of General, Visceral and Vascular Surgery, Marien Hospital Herne, University Hospital Ruhr-University Bochum, Herne, Germany

Henry Hoffmann Center for Hernia Surgery and Proctology, ZweiChirurgen GmbH, Basel, Switzerland

Katrin Hoffmann Department of General, Visceral and Transplant Surgery, University Hospital Heidelberg, Heidelberg, Deutschland

Kim C. Honselmann Department of Surgery, University Hospital Schleswig-Holstein, Luebeck, Germany

Jens Höppner Department of Surgery, University Hospital Schleswig-Holstein, Luebeck, Germany

Bernd Jänigen Department of General, Visceral and Transplant Surgery, University Hospital Freiburg, Freiburg, Germany

Karsten Junge Department of General, Visceral and Minimally-invasive Surgery, Rhein-Maas Hospital, Würselen, Germany

Tobias Keck Department of Surgery, University Medical Center Schleswig-Holstein, Luebeck, Germany

Christoph Kettelhack Clarunis—Universitäres Bauchzentrum Basel, University Hospital Basel, Basel, Switzerland

Thorsten Lindenau Department of General, Visceral and Minimally-invasive Surgery, Rhein-Maas Hospital, Würselen, Germany

Robert Mechera Clarunis—Universitäres Bauchzentrum Basel, University Hospital Basel, Basel, Switzerland

Heidi Misteli Department of Surgery, Hospital Uster, Uster, Switzerland

Didier Mutter Department of Digestive and Endocrine Surgery, NHC, Pôle Hépato-Digestif, University Hospital Strasbourg, Strasbourg, France

Christian A. Nebiker Department of General Surgery, Hospital Aarau, Aarau, Switzerland

Debora Nowakowski Department of Surgery, Hospital Baselland, Basel, Switzerland

Daniel Oertli Department of General Surgery, University Hospital Basel, Basel, Switzerland

Jens Otto Department of General, Visceral and Minimally-invasive Surgery, Rhein-Maas Hospital, Würselen, Germany

Jörg Pelz Department of General, Visceral and Oncological Surgery, St. Bernward Hospital, Hildesheim Hospital, Hildesheim, Germany

Przemyslaw Pisarski Department of General, Visceral and Transplant Surgery, University Hospital Freiburg, Freiburg, Germany

Maren Rudat Interdisciplinary Intensive Care Unit, Sana Kliniken Ostholstein, Eutin Hospital, Eutin, Germany

Peter Schemmer Department of General, Visceral and Transplant Surgery, University Hospital Graz, Graz, Austria

Sebastian Stehr Department of Anesthesiology and Intensive Care Medicine, University Hospital Leipzig, Leipzig, Germany

Athanasios Tampakis Clarunis—Universitäres Bauchzentrum Basel, University Hospital Basel, Basel, Switzerland

Oliver Thomusch Department of General, Visceral and Transplant Surgery, University Hospital Freiburg, Freiburg, Germany

Robert Udelsman Miami Cancer Institute, Miami, FL, USA

Jens Wannenmacher Surgical Department A, Ludwigshafen Hospital, Ludwigshafen, Germany

Benjamin Weixler Department of General and Visceral Surgery, Campus Benjamin Franklin, Charité—University Hospital Berlin, Berlin, Deutschland

Stefan Willis Surgical Department A, Ludwigshafen Hospital, Ludwigshafen, Germany

Abbreviations

γGT	γ-Glutamyl transferase
^{18}F-FDG-PET	^{18}F-fluorodeoxyglucose positron emission tomography
5-ASA	5-aminosalicylic acid
5-FU	5-Fluorouracil
5-HIAA test	5-Hydroxyindolacetic acid test
^{99m}Tc-MIBI	^{99m} Technetium methoxyisobutyl isonitrile
a. a.	From anocutaneous line
AAA	Abdominal aortic aneurysm
AAGBI	Association of Anesthetists of Great Britain and Ireland
Ab	Antibody
ABBA	Axillo-bilateral-breast approach
ABCDE	Airway, breathing, circulation, disability, exposure sequence
ACDC	Acute cholecystitis: early versus delayed cholecystectomy (study)
ACE	Angiotensin-converting enzyme
ACS	Abdominal compartment syndrome
ACTH	Adrenocorticotropic hormone
AD	Autosomal dominant
AEG	Adenocarcinoma of the esophagogastral junction, adenocarcinoma of the esogastric junction
AIDS	Acquired immunodeficiency syndrome
AIS	Abbreviated injury scale
AJCC	American Joint Committee on Cancer
AKS	Abdominal compartment syndrome
ALM	Adenoma like mass
ALT	Atypical lipomatous tumor
AMI	Acute mesenteric ischemia
AMS	Superior mesenteric artery
ANCA	Antineutrophil cytoplasmic antibody
AP	Alkaline phosphatase
APC	Adenomatous colonic polyposis, adenomatous polyposis coli
APP	Abdominal perfusion pressure
Approx.	Approximatively
ASA	American Society of Anesthesiologists
ASCA	Anti-Saccharomyces cerevisiae antibody
ASS	Acetylsalicylic acid
AT II	Angiotensin II
ATA	American Thyroid Association

ATLS	Advanced trauma life support
ATN	Acute tubular necrosis
AVPU Scheme	Alert, voice, pain, unresponsive scheme
AWMF	Arbeitsgemeinschaft der Wissenschaftlichen Medizinischen Fachgesellschaften
BC	Before christ
BDA	Berufsverband Deutscher Anästhesisten
BG	Blood glucose
BIS	Bispectral index
BMI	Body mass index
BPD	Biliopancreatic diversion
BPD/DS	Biliopancreatic diversion with duodenal switch
BS	Blood sugar
BSA	Body surface area
BSR	Blood sedimentation rate
BUN	Blood urea nitrogen
BW	Body weight
CAD	Coronary artery disease
CAEK	Surgical Working Group Endocrinology
CAM-ICU	Confusion Assessment Method/Intensive Care Unit
CAPD	Continuous ambulatory peritoneal dialysis
CAr	Cardiac arrhythmia
CASH	Chemotherapy-Associated Steato Hepatitis
CaSR	Calcium-sensing receptor
CASTLE	Carcinoma with thymus-like differentiation
CC Score	Completeness of cytoreduction score
CCC (or CC)	Cholangiocarcinoma
CCDS	Color-coded Doppler sonography
CCE (also CHE)	Cholecystectomy
CCIS	Cleveland clinic incontinence score
CDD	Classification of diverticular disease
CDUS	Color Doppler ultrasound
CEA	Carcinoembryonic antigen, carcinoembryonal antigen
CEEA	Circular end-to-end anastomosis
CHD	Coronary heart disease
CIBD	Chronic inflammatory bowel disease
CLL	Chronic lymphocytic leukemia
CM	Contrast medium
CME	Complete mesocolic excision
CMI	Chronic mesenteric ischemia
CMS	Circulation, motor function, sensory function
CMV	Cytomegalovirus
CNS	Central nervous system
CO	Cardiac output
COPD	Chronic obstructive pulmonary disease
CRC	Colorectal cancer
CRH	Corticotropin-releasing hormone
CRM	Circumferential resection margin
CRP	C-reactive protein
CRS	Cytoreductive surgery
CSC	Chronic sclerosing cholangitis
CT	Computer tomography
CUSA	Cavitron ultrasonic surgical aspiration
CVC	Central venous catheter
CVD	Cardiovascular disease
CVI	Chronic venous insufficiency
CVL	Central venous line
CVP	Central venous pressure
DALM	Dysplasia-associated lesion or mass
DD	Differential diagnosis
DES	Drug eluting stent
DGF	Delayed graft function
DJ	Double J catheter

DOACs	Direct-acting oral anticoagulants
DPAM	Disseminated peritoneal adenomucinosis
DPPHR	Duodenum preserving pancreas head resection
DSO	German foundation for organ transplantation
Dx	Diagnosis
E.g.	Exempli gratia (for example)
EBV	Ebstein–Barr virus
ECOG	Eastern Cooperative Oncology Group
EDTA	Ethylenediaminetetraacetic acid
EEG	Electroencephalogram
EGAPP	Evaluation of genomic applications in practice and prevention
EGD	Esophagogastroduodenoscopy
EGFR	Epidermal-growth-factor receptor
EMR	Endoscopic mucosal resection
EndoVAC	Endoscopic vacuum therapy
ENETS	European Neuro-Endocrine Tumor Society
EPCAM	Epithelial cell adhesion molecule
ERC	Endoscopic retrograde cholangiography
ERCP	Endoscopic retrograde cholangiopancreaticography
ERD	Erosive reflux esophagitis, erosive reflux disease
ESBL	Extended-spectrum beta-lactamase
ESC	European Society of Cardiology
ESD	Endoscopic submucosal dissection
ESDR	End-stage renal disease
ESMO	European Society for Medical Oncology
ESP	Eurotransplant senior program
ESR	Erythrocyte sedimentation rate
ET	Eurotransplant
etc.	et cetera
ETKAS	Eurotransplant kidney allocation system
EUS	Endoscopic ultrasound
FAMMM Syndrome	Familial atypical multiple birthmark melanoma syndrome
FAP	Familial adenomatous polyposis
FAST	Focused assessment with sonography in trauma
FB	Finger breadth
FHH	Familial hypocalciuric hypercalcemia
Fig.	Figure
FISH	Fluorescence in situ hybridization
FLR	Functional liver volume after resection
FMTC	Familial medullary thyroid cancer
FNA	Fine needle aspiration cytology
FNCLCC	Fédération Nationale des Centres de Lutte Contre le Cancer
FNH	Focal nodular hyperplasia
FNMTC	Familial non-medullary thyroid cancer
FOBT	Fecal occult blood test
FPTC	Familial papillary thyroid cancer
Fri	French (= Charriere)
fT3, fT4	Free triiodothyronine (fT3), free thyroxine (fT4)
FTC	Follicular thyroid carcinoma, follicular thyroid cancer
G6PD	Glucose-6-phosphate dehydrogenase
GC	General condition
GERD	Gastroesophageal reflux disease
GFR	Glomerular filtration rate

GI tract	Gastrointestinal tract
GIA	Gastrointestinal anastomosis
GIST	Gastrointestinal stromal tumors
GLP-1	Glucagon-like peptide 1
GM-CSF	Granulocyte macrophage colony-stimulating factor
GOT	Glutamate oxaloacetate transaminase = aspartate aminotransferase, AST or ASAT
GPT	Glutamate pyruvate transaminase = Alanine aminotransferase, ALT or ALAT
HAL	Hemorrhoidal artery ligation
HBV	Hepatitis B virus
HCC	Hepatocellular carcinoma
HCV	Hepatitis C virus
HD	High definition
HDi	Hemodialysis
HIPEC	Hyperthermic intraperitoneal chemotherapy
HIT	Heparin-induced thrombocytopenia
HIV	Human immunodeficiency virus
HLA	Human leucocyte antigen
HNF-1alpha	Hepatocyte nuclear factor 1alpha
HNPCC	Hereditary non-polyposis colorectal cancer
HP	Helicobacter pylori
HPF	High power field
HPT-JT	Hyperparathyroidism-jaw tumor syndrome
HPV	Human papillomaviruses
HSV	Herpes simplex virus
HTK	Histidine tryptophan ketoglutarate
HU	High urgency
HUS	Hemolytic uremic syndrome
IAD	Intra-abdominal pressure
IAH	Intra-abdominal hypertension
IAP	Intra-abdominal pressure
IBD	Inflammatory bowel disease, chronic inflammatory bowel disease
IC	Incontinence index
ICS	Intercostal space
ICU	Intensive care unit
ICV	Ileocecal valve
IDC	Indwelling urinary catheter
IDDM	Insulin-dependent diabetes mellitus
IEN	Intraepithelial neoplasia
IFN	Interferon
IH	Inguinal hernia
ILP	Isolated limb perfusion
IMC	Intermediate care
INR	International normalized ratio
IORT	Intraoperative radiotherapy
IPMN	Intraductal papillary-mucinous neoplasia
IPOM	Intraperitoneal onlay mesh
IPST	Intraperitoneal stoma mesh
IRE	Irreversible electroporation
ISGLS	International Study Group of Liver Surgery
ITP	Idiopathic thrombocytopenic purpura
KCl	Potassium chloride
KLLN	Killin
KT	Kidney transplantation
KTx	Kidney transplantation
LAD	Lymphadenectomy
LAGB	Laparoscopic adjustable gastric banding
LAR	Low anterior resection
LARR	Low anterior rectal resection
LDH	Lactate dehydrogenase
LDL	Low density lipoprotein
LDP	Lloyd Davis position, modified Lloyd Davis position

LIFT	Ligation of intersphincteric fistula tract
Lig.	Ligament
LMWH	Low molecular weight heparin
LN	Lymph nodes
LRFS	Local relapse-free survival
MALS	Median arcuate ligament syndrome
MALT	Lymphoid tissue of the mucosa-associated type, mucosa-associated lymphoid tissue
MAO	Monoaminooxidase
MAP	Mean arterial pressure
MCN	Mucinous cystadenoma, mucinous cystic neoplasm
MCP	Metoclopramide
MELD	Model for end-stage liver disease
MEN 1	Multiple endocrine neoplasia type 1
MET	Metabolic equivalent of task
MFH	Myxoid fibrous histiocytoma
Min.	Minute(s)
MIVAP	Minimally invasive video-assisted parathyroidectomy
MIVAT	Minimally invasive video-assisted thyroidectomy
MMP	Mismatch probability
MMR	Mismatch repair
Mod.	Modified
MODY	Maturity onset diabetes of the young
MPNST	Malignant peripheral nerve sheath tumor
MRCP	Magnetic resonance cholangiopancreatography
MRI	Magnetic resonance imaging
MRSA	Methicillin-resistant Staphylococcus aureus
MRSE	Methicillin-resistant Staphylococcus epidermidis
MSH	Melanocyte-stimulating hormone
MSI	Microsatellite instability
MTC	Medullary thyroid cancer
NAFLD	Non-alcoholic fatty liver disease
NASH	Non-alcoholic fatty liver hepatitis, non-alcoholic steatohepatitis
NCCN	National comprehensive cancer network
NCH/ NSY	Neurosurgery
NEN	Neuroendocrine neoplasia
NERD	Non-erosive reflux disease
NET	Neuroendocrine tumor
NF-NET	Non-Functional NET
NIBPM	Non-invasive blood pressure measurement
NMTC	Non-medullary thyroid cancer
NOA/ NOACs	New oral anticoagulants
NOMI	Non-occlusive mesenteric ischemia
NOTES	Natural orifice transluminal endoscopic surgery
NRS	Numerical rating scale
NSAID	Non-steroidal anti-inflammatory drugs
NSHPT	Neonatal severe hyperparathyroidism
Nu-DESC	Nursing delirium screening scale
NYHA	New York Heart Association
OAD	Oral antidiabetics
ODS	Obstructive defecation syndrome
OGTT	Oral glucose tolerance test
OPSI	Overwhelming post-splenectomy infection
OSAS	Obstructive sleep apnea syndrome
OTSC	Over-the-scope-clip
P_aO_2	Arterial oxygen partial pressure
PACU	Post-anesthesia care unit

PAD	Peripheral artery disease
p-ANCA	Perinuclear anti-neutrophil cytoplasmic antibody, perinuclear cytoplasmic antibody
PAOD	Peripheral arterial occlusive disease
PAP	Perioperative antibiotic prophylaxis
PBC	Primary biliary cirrhosis
PCI	Peritoneal cancer index
PCR	Polymerase chain reaction
PCT	Procalcitonin
PDC	Peridural catheter
PDGFRA	Platelet-derived growth factor receptor α
PDS	Polydioxanone
PE	Physical exam
PEEP	Positive end-expiratory pressure
PEI	Percutaneous Ethanol Injection
PET	Positron emission tomography
PG	Parathyroid gland
PHLF	Posthepatectomy liver failure
pHPT	Primary hyperparathyroidism
PICCO	Pulse index continuous cardiac output
PIPAC	Pressurized intraperitoneal aerosol chemotherapy
PMCA	Peritoneal mucinous carcinomatosis
PME	Partial mesorectal excision
PNE	Percutaneous nerve evaluation
pNET	Neuroendocrine tumor of the pancreas
PNET	Primitive neuroectodermal tumor
POCD	Postoperative cognitive deficit
POEM	Peroral endoscopic myotomy
POMC	Proopiomelanocortin
PONV	Postoperative nausea and vomiting
POPF	Postoperative pancreatic fistula
PostR	Postoperative radiotherapy
PPH	Post-pancreatectomy hemorrhage
PPI	Proton pump inhibitor
PPNAD	Primary pigmented nodular adrenocortical disease
PPPD	Pylorus-preserving pancreaticoduodenectomy (pancreatic head resection)
PRA	Panel reactive antibodies
PRBCs	Packed red blood cells
PrR	Preoperative radiotherapy
PSA	Prostate-specific antigen
PSC	Primary sclerosing cholangitis
PSDSS	Peritoneal surface disease severity score
PT	Prothrombin time
PTA	Percutaneous transluminal angioplasty
PTC	Papillary thyroid cancer
PTCD/PTBD	Percutaneous transhepatic cholangiodrainage/Percutaneous transhepatic biliary drainage
PTEN	Phosphatase and tensin homolog
PTH	Parathormone
PTHC	Percutaneous transhepatic cholangiography
PTHrP	Parathyroid hormone-related peptide
PTT	Partial thromboplastin time, partial thromboplastin time
PTU	Propylthiouracil
PUMP	Preperitoneal umbilical hernia mesh plasty
R status	Residual status
RAMPS	Radical antegrade modular pancreatosplenectomy
RCR	Revised cardiac risk

RET gene	Rearranged-during-transfection gene
RFA/RFTA	Radiofrequency ablation/radiofrequency thermoablation
RPS	Retroperitoneal sarcoma
RR	Recovery room
RYGB	Roux-en-Y Gastric Bypass
SADI-S	Single anastomosis duodeno-ileal bypass with sleeve gastrectomy
SB-NET	Small bowel neuroendocrine tumor
SBO	Small bowel obstruction
SCM	Sternocleidomastoid muscle
SCN	Serous cystadenoma, serous cystic neoplasm
SDH	Succinate dehydrogenase
Sect.	Section
SEER	Surveillance, epidemiology, and end results program
SETTLE	Spindle epithelial tumor with thymus-like differentiation
sFLR	Standardized functional liver volume, standardized future liver remnant
SG	Sleeve gastrectomy
sHPT	Secondary hyperparathyroidism
SIBO	Small intestinal bacterial overgrowth
SIRS	Systemic inflammatory response syndrome
SIRT	Selective internal radiotherapy
SLAF	Subcutaneous linea alba fasciotomy
SMA	Smooth muscle actin
SNM	Sacral nerve modulation
SNS	Sacral nerve stimulation
SPECT	Single photon emission computed tomography
SPN	Solid pseudopapillary neoplasia
SpO_2	Pulsoximetric oxygen saturation
SPPT	Solid pseudopapillary neoplasia, solid pseudopapillary tumor (of the pancreas)
SSI	Infection of a surgical site, surgical site infection
STARR	Stapled transanal rectal resection
STIKO	Ständige Impfkommission (Robert Koch Institut)
STS	Soft tissue sarcoma
SUDD	Symptomatic uncomplicated diverticular disease
SUV	Standardized uptake value
T3	Triiodothyronine
T4	Thyroxine
TACE	Transarterial chemoembolization
TAMIS	Transanal minimally invasive surgery
TAPP	Transabdominal preperitoneal plasty
TaTME	Transanal Total Mesorectal Excision
TEM/TEO	Transanal endoscopic microsurgery/surgery
TEP	Total extraperitoneal plasty
Tg	Thyroglobulin
TgAb	Thyroglobulin antibody
tHPT	Tertiary hyperparathyroidism
Thyroid	Thyroid gland
TLV	Total liver volume
TME	Total mesorectal excision

TNF	Tumor necrosis factor
TNM	Tumor node metastasis (classification)
TPG/GTA	German transplant act
TPHA	Treponema pallidum hemagglutination assay, test for infection with the causative agent of syphilis (lues)
TPIAT	Total pancreatectomy with autologous islet cell transplantation
TPO-MAb = TPO-Ab = MAb	Thyroid peroxidase antibodies = microsomal antibodies
TRAb	TSH receptor autoantibodies
TRF	Thyrotropin = TSH-releasing factor
TRH	Thyrotropin-releasing hormone
TSH	Thyroid-stimulating hormone
TTR amyloidosis	Transthyretin amyloidosis
TTR	Transthyretin
UCSF	University of California San Francisco
UFH	Unfractionated heparin
UGI	Upper gastrointestinal
UGIT	Upper gastrointestinal tract
UICC	Union for International Cancer Control
US	Ultrasound, sonography
USD	US Dollar
VAS	Visual analogue scale
VATS	Video-assisted thoracoscopy
VBG (VBP)	Vertical banded gastroplasty (Vertical banded Gastro plasty)
VRAM	Vertical rectus abdominis myocutaneous flap
VRE	Vancomycin-resistant enterococci
VZV	Varicella-Zoster virus
WBC	White blood cell count
WDTC	Well-differentiated thyroid cancer
WHO	World Health Organization
WSACS	World Society of Abdominal Compartment Syndrome

Esophagus, Stomach and Duodenum

Torben Glatz and Jens Höppner

Contents

F. Billmann, T. Keck (eds.), *Essentials of Visceral Surgery*,
https://doi.org/10.1007/978-3-662-66735-4_1

1.1 Anatomy and Physiology

1.1.1 Esophagus

- Cervical, thoracic and abdominal esophagus (total length approx. 25–28 cm)
- Physiological esophageal constrictions at the upper esophageal sphincter, tracheal bifurcation and lower esophageal sphincter
- Transition from the hypopharynx with striated, voluntarily innervated musculature to the esophagus with smooth musculature
- Histologically lined with squamous epithelium
- Transport function for food pulp and saliva

1.1.2 Stomach

- The cardia, fundus, corpus and antrum form the stomach (◘ Fig. 1.1)
- Sphincter muscle at the stomach outlet (pylorus)
- Histologically lined with cylindrical epithelium
- Blood supply via arcade from right and left gastric artery (small curvature), arcade from left and right gastroomental artery (large curvature) as well as short gastric vessels
- Reservoir function for food pulp
- Production of pepsin and hydrochloric acid for digestion
- Production of intrinsic factor (vitamin B_{12} absorption in the terminal ileum)

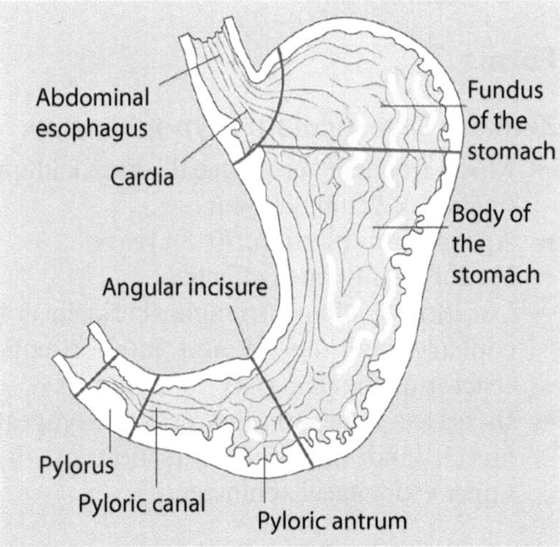

◘ **Fig. 1.1** Classification of the stomach according to external shape. (Mod. according to von Lanz and Wachsmuth 2004)

1.1.3 Duodenum

- Superior part, descending part, inferior part, ascending part of the duodenum (pars I–IV duodeni)
- Common orifice of bile duct and pancreatic duct at the major duodenal papilla (papilla Vateri) in the descending part, sometimes accessory pancreatic duct with separate orifice into the duodenum (minor duodenal papilla)
- Histologically lined with cylindrical epithelium
- Blood supply via gastroduodenal artery as well as branches of the superior mesenteric artery (sup. and inf. pancreatoduodenal artery, Rio-Branko arcade to gastroduodenal artery)
- Mixture of food pulp with bile and pancreatic secretions

1.2 Leading Symptoms and Diagnosis

1.2.1 Leading Symptoms

- Different for esophagus and stomach/duodenum

Esophagus
- Swallowing disorders/dysphagia
- Regurgitation of food
- Retrosternal pain
- Weight loss

Stomach
- Upper abdominal pain
- Regurgitation
- Weight loss

Upper GI Bleeding

- Vomiting blood (hematemesis)/tarry stools (hematochezia)/anemia

1.2.2 Diagnosis

Endoscopy

- Esophagogastroduodenoscopy (EGD)
- Endosonography for staging examination of neoplasms
- Manometry for the diagnosis of the movement disorders of the esophageal musculature
- 24 h-pH-metry, impedance measurement for the diagnosis of gastroesophageal reflux disease

Radiology/Nuclear Medicine

- Contrast esophagogram
- Computed tomography chest/abdomen
- MRI and PET-CT for special indications
- Gastric emptying scintigraphy

1.2.3 Therapeutic Principles

- Conservative
- Endoscopic
- Surgical

1.3 Benign Diseases of the Esophagus

Summary

- Diverticular disease:
  - Zenker's diverticulum
  - Midesophageal diverticulum
  - Epiphrenic diverticulum
- Achalasia:
  - Endoscopic and surgical therapy
- Gastroesophageal reflux disease (GERD)/hiatal hernias
  - Axial hiatal hernia
  - Paraesophageal hiatal hernia
  - Gastroesophageal reflux disease—Diagnosis
  - Gastroesophageal reflux disease—pharmacological and surgical therapy
- Esophageal perforations

1.3.1 Diverticular Diseases of the Esophagus

Etiology

Zenker's Diverticulum and Epiphrenic Diverticulum (Pulsion Diverticulum)

- Due to a mismatch between increased intraluminal pressure and anatomical muscle gap; preferentially at predilection sites above the esophageal sphincter
- Pseudodiverticulum (diverticular sac consists only of mucosa and submucosa)

Midesophageal Diverticulum (Traction Diverticulum)

- Diverticulum includes all wall layers of the esophagus
- Due to traction on the esophagus from outside, e.g. due to residual embryonic tissue connections between trachea and esophagus or also in the context of inflammatory processes in the mediastinum
- Located mostly in the middle esophagus
- Overall very rare

Forms

Zenker's Diverticulum (Hypopharynx)

- Most frequent esophageal diverticulum (incidence 2:100,000/year)
- Age of manifestation: 70–80 years
- Predominantly men affected
- Location: Killian's triangle (between cricopharyngeal muscle and inferior constrictor of the pharynx)
- Increased tone of the cricopharyngeal muscle and impaired relaxation of the upper esophageal sphincter

Killian-Jamison Diverticulum

- Pulsion diverticulum
- Origin immediately below the upper sphincter

- Localization ventrolaterally under the cricopharyngeal muscle or
- Localization dorsal through the Laimer triangle
- Mostly small and asymptomatic diverticula

Epiphrenic Diverticulum

- Pulsion diverticulum
- Localized up to 10 cm above the Z-line
- Much rarer than Zenker's diverticulum
- Development due to increased intraluminal pressure
- Usually associated with achalasia or diffuse esophageal spasm

Symptoms

- Dysphagia
- Regurgitation of undigested food
- Foetor ex ore
- Chronic cough and aspiration of food debris
- Recurrent pneumonias
- Lump feeling in the throat
- Cervical borborygmi (pathognomonic in Zenker diverticulum)
- Retrosternal pain and heartburn (epiphrenic diverticula)

Therapy

Zenker-Diverikel

- Cervical diverticular resection and myotomy of the cricopharyngeal muscle
- Cervical diverticulopexy and myotomy of the cricopharyngeal muscle
- Endoscopic interventional transoral splitting (stapler, laser, needle knife)

Epiphrenic Diverticulum

Caution

Treatment of the underlying esophageal motility disorder required.

- Laparoscopic diverticulotomy and myotomy of the lower esophageal sphincter (+/– fundoplication)
- Transthoracic diverticulotomy and myotomy of the lower esophageal sphincter

1.3.2 Achalasia

- Incidence = 1/100,000 population/year

Etiology

Pathogenesis

- Degeneration of the myenteric plexus
- Lack of relaxation of the lower esophageal sphincter

Forms

Primary Achalasia

- Etiology unknown

Secondary Achalasia

- Chagas disease
- Gastric Cancer
- Esophageal Cancer

Symptoms

- Dysphagia
- Regurgitation of food
- Retrosternal pain
- Aspiration

Complications

- Aspiration pneumonia
- Esophageal cancer (increased incidence in achalasia)

Staging

- Stage I: Hypermotile form
- Stage II: Hypomotile form
- Stage III: Amotile form

Diagnosis

Esophagogastroduodenoscopy (EGD)

- Exclusion of malignancy and benign stenosis

Manometry

- Pressure measurement in the esophagus via probe
- Slow retraction of the probe during the swallowing act and digital recording and evaluation of peristalsis

1

- Highest sensitivity for the diagnosis of achalasia
- Findings: Combination of hypermotility/hypomotility/peristalsis and lack of relaxation of the lower esophageal sphincter

X-Ray (Esophagogram)/Computed Tomography

- Classic "champagne glass" shape of the esophagus with prestenotic dilatation

Therapy

Medical Therapy

Principle

- Drug-induced relaxation of the smooth muscle fibers of the lower esophageal sphincter

Preparations

- Calcium channel blockers (e.g. nifedipine)
- Long-acting nitrates
- Phosphodiesterase-5 inhibitor (sildenafil)

Drug Therapy

- Best results with nifedipine (10–30 mg) sublingually approx. 30 min before a meal (leads to a relaxation of the lower oesophageal sphincter lasting approx. 60 min).
- Overall, the effect of drug therapy is usually not satisfactory: persistence of symptoms and side effects of the drugs (headache, hypotension, etc.).

Endoscopic Therapy

Pneumatic Dilatation

- Dilatation with special balloon under fluoroscopy or under endoscopic guidance
- Disruption of the muscle fibers of the lower esophageal sphincter
- Multiple applications are often necessary, but long-term alleviation of symptoms is possible in up to 50–80% of patients
- Risk of esophageal perforation due to dilatation

Endoscopic Injection of Botulinum Toxin

- Low risk procedure
- High initial response rate (>75%)
- Frequent early recurrences (50%)

Peroral Endoscopic Myotomy (POEM)

- Endoscopic alternative to surgical myotomy
- Procedure:
  - Endoscopic incision of the mucosa, then submucosal tunnelling and long-stretch myotomy by diathermy
- In the short-term follow-up results comparable with the surgical procedure
- Centre-based expertise

Surgical Therapy

Surgical Therapy Options

- Myotomy of the lower esophageal sphincter possible via laparoscopy, laparotomy or thoracotomy (Vaezi et al. 2013) or robotically-assisted
- Gold standard: Laparoscopic Heller myotomy + fundoplication
- For stage III: discuss esophagectomy with gastric tube reconstruction

Results After Myotomy

- Partial or complete relief of symptoms in 90% of patients
- 30% of the patients develop reflux symptoms postoperatively, therefore an additional fundoplication is mandatory

Surgical Procedure

Laparoscopic Heller Myotomy

- Supine position with spread legs
- Insertion of the camera trocar, insertion of the pneumoperitoneum; operation may be robotically assisted
- Exposure of the esophageal hiatus by means of a liver retractor and positioning of the patient
- Ventral mobilization of the esophagus into the lower mediastinum
- Identification and protection of the vagus nerve
- Longitudinal severing of the muscle fibres of the lower oesophageal sphinc-

ter including cardia while sparing the mucosal tube
- Covering the defect with an anterior fundoplication (► Sect. 1.3.5), or Nissen fundoplication

1.3.3 Esophageal Perforation

Summary

- Different etiologies (malignant, spontaneous, iatrogenic)
- Life-threatening disease
- Therapy today mostly endoscopic (stent or endoluminal vacuum therapy EndoVAC)
- Surgical therapy (primary suture + fundoplication or muscle flap) as effective therapy option

Etiology

- Iatrogenic:
  - As a result of endoscopic procedures (EGD, ERCP, endosonography)
  - Complication of cardiothoracic surgery
  - Gastric tube
- Malignant:
  - Tumor perforation due to esophageal cancer
- Spontaneous:
  - Boerhaave Syndrome
  - Often as a result of sudden vomiting
  - Lower/middle third esophageal rupture

Symptoms

- Acute chest pain:
  - Differential Diagnosis:
    - Myocardial Infarction
    - Pulmonary Embolism
    - Aortic dissection
  - Frequently misdiagnosed
- Hematemesis
- Dyspnea
- Fever
- Complications:
  - Mediastinitis
  - Pleural effusion/empyema
  - Pneumothorax
  - Septic shock

Diagnosis

Endoscopy (EGD)

- Localization of the perforation
- Assessment of the size of the perforation

Computed Tomography of the chest

- Oral and intravenous contrast agent
- Confirmation of transmural perforation
- Detection of pleural empyema/mediastinal abscess

Therapy

- Closure of the perforation
- Endoluminal vacuum therapy
- Drainage of the contaminated cavities (mediastinum, pleura)

Surgical Therapy

- Primary suture of the esophageal perforation
- Additional coverage by means of fundoplication or muscle flap
- Insertion of mediastinal drains
- Insertion of chest drain(s)
- Video-assisted thoracoscopy (VATS) for pleural empyema
- Ultima Ratio: Esophageal resection and reconstruction via gastric tube or diversion

Endoscopic Therapy

- Actually Gold standard
- Less invasive and comparably effective
- Endoscopic insertion of a partially coated metal stent
- Endoscopic vacuum therapy-EndoVAC
- Over-the-scope clip (OTSC) only for small and recent perforations

Conservative Therapy

- Indicated only in palliative situation or very old perforation without sepsis
- Transcutaneous or endoluminal drainage of the contaminated cavity

1

Prognostic Factors

- Delayed therapy (>48 h) unfavourable
- Septic shock at the time of therapy
- Spontaneous esophageal perforation (Boerhaave syndrome; Connelly et al. 2013)
- Size and localization of the perforation not prognostically relevant

1.3.4 Hiatal Hernias

Etiology

- Acquired pathology in the majority of patients
- Risk factors:
  - Overweight
  - Pregnancy
  - Connective tissue aging

Types of Hiatal Hernias (■ Fig. 1.2)

Cardiofundal Malposition

- Mildest type
- Often incidental finding

Axial Sliding Hernia

- 90% of all hernias
- Intrathoracic position of the gastric cardia

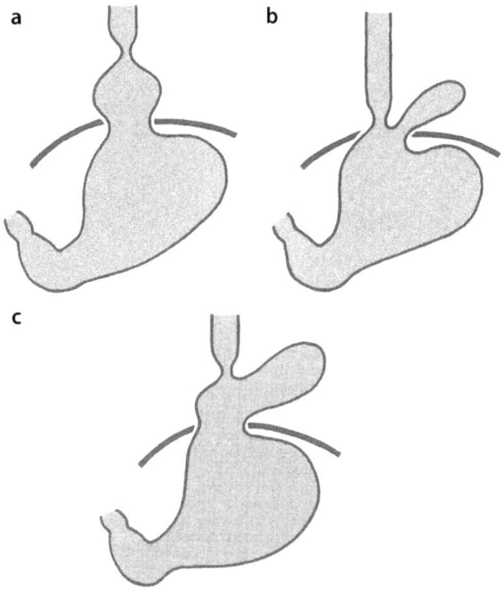

■ Fig. 1.2 Types of hiatal hernia. (a) Axial sliding hernia. (b) Paraesophageal hernia. (c) Mixed Hernia. (From von Lanz and Wachsmuth 2004)

Paraesophageal Hernia

- Lower esophageal sphincter intraabdominal
- Partial or complete intrathoracic stomach (upside-down stomach)

Mixed Forms

- Rarely, additional herniation of omentum, small or large intestine

Symptoms

Axial Hernias

- Often asymptomatic (90%)
- But predisposition for gastroesophageal reflux with insufficient function of the lower esophageal sphincter

Paraesophageal Hernias

- Initially often asymptomatic as well
- Possibly postprandial unspecific abdominal or thoracic complaints
- Complications:
  - Dysphagia
  - Incarceration
  - Ulceration
  - Chronic anemia
  - Dyspnea

Therapy

Symptomatic Therapy

- Proton-pump inhibitors
- See below: Therapy of reflux disease (► Sect. 1.3.5)

Surgical Therapy

- Strategy: Reduction of the hernia, anterior and/or posterior hiatoplasty, fundoplication or gastropexy
- Indication:
  - In axial hernia only in case of symptomatic reflux (GERD, 24 h pH-metry, volume reflux, metaplasia)
  - Indication for elective surgical intervention for paraesophageal hernia
  - Emergency indication for incarcerated hernias (usually paraesophageal)

Reinforcement of hiatoplasty by reinforcement with non-resorbable or bioresorbable mesh possible, benefit not proven. Risk of injury of esophagus or severe complications.

1.3.5 Gastroesophageal Reflux Disease (GERD)

Summary

- GERD subsumes different disease entities
- Prevalence: 15% of the western population
- Multifactorial pathophysiology
- Therapy initially conservative with proton pump inhibitors (PPI)
- Laparoscopic fundoplication as an effective therapeutic option in case of failure of drug therapy or patient preference

Definition

- "GERD" = "gastroesophageal reflux disease"
- The term subsumes the following entities:
  - Erosive reflux esophagitis of various degrees of severity (ERD)
  - Non-erosive reflux disease (NERD)
  - Hypersensitive esophagus
  - Extraesophageal manifestations
  - Complications of GERD
  - Functional reflux complaints

Etiology

Demographics

- Prevalence: about 15% with increasing incidence
- Approximately 50% of patients with GERD do not have endoscopically definable lesions (NERD)
- Approx. 5% of GERD patients develop Barrett's esophagus = intestinal metaplasia of the epithelium in the (distal) esophagus

Pathophysiology and Risk Factors

- Pathophysiology:
  - Primary GERD: Unclear dysfunction of the lower esophageal sphincter
  - Secondary GERD: in the context of other diseases or as a consequence of surgical treatment (esophageal cancer, post-heller myotomy)
- Predisposing factors (due to dysfunction of the lower esophageal sphincter):
  - Pregnancy
  - Obesity
  - Hiatal Hernia
  - Nutritional factors
- Predisposing factors (due to irritating reflux):
  - Overproduction of gastric acid, e.g. due to Helicobacter pylori
  - Alkaline reflux (e.g. bile reflux after gastrectomy)
  - Alcohol, coffee, nicotine, various drugs affect both the lower esophageal sphincter and gastric content
- Frequently increased symptoms postprandially and due to bending or pressing

Symptoms

- Chief complaint = heartburn
- Other symptoms:
  - Diffuse epigastric pain
  - Retrosternal pain
  - Belching
  - Volume reflux with regurgitation of food residues
  - Dysphagia
  - Irritative cough, hoarseness

Diagnosis

Esophagogastroduodenoscopy (EGD)

- Detection of erosive lesions
- Classification according to the Los-Angeles classification (◘ Table 1.1)
- Often no correlation between intensity of complaints and endoscopic findings

◘ **Table 1.1** Los-Angeles classification of gastroesophageal reflux disease

Stage	Findings
A	Erosions <5 mm
B	Erosions >5 mm
C	Confluent erosions <75% of circumference
D	Confluent erosions >75% of circumference

1

- Exclusion of complication:
  - Stenosis
  - Barrett's Esophagus
  - Dysplasia
  - Ulceration
  - Esophageal Cancer

24 h pH-Metry/Impedance Measurement

- Quantification of gastroesophageal reflux via probe
- Prior discontinuation of PPI
- Highest sensitivity and specificity for the detection of GERD

With pH-metry only acid reflux is detected, with impedance measurement: detection of any type of reflux.

Manometry

- Relevant for the exclusion of motility disorders, especially before surgical therapy (fundoplication, magnetic sphincter augmentation)
- Hypomotility of the distal esophagus often associated with long-lasting GERD
- Details ► Sect. 1.3.2

Therapy

Conservative Therapy

- Changes in "life style": weight loss, avoidance of noxious substances, sleeping with the upper body elevated, discontinuation of triggering medications
- Medical: Proton pump inhibitors (PPI)
- Objective: Symptom control and healing of existing erosions
- Therapy failure of PPI: always detailed diagnosis with endoscopy and pH-metry/impedance measurement
- Asymptomatic erosive reflux esophagitis: therapy indicated

Surgical Therapy

- Indication:
  - Long-term need for therapy
  - Inadequate symptom control with PPI
  - Volume reflux
  - Side effects of drug therapy
  - Patient preference
- Operation of choice = laparoscopic fundoplication:
  - 360°—Nissen, 270° posterior—Toupet
  - Always with hiatoplasty (if necessary reduction of a hiatal hernia)
- Results:
  - Success rate approx. 85% with thorough patient selection
  - Lower success rate for re-operation (re-fundoplication)

! Even after surgical treatment, endoscopic controls are recommended for pre-existing Barrett's esophagus.

Surgical Procedure

Laparoscopic Fundoplication 360° According to Nissen

- Supine split-legs position (french position)
- Insertion of the camera trocar, insertion of the pneumoperitoneum; robot-assisted operation possible
- Exposure of the esophageal hiatus by means of a liver retractor and positioning of the patient
- Visualisation of the left and right diaphragmatic crus
- Mobilization of the esophagus into the lower mediastinum, with creation retroesophageal window
- Identification of the vagal nerve
- Partial mobilization of the gastric fundus (division short gastric vessels)
- Calibration of the esophagus with large lumen gastric tube (bougie)
- Posterior hiatoplasty with non-absorbable suture material
- Retroesophageal pulling of the fundus
- Creation of the wrap: suture of the retroesophageal fundus anterior to additional part of fundus with 2–3 non-absorbable sutures
- Fixation of the wrap to the esophagus with distal suture

1.3.6 Guidelines

AWMF guideline registry: gastroesophageal reflux disease (German Society of Gastroenterology, Digestive and Metabolic Diseases, AWMF), 2014, AWMF registration number: 021/013—valid until May 31, 2019 currently under revision (7/2020).

1.4 Malignant Diseases of the Esophagus

1.4.1 Overview

Esophageal Cancer

- Squamous cell carcinoma
- Adenocarcinoma
- Adenosquamous carcinomas, undifferentiated carcinomas

Adenocarcinoma of the Gastroesophageal Junction (AEG)

- AEG 1, AEG 2 and AEG 3 with esophageal infiltration are classified as esophageal carcinoma according to UICC TNM 8th version (2017). Differentiation AEG 1–3: according to the epicenter of the tumor, not the upper margin.

1.4.2 Esophageal Carcinoma (Including AEG)

Summary

- Squamous cell carcinoma vs. adenocarcinoma: different etiology and tumor biology
- Leading symptoms: Dysphagia, weight loss, hematemesis
- Pretherapeutic staging: EGD/endosonography/CT (cTNM + histology)
- Neoadjuvant therapy for T3 or any T with N+: Neoadjuvant radiochemotherapy (adenocarcinoma and squamous cell carcinoma) or perioperative chemotherapy for adenocarcinoma
- Operative standard: Thoracoabdominal esophagectomy with 2-field lymphadenectomy and advancement of stomach into right chest and esophagogastric anastomosis
- High rate of postoperative complications after esophagectomy
- Minimally invasive laparoscopic and robotic-assisted procedures with potential benefits in terms of postoperative morbidity
- Minimally invasive abdominal gastric mobilisation/advancement (hybrid OP) with evidence-based (Ib) advantages
- In case of functional or oncological inoperability definitive radiochemotherapy or systemic chemotherapy, if necessary palliative insertion of esophageal stents

Definition

- All epithelial malignancies between upper and lower esophageal sphincter
- Adenocarcinomas of the gastroesophageal junction with infiltration of the esophagus are defined as esophageal carcinoma (UICC TNM 8)

Types

Adenocarcinoma

- 95% in the distal esophagus

Adenocarcinoma of the Gastroesophageal Junction (AEG)

- Definition: All adenocarcinomas with tumor center 5 cm proximal to 5 cm distal to the gastroesophageal junction. Definition by tumour epicentre, not upper margin (UICC 8th version)
- Classification according to Siewert:
  - AEG 1: Tumour centre 1–5 cm proximal to the gastro-esophageal junction
  - AEG 2: Tumour centre from 1 cm proximal to 2 cm distal to the gastroesophageal junction
  - AEG 3: Tumour centre 2–5 cm distal to the gastro-esophageal junction

Squamous Cell Carcinoma
- May occur throughout the esophagus

Adenosquamous Carcinomas, Undifferentiated Carcinomas
- Rare entities

Epidemiology and Etiology

Occurrence
- Approx. 6000 new cases in Germany/year
- Significant increase in the incidence of adenocarcinoma in Europe and the USA
- 80% men, 20% women

Risk Factors
Squamous Cell Carcinoma
- Nicotine abuse
- Alcohol abuse
- Achalasia
- History of radiation therapy in the head and neck region

Adenocarcinoma
- Gastroesophageal reflux disease
- Barrett's Esophagus
- Nicotine abuse
- Achalasia

Tumor Spread

Continuous Spread
- Intramural
- Direct organ infiltration (pericardium, pleura, aorta)

Lymphogenous Spread
- Lymph node levels: cervical, mediastinal and abdominal

Hematogenous Spread
- Hepatic: via portal vein
- Pulmonary, osseous or cerebral: via vena cava or liver

Classification
UICC/AJCC TNM 8 Classification (2017)
- T (Tumor)
  - TX Tumor cannot be assessed
  - T0 No primary tumor detectable
  - Tis High-grade dysplasia (malignant cells above the basement membrane)
  - T1a Infiltration of the lamina propria and muscularis mucosa
  - T1b Infiltration of the tela submucosa (further subcategories)
  - T2 Infiltration of the tunica muscularis
  - T3 Infiltration of the adventitia
  - T4a Infiltration of pleura, pericardium, peritoneum, azygos vein or diaphragm
  - T4b Infiltration of other organs, such as aorta, vertebral body or trachea
- N (Lymph nodes)
  - NX Regional lymph nodes cannot be assessed
  - N0 No metastases in the lymph nodes
  - N1 Metastases in 1–2 regional lymph nodes
  - N2 Metastases in 3–6 regional lymph nodes
  - N3 Metastases in 7 or more regional lymph nodes
- M (Metastases)
  - M0 No Distant Metastasis
  - M1 Distant Metastasis(es)

UICC Stages According to the TNM Classification 8th Version (2017)

Stage 0	Tis	N0	M0
Stage I	T1	N0	M0
Stage IIa	T1	N1	M0
Stage IIb	T2	N0	M0
Stage III	T2	N1	M0
	T3–4a	N0–1	M0
Stage IVa	T1–4a	N2	M0
	T4b	N0–2	M0
	T1–4	N3	M0
	Any T	N3	M0
Stage IVb	Any T	Any N	M1

Symptoms
- Weight loss
- Retrosternal pain
- Hematemesis/melena/anemia

Diagnosis

Esophagogastroduodenoscopy (EGD)

- Biopsy
- Confirmation of tumor diagnosis
- Localization of the tumor

Endosonography

- Infiltration depth
- Assessment of T- and N-stage

Thoracic CT, Abdominal CT

- Assessment of primary tumor and lymph node involvement
- Distant metastases

Bronchoscopy

- For squamous cell carcinoma to exclude second carcinoma
- If the tumor is closely located to the central airways (tracheal infiltration, bronchial infiltration)

Panendoscopy

- In the case of squamous cell carcinoma to exclude second carcinoma in the ENT area

PET-CT, MRI Abdomen

- Not required for primary diagnosis
- Only to exclude metastases in rare and special indications
- Helpful in recurrence diagnosis

Therapy

Indication

- Therapeutic approach according to guideline (AWMF 021/023OL: 12/2018) depending on preoperative staging (◘ Figs. 1.3 and 1.4)
- Surgical therapy in specialized centers with high case load
- In early stages (T1a) consider endoscopic local therapy

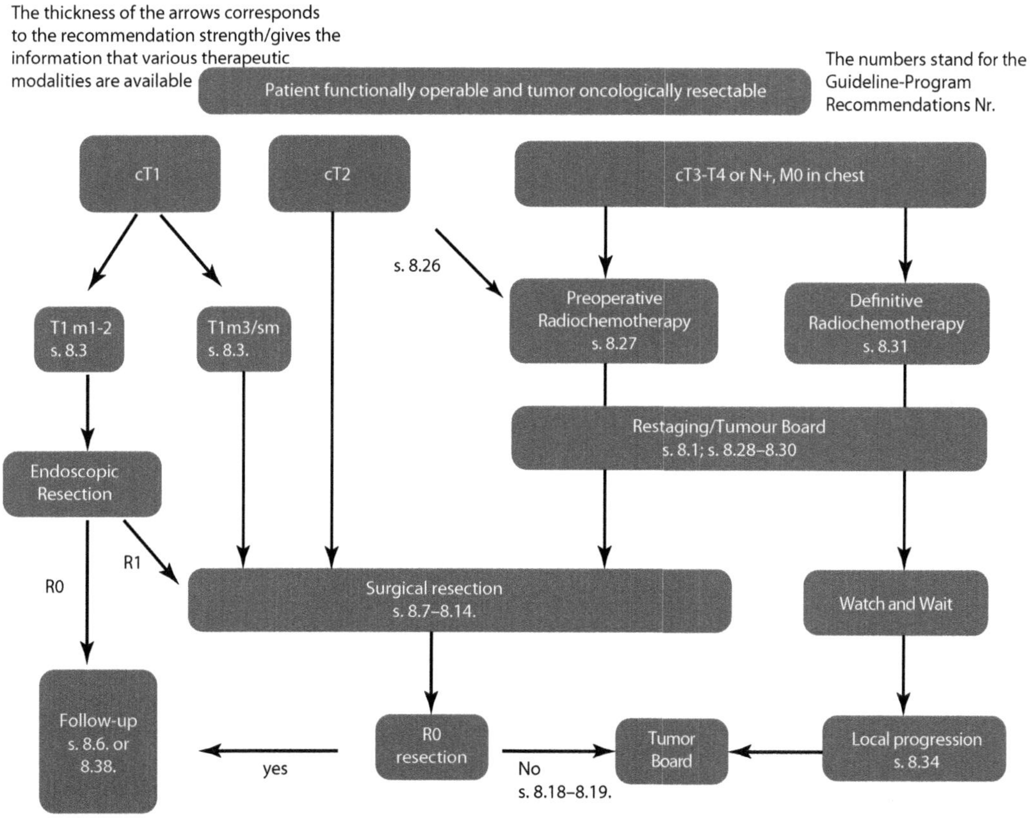

◘ **Fig. 1.3** Treatment algorithm for functionally operable and oncologically resectable squamous cell carcinoma of the esophagus. (From Guideline Program in Oncology 2018; courtesy)

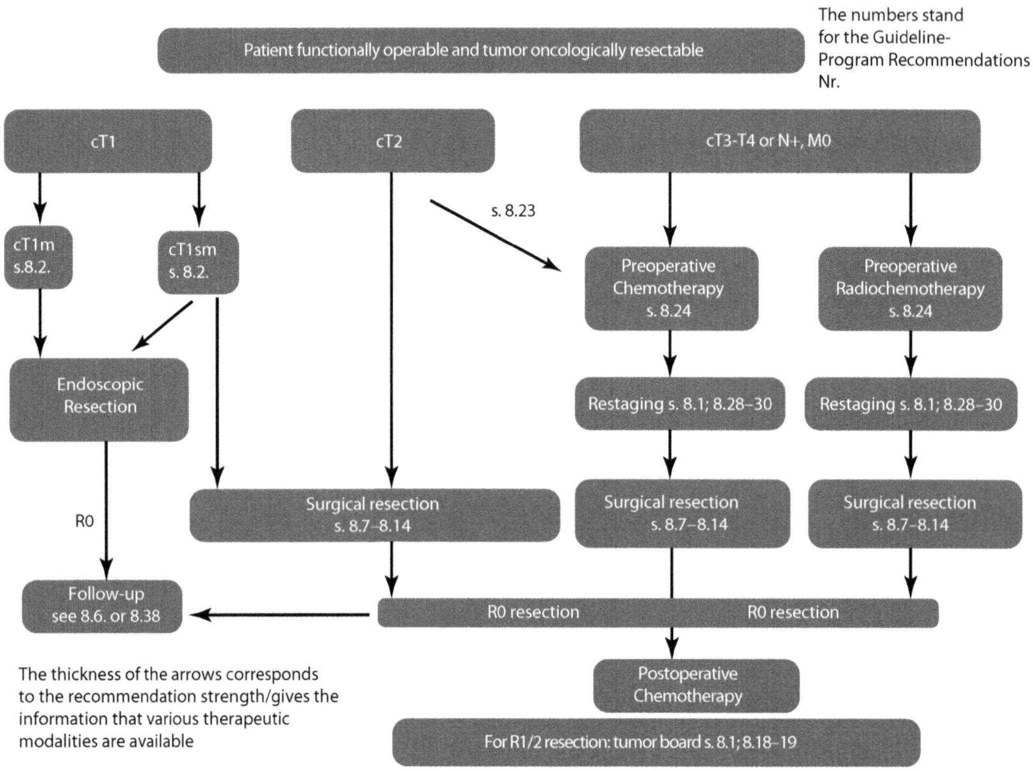

Fig. 1.4 Treatment algorithm for functionally operable and oncologically resectable adenocarcinomas of the esophagus and gastroesophageal junction. (From Guideline Program in Oncology 2018; courtesy)

- In case of planned two-cavity procedure, consider general operability, especially cardiac and pulmonary comorbidity
- In case of inoperability, severe comorbidity or patient preference: definitive radiochemotherapy

Multimodal Therapy

Principles

- Improved local and systemic tumor control
- Indication usually for tumor stage T3/4 and/or positive lymph node status
- Down staging of primary inoperable tumors
- Increased R0 resection rates
- Reduced recurrence rate
- Prolonged overall survival
- After neoadjuvant therapy: re-staging (endoscopy and CT)
- Surgery: usually at time interval of 4–6 weeks after neoadjuvant therapy

Neoadjuvant Radiochemotherapy

- For squamous cell carcinoma and adenocarcinoma
  - 36–54 Gy radiation dose with simultaneous chemotherapy
  - Currently different protocols (e.g. CROSS protocol: 41.4 Gy divided into 23 single doses of 1.8 Gy each plus chemotherapy with carboplatin and paclitacel)

Perioperative Chemotherapy

- Alternative treatment protocol for adenocarcinoma of the gastroesophageal junction
- Protocol analogous to multimodal therapy for gastric carcinoma (▶ Sect. 1.6)
- Advantages over neoadjuvant radiochemotherapy possibly due to improved systemic tumor control and reduced perioperative morbidity

Additive/Palliative Therapy

Principles

- Endoscopic stent insertion
- Installation of percutaneous endoscopic gastrostomy or catheter jejunostomy for enteral feeding
- Palliative radiochemotherapy
- Palliative chemotherapy

Strategy

- In case of locally inoperable tumor or functionally inoperable patient: definitive radiochemotherapy (long-term survival >10–35% in stage II/III)
- In case of R1/R2 resection and lack of possibility for surgical resection: postoperative radiochemotherapy
- In case of recurrence or tumor persistence after definitive radiochemotherapy: salvage esophagectomy may be necessary (**caution**: increased postoperative morbidity)
- In metastatic adenocarcinoma: palliative chemotherapy
- In metastatic squamous cell carcinoma: palliative chemotherapy
- In case of pronounced dysphagia and weight loss: endoscopic implantation of a self-expanding metal stent recommended, also possible prior to neoadjuvant therapy

Operative Therapy Principles

Local Endoscopic Interventional Procedures

- Indication:
  - If there is evidence of high-grade intraepithelial neoplasia or mucosal carcinoma (<2 cm, no lymphatic invasion L0, no venous invasion V0, no ulceration, grading G1/G2) in Barrett's esophagus
  - In case of lymphatic or blood vessel infiltration, poor degree of differentiation (≥G3), submucosal infiltration or tumor remnant at the basal resection margin: indication for esophageal resection
- Disadvantages:
  - No reliable assessment of the lymph node status
  - No certainty of R-status for extended resections in piece-meal technique
  - High risk of stenosis after (circular) resection of extensive findings
- Principle and Endoscopic Procedure:
  - Endoscopic resection depending on the extent and localization of the tumor
  - In case of Barrett's mucosa additional thermoablation of the complete area
  - Endoscopic mucosal resection (EMR)
  - Endoscopic submucosal dissection (ESD)

Esophagectomy

- Principles of resection:
  - For AEG 3: transhiatal extended gastrectomy (► Sect. 1.6)
  - For AEG 2 alternatively:
    - Transhiatal extended gastrectomy or
    - Esophagectomy
    - For tumors with massive infiltration on the stomach: esophagogastrectomy
  - For AEG 1: always abdominothoracic esophagectomy
  - Standard procedure = Ivor-Lewis esophagectomy (see "Operative Procedure"):
    - Mobilization and resection of the esophagus via right thoracotomy or thoracoscopy with mediastinal en bloc lymphadenectomy
    - Dissection of the esophagus at the level of the azygos arch or in the upper thoracic aperture
    - Lymphadenectomy in the abdominal compartment and gastric mobilization and advancement via upper abdominal laparotomy or laparoscopy
  - Alternatively, thoracic and abdominal parts can each be minimally invasive
    - Hybrid laparoscopic/thoracotomic or laparotomic/thoracoscopic procedure widely used
    - Complete laparoscopic and thoracoscopic (if necessary, with robotic-assisted technique)
    - Potential reduction of pulmonary complications
    - Less blood loss, faster recovery

- For squamous cell carcinoma: resection of the esophagus into the upper thoracic aperture with cervical lymphadenectomy if necessary
  - One-stage resection-reconstruction as a standard procedure
  - Two-stage resection-reconstruction: with temporary cervical diversion of the esophagus and gastric blind closure, interval reconstruction in septic patients after (tumor) perforation
- Principles of Reconstruction:
  - Preferred Reconstruction via gastric mobilization, advancement and intrathoracic anastomosis
  - Alternatively cervical anastomosis via separate left cervical incision
  - Reconstruction with colonic interposition for tumor infiltration of the stomach
  - Reconstruction in the posterior mediastinum, alternatively retrosternal
- Postoperative complications:
  - High rate of perioperative complications (morbidity up to 70%)
  - Pulmonary complications (pneumonia, pleural effusion, pneumothorax)
  - Anastomotic leak (therapy by stent insertion or ENDOVAC, surgical revision)
  - Chyle Leak due to injury of the thoracic duct
  - Delayed gastric emptying
  - Wound infections, post-operative bleeding, etc.
  - Cardiac complications (high rate of arrhythmias, pericardial effusion)
- Perioperative management:
  - Preoperative respiratory therapy, exercise and nutrition program
  - Treatment of patients in specialized centers
  - Optimized anaesthetic and intensive care management
  - Peridural catheter for postoperative analgesia
  - Postoperative nutrition via catheter jejunostomy, alternatively parenteral nutrition
  - Aspiration prophylaxis, if necessary scheduled postoperative bronchoscopies

Surgical Procedure

Ivor Lewis Esophagectomy

- Preoperative colonoscopy: if colon interposition necessary!
- Anaesthetic preparation: Peridural catheter, central venous catheter, continuous arterial blood pressure measurement, double lumen endotracheal tube
- Positioning of the patient in a semi-lateral position, right thoracic elevation
- Alternative: Intraoperative repositioning Left lateral position → Supine position
- Right thoracotomy
- Division of the azygos vein
- Mobilization of the esophagus including the periesophageal lymphatic and fat tissue and the peribronchial lymph nodes. **Caution**: thoracic duct!
- Upper abdominal median laparotomy
- Mobilization of the stomach while sparing the gastroepiploic arcade
- Division of the left gastric artery and short gastric vessels
- Abdominal lymphadenectomy (hepatic artery, coeliac trunk, splenic artery)
- Resection of the esophagus and the proximal stomach
- Mobilization of the stomach (stapler-resection)
- Transhiatal advancement of the stomach into the posterior mediastinum
- End-to-side anastomosis using a circular stapler
- Insertion of chest tubes
- Alternatively, minimally invasive procedure

Prognostic Factors

- Postoperative staging (UICC)
- Lymph node ratio (quotient of affected and removed lymph nodes)
- Lymphatic/venous invasion
- Response to neoadjuvant therapy (clinical and histopathological regression)
- R status (residual status)

Follow-Up

Purpose

- Symptom-oriented follow-up
- Diagnosis and treatment of functional disorders (recurrence or benign complications of treatment)
- Nutritional medical follow-up, additional nutrition if necessary
- Early detection of potentially curable local recurrences

Implementation

- After successful endoscopic therapy of a high-grade intraepithelial neoplasia or an early carcinoma, regular control endoscopies (after 3 months, then every 6 months for 2 years and thereafter annually)
- After oesophagectomy, no predefined scheme, e.g. history, physical examination and computed tomography of abdomen/thorax every 6 months

1.5 Benign Diseases of the Stomach

1.5.1 Gastroduodenal Ulcer Disease

Summary

- Mostly due to Helicobacter pylori positive gastritis
- Non-specific symptoms or upper abdominal pain
- Complications: Hemorrhage, penetration, perforation, stenosis, neoplasia
- Differential diagnosis: gastric cancer
- Conservative therapy of the underlying pathology + proton-pump inhibitors
- Endoscopic therapeutic options for complications: Injection or clipping of bleedings, dilation of stenoses
- Surgical interventions for complicated ulcer disease:
  - Surgical hemostasis in case of endoscopically uncontrollable bleeding
  - Excision and suturing for perforation
  - Distal gastric resection for perforation or stenosis

Etiology

Appearance

- Incidence approx. 200/100,000
- Ratio men:women = 3:1
- Localization mostly at the small curvature, antrum and in first part of duodenum

Risk Factors

- Chronic gastritis due to Helicobacter pylori
- Genetic predisposition (blood group 0, HLA B-5)
- Use of NSAIDs (ASS, diclofenac, ibuprofen): increased risk especially in combination with glucocorticosteroids
- Smoking
- Zollinger-Ellison syndrome (gastrinoma)
- Hypercalcemia, usually with parathyroid adenoma
- Acute stress ulcer: risk factor independent etiology (after polytrauma, long intensive care stay, major operations, etc.)

Symptoms

- Epigastric pain
- Fasting pain: for duodenal ulcer
- Postprandial pain: for gastric ulcer
- Upper gastrointestinal bleeding
- Perforation with rapid onset (chemical) peritonitis. **Caution**: masked symptoms with occult perforation

Diagnosis

Endoscopy (EGD)

- Confirmation of diagnosis and biopsy to exclude malignancy
- With conservative therapy always re-endoscopy to record complete healing of the ulcer (DD cancer!)

Radiology

- Computed tomography with oral contrast medium: only indicated to exclude penetration or perforation

Further Diagnosis

- Diagnosis of Helicobacter pylori
- Determination of gastrin, calcium and parathormone to exclude a hormonal cause

Complications

- Bleeding
- Perforation/penetration
- Stenosis
- Neoplasia

Therapy

Conservative Therapy

- For Helicobacter-positive gastritis: eradication with proton-pump inhibitor and clarithromycin + amoxicillin (French triple therapy) or metronidazole (Italian triple therapy) for 7 days
- Avoidance of noxious substances (NSAR, smoking, coffee, alcohol, stress)
- Proton pump inhibitors

Interventional Therapy

- In case of ulcer bleeding: bleeding control by injection with adrenalin/histoacryl or clipping
- In case of endoscopically uncontrollable ulcer bleeding or high risk of recurrent bleeding after primary successful endoscopic hemostasis: Interventional angiography with endovascular hemostasis (coiling of gastroduodenal artery)
- In case of stenosis: endoscopic dilation (bougie) possible

Surgical Therapy

- In gastrinoma or parathyroid adenoma: surgical therapy of the underlying pathology (► Chaps. 6 and 9).
- Surgical therapy of ulcer complications:
  - Ulcer perforation: if possible excision and primary suture of the ulcer, otherwise distal gastric resection
  - Gastric stenosis: distal gastric resection or gastroenterostomy, if malignant cause of stenosis can be ruled out
- 2/3 gastric resection (Billroth I with gastroduodenostomy or Bilroth II with gastrojejunostomy) and the vagotomy procedures for the treatment of ulcer disease: obsolete today due to effective conservative treatment options—PPI, HP (Helicobacter pylori) eradication.
- In case of ulcer bleeding in the first part of duodenum: extra- and intraluminal (duodenum) closure of the gastroduodenal artery.

Surgical Procedure

Distal Gastric Resection Analogous to Billroth II

- Anesthesiology preparation: peridural catheter, central venous catheter, continuous arterial blood pressure measurement
- Supine position
- Upper abdominal median laparotomy, alternatively upper abdominal transverse laparotomy
- Distal gastric mobilization of the stomach
- Resection of approx. 2/3 of the distal stomach by transection of the postpyloric duodenum
- Closure of the duodenal stump with stapler, if necessary additional sutures
- Reconstruction using a small bowel loop (Y-Roux technique or classical omega reconstruction)

1.5.2 Guidelines

AWMF Guideline Register: Helicobacter pylori and gastroduodenal ulcer disease (German Society of Gastroenterology, Digestive and Metabolic Diseases, AWMF), 2014, AWMF registration number: 021/001, ► http://www.awmf.org/leitlinien.html

1.6 Malignant Diseases of the Stomach

1.6.1 Gastric Adenocarcinoma

Summary

- Frequent tumor worldwide, decreasing incidence in the western population
- Intestinal or diffuse histological differentiation according to Lauren
- Early lymphogenic, hematogenic and peritoneal spreading
- Tumour stage is often advanced at the time of diagnosis
- For T3/4 or N+: Multimodal therapy concept consisting of perioperative chemotherapy and surgical resection
- Therapeutic standard: Total gastrectomy with D2 lymphadenectomy
- For distal tumors: Subtotal gastrectomy possible

Definition

- All tumors of the gastric antrum, corpus and cardia with distance >5 cm from the Z-line
- AEG 3 tumors without esophageal infiltration (UICC TNM 7, 2010)
- Tumors of the gastroesophageal junction with esophageal infiltration are classified as esophageal cancers (UICC TNM 7, 2010)

Forms

- According to histology (Lauren classification)
  - Intestinal type
  - Diffuse type (signet ring cells)
- According to localization
  - Antrum
  - Corpus/Fundus
  - Subcardial (AEG 3)

Epidemiology and Etiology

Occurrence

- Approx. 15,000 new cases in Germany per year
- Predominantly men (ratio men:women = 3:2)
- Older patients
- Incidence varies considerably from region to region (increased incidence mainly in Asia, but also in South America, Southern and Eastern Europe)
- In the western population, decreasing incidence of gastric cancer, but increasing incidence of gastroesophageal junction tumors

Risk Factors

- Helicobacter pylori
- Age
- Low socioeconomic status
- Nicotine and alcohol abuse
- Family history
- Previous gastric surgery
- Pernicious anaemia
- Nutritional and environmental factors

Tumor Spread

- Continuous
  - Intramural
  - Direct organ infiltration (spleen, pancreas, colon, duodenum)
- Lymphogenic (◘ Fig. 1.5)
  - Early lymphogenic metastasis
  - Lymph node compartments D1–D4
- Hematogenic
  - Hepatic via portal vein
  - Pulmonary, osseous, cerebral
- Peritoneal carcinomatosis
  - Often early peritoneal seeding
  - Ovarian metastasis: "Krukenberg tumor"

Classification

TNM 7 Classification (2010)

- T (Tumor)
  - T0 No primary tumor detectable
  - Tis carcinoma in situ
  - T1a Infiltration of the lamina propria or muscularis mucosae
  - T1b Infiltration of the tunica submucosa
  - T2 Infiltration of the muscularis propria
  - T3 Infiltration of the subserosa

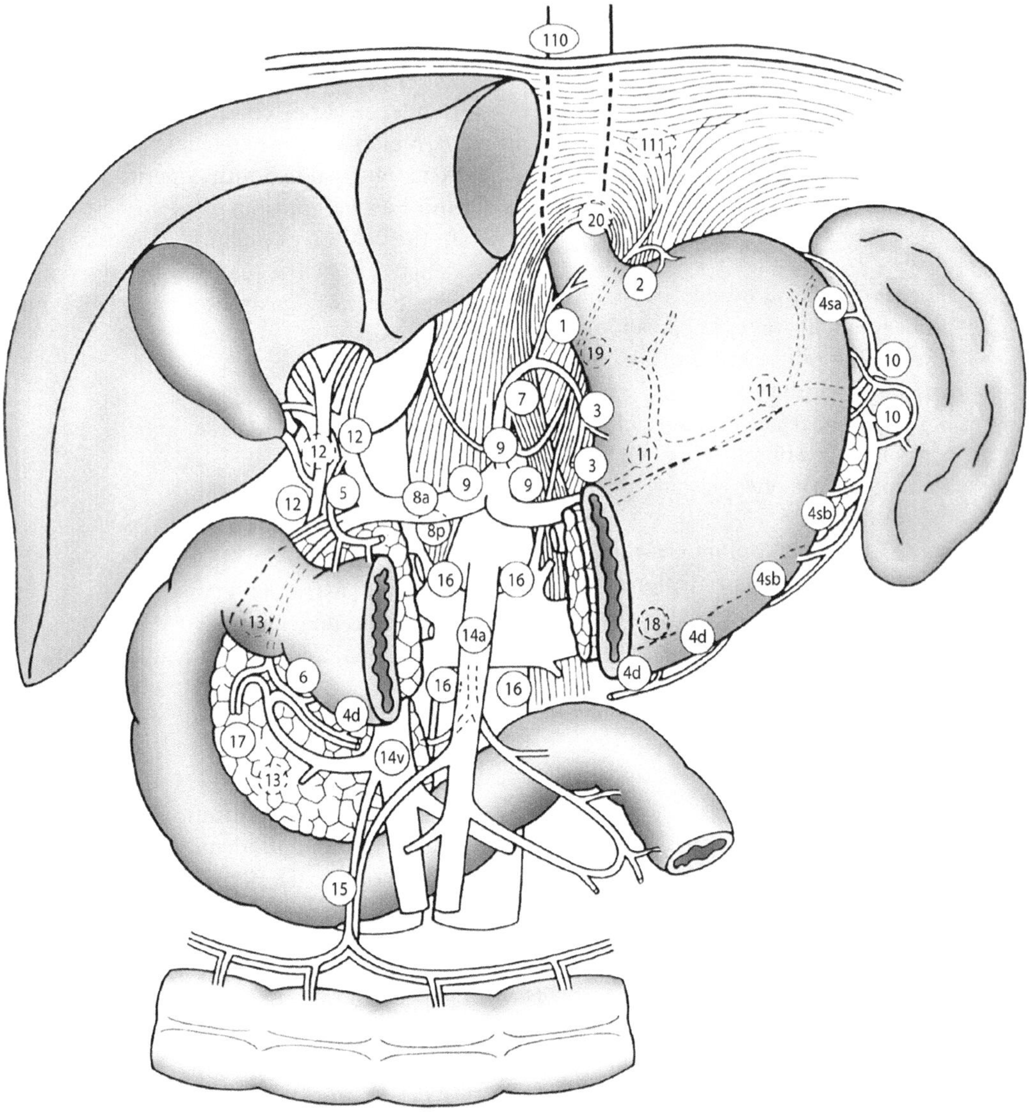

Fig. 1.5 Regional and distant lymph nodes of the stomach. Lymph node compartment D1: *1–6*, lymph node compartment D2: *7–11*, lymph node compartment D3: *12–14*, lymph node compartment D4: *15–16*. (According to Siewert et al. 2010)

  - T4a Penetration of the visceral peritoneum **without** infiltration of adjacent organs
  - T4b Penetration of the visceral peritoneum **with** infiltration of adjacent organs (pancreas, spleen, liver)
- N (Node)
  - N0 No metastases in the lymph nodes
  - N1 Metastases in 1–2 regional lymph nodes
  - N2 Metastases in 3–6 regional lymph nodes
  - N3a Metastases in 7–15 regional lymph nodes
  - N3b Metastases in 16 or more regional lymph nodes
- M (Metastasis)
  - M0 No distant metastases
  - M1 distant metastasis(s)

UICC Stages According to the TNM Classification

Stage 0	Tis	N0	M0
Stage Ia	T1	N0	M0
Stage Ib	T1	N0	M0
	T2	N0	M0
Stage IIa	T1	N2	M0
	T2	N1	M0
	T3	N0	M0
Stage IIb	T1	N3	M0
	T2	N2	M0
	T3	N1	M0
	T4a	N0	M0
Stage IIIa	T2	N3	M0
	T3	N2	M0
	T4a	N1	M0
Stage IIIb	T3	N3	M0
	T4a	N2	M0
	T4b	N0/1	M0
Stage IIIc	T4a	N3	M0
	T4b	N2/3	M0
Stage IV	Each T	Each N	M1

Symptoms

- Often unspecific
- Inappetence/weight loss
- Nonspecific upper abdominal pain
- Recurrent vomiting
- Hematemesis/melena/anaemia

Diagnosis

Esophagogastroduodenoscopy/ Endosonography

- Biopsy
- Confirmation of tumor diagnosis
- Localization of the tumor
- Infiltration depth
- Assessment of T- and N-stage

Thoracic CT, Abdominal CT

- Assessment of the primary tumor and lymph node involvement
- Distant metastases

Diagnostic Laparoscopy

- Staging of peritoneal carcinomatosis
- Biopsy if necessary
- Laparoscopy is an important diagnostic step prior to preoperative therapy

PET-CT, MRI Abdomen, Bone Scintigraphy

- Not required for primary diagnosis
- Only to exclude metastases in rare and special indications
- Helpful in recurrence diagnosis

Therapy

Indication

- Therapeutic procedure according to the guideline depending on the preoperative staging (◘ Table 1.2 and ◘ Fig. 1.6)
- Consider endoscopic mucosal resection at T1a stage

◘ **Table 1.2** Therapeutic strategy for gastric cancer depending on preoperative staging; T1 and T2 see Fig. 1.6

Tumor stage	Therapy
T2 N0 M0	Primary resection
T3/4 N0 M0 Tx N+ M0	Perioperative chemotherapy + resection
Tx Nx M1	Palliative therapy: palliative gastrectomy, gastroenterostomy, palliative chemotherapy Consider resection + peritonectomy + HIPEC for limited peritoneal carcinomatosis and good response to perioperative chemotherapy

HIPEC hyperthermic intraperitoneal chemoperfusion

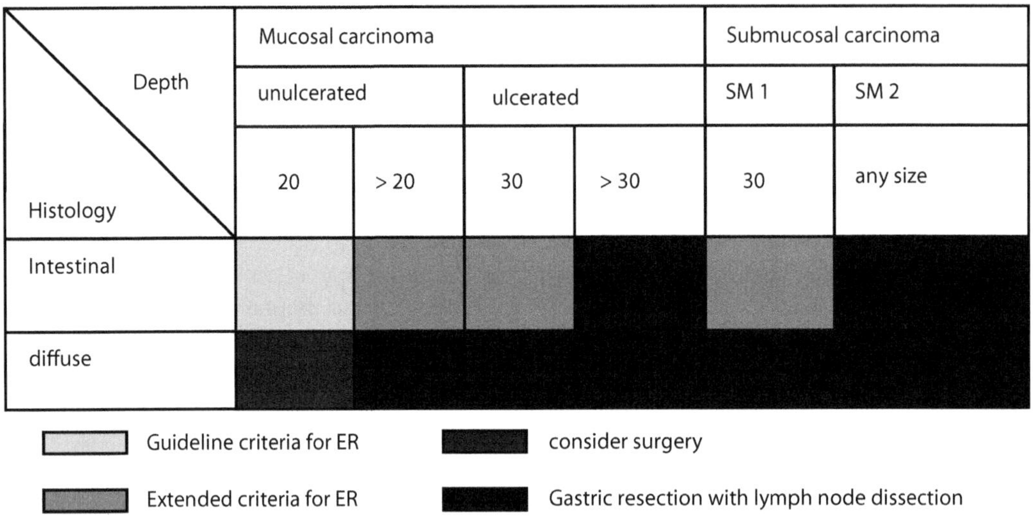

Fig. 1.6 Guideline criteria and expanded criteria for early gastric cancer. (From Guideline Program in Oncology 2019; used with permission)

- Curative therapy for localized and locally advanced tumors
- In case of inoperability, severe comorbidity or patient request palliative chemotherapy
- Palliative gastrectomy for limited metastasis in the young and/or low comorbid patient
- Palliative gastrectomy for tumor hemorrhage and tumor perforation

Multimodal Therapy

Principles

- Improved local and systemic tumor control
- Prognostic improvement in locally advanced tumors
- Indication usually for tumor stage T3/4 and/or positive lymph node status
- Down staging of inoperable tumors
- Increased R0 resection rates
- Reduced recurrence rate
- Prolonged overall survival
- After neoadjuvant therapy: re-staging (endoscopy, computed tomography)
- Surgery at intervals of 4–6 weeks after neoadjuvant therapy

Perioperative Chemotherapy

- Combination of pre- and postoperative chemotherapy
- Various platinum-based chemotherapy protocols:
  - ECF (epirubicin, cisplatin and 5-fluorouracil)
  - ECX (epirubicin, cisplatin, capecitabine)
  - EOX (epirubicin, oxaliplatin, capecitabine)
  - FLOT (docetaxel, folic acid, 5-fluorouracil, oxaliplatin)
  - DCF (docetaxel, cisplatin, 5-fluorouracil)
  - Cisplatin + 5-fluorouracil

Adjuvant Radiochemotherapy

- Widely used in the USA, in Europe only for limited lymphadenectomy (≤D1) or R1/2 resection according to interdisciplinary board recommendation.
- Consider in lymph node positive patients without preoperative chemotherapy even after D2 lymphadenectomy.

Additive/Palliative Therapy

Principles

- Palliative gastrectomy for bleeding tumors or limited metastatic tumors with obstructive symptoms
- Gastroenterostomy for stenosis and inoperable tumor
- Palliative chemotherapy
- Definitive radiochemotherapy

Strategy

- In case of R1/R2 resection and no possibility of further surgical resection: adjuvant radiochemotherapy
- In case of locally inoperable tumor or distant metastasis: palliative chemotherapy
- Palliative gastrectomy only for bleeding tumors after exhaustion of endoscopic and angiographic methods
- Bypass procedure: for clinically manifest gastric outlet stenosis

Operative Therapy Principles

- Local endoscopic interventional procedures:
  - Indication:
    - Intraepithelial neoplasms of any size as well as early gastric cancers that meet all four of the following criteria **should be** resected endoscopically en-bloc: <2 cm in diameter, not ulcerated, mucosal carcinoma, intestinal type/grade of differentiation good to moderate "(G1/G2)"
    - Early gastric cancers with a maximum of one "extended criterion" can be endoscopically resected curatively. Extended criteria are; differentiated mucosal carcinoma (G1/2) without ulceration and size >2 cm; differentiated mucosal carcinoma with ulceration <3 cm; well-differentiated carcinoma with submucosal invasion <500 µm and size <3 cm; undifferentiated mucosal carcinoma <2 cm in diameter (provided there is no biopsy evidence of tumor cells <1 m)
    - Indication for gastric (partial) resection plus lymphadenectomy in the presence of risk criteria or residual tumor at the basal resection margin
  - Disadvantages:
    - No reliable assessment of the lymph node status
    - No assessment of R-status for extended resections in piece-meal technique
  - Principle and endoscopic procedure:
    - Endoscopic resection depending on extension and localization
    - Endoscopic mucosal resection (EMR)
    - Endoscopic submucosal dissection (ESD)
    - Goal: En-bloc resection
- Gastrectomy/Gastric Resection:
  - Principles of resection:
    - A safe resection distance of 5 cm for the intestinal type and 8 cm for the diffuse type should be achieved
    - Gastrectomy with lymphadenectomy of the compartments D1 and D2 is standard
    - For distal tumors, subtotal (4/5) gastrectomy is sufficient, leaving a small proximal gastric remnant
    - In case of subcardial gastric cancer (AEG 3) a transhiatal extended gastrectomy including the distal esophagus is necessary
    - In case of limited peritoneal carcinomatosis, gastrectomy with local peritonectomy and, if necessary, hyperthermic intraoperative chemotherapy can be performed with curative intention
    - Laparoscopic and robotic-assisted surgery can be performed in a specialized center
  - Principles of Reconstruction:
    - No clear recommendation, procedure depending on the experience of the surgeon
    - Classical Roux-en-Y reconstruction
    - Different techniques of jejunum pouch reconstruction, e.g. J-pouch (possible quality of life advantage)
  - Postoperative complications:
    - Duodenal Stump Insufficiency
    - Anastomotic leak of the esophagojejunostomy
    - Pulmonary and cardiac complications
    - Pancreatic fistula after D2 lymphadenectomy
    - Cachexia

1

Surgical Procedure
Gastrectomy
- Anaesthesiological preparation: Peridural catheter, central venous catheter, continuous arterial blood pressure measurement
- Supine position
- Upper abdominal median laparotomy, alternatively upper abdominal transverse laparotomy
- Incision of gastrocolic ligament and opening of lesser sac (great omentum resected en-bloc with gastric specimen)
- Transection of the gastro-splenic ligament and short gastric vessels near the spleen
- Division of the gastroomental artery close to the pancreatic head
- Transection of the right gastric artery
- Division of the postpyloric duodenum and closure of the duodenal stump
- D2 lymphadenectomy including the lymph nodes around the hepatic, celiac and splenic arteries, and division of left gastric artery at its origin near the coeliac trunk
- Division of the vagal nerve at the abdominal esophagus
- Dissection/Mobilisation of the abdominal esophagus
- Roux-en-Y Reconstruction using a small bowel loop (Jejunum)

Prognosis

Prognostic Factors
- Postoperative stage (UICC TNM)
- Lymph node ratio (quotient of affected and removed lymph nodes)
- Lymphatic/venous invasion
- Response to neoadjuvant therapy (clinical and histopathological regression according to Becker et al. 2011)
- R status (residual status)

Follow-Up

Goals
- Symptom-oriented follow-up
- Rule out functional disorders as a result of recurrence or as benign complications of treatment
- Nutritional medical follow-up, additional nutrition if necessary
- Early detection of potentially curable local recurrences
- Early detection of distant metastases

Implementation
- After successful endoscopic therapy of a high-grade intraepithelial neoplasia or an early cancer, regular control endoscopies (every 3 months in the first year, every 6 months in the second year, thereafter annually)
- After gastrectomy, so-called symptom-oriented follow-up without a predefined scheme, e.g. anamnesis, physical examination and computer tomography of abdomen/thorax every 6 months

1.6.2 Gastrointestinal Stromal Tumours (GIST)

► Chapter 14

1.6.3 Guidelines

Guideline program oncology (German Cancer Society, German Cancer Aid, AWMF): “Gastric carcinoma”—Diagnostics and therapy of adenocarcinomas of the stomach and esophagogastric junction, long version 2.0, 8/2019, AWMF registration number: 032-009OL

1.7 Diseases of the Duodenum

Summary

- Duodenal diverticulum: Common finding usually not requiring any treatment
- Duodenal ulcer: ► Sect. 1.5
- Duodenal cancer

- Rare tumor disease
- FAP (familial adenomatous polyposis)/duodenal polyps as risk factors

1.7.1 Diverticular Disease of the Duodenum

Incidence

- Approximately 10–20%

Types

- Duodenal diverticula are mostly found near pancreas head
- Rarely intraluminal or intramural duodenal diverticula, as congenital malformations, originating from a mucosal duplication

Symptoms

- Mostly incidental finding during ERCP
- Mostly asymptomatic and without need for therapy

Therapy

- Very rarely duodenal diverticula require surgery

Complications

- Rarely upper GI bleeding and perforation.
- Very rarely obstruction of bile duct (jaundice) and pancreatic duct (pancreatitis) due to compression.

1.7.2 Duodenal Cancer

Etiology and Tumor Manifestation

Appearance

- Rare tumor disease
- Duodenal adenoma as a precancerous condition
- Frequently in the context of hereditary tumor syndromes: FAP, HNPCC ("hereditary non-polyposis colorectal cancer"), Peutz-Jeghers syndrome, Gardner syndrome
- Other risk factors: Crohn's disease, celiac disease
- Up to 90% of patients with FAP develop duodenal polyps; lifetime risk of duodenal cancer is 3–4%

Symptoms

- Often asymptomatic
- Hematemesis/anaemia
- Stenosis/inappetence/weight loss/vomiting
- Obstructive jaundice or pancreatitis if infiltration of the duodenal papilla

Diagnosis and Therapy

Diagnosis

- Endoscopic diagnosis with biopsy: always + immediately in case of suspected tumor
- In case of tumor detection: CT abdomen/thorax and if necessary endosonography for reliable staging

Endoscopic Therapy

- Duodenal polyps are removed endoscopically analogous to colon polyps
- In the case of larger, flat polyps, consider ablation using the piece-meal technique with additional thermal ablation of the affected area, if necessary
- For duodenal polyposis, determine Spigelman score (polyp number, polyp size, histologic type, grading of intraepithelial neoplasia): Stage I–IV
  - In stage I–III regular endoscopic controls
  - In stage IV, consider surgical therapy

Surgical Therapy

- Surgical excision with transverse closure of the excision site: for adenomas that cannot be removed by endoscopy
- Transduodenal papillary excision with re-insertion of the main pancreatic duct and bile duct: in case of papillary adenomas
- Pancreas sparing duodenectomy (caution: morbidity): for benign tumors (e.g. duodenal polyposis)
- Radical oncological resection (pylorus preserving pancreatoduodenectomy or Whipple operation): in the case of duodenal cancer

1

Multimodal Therapy

- No recommendations due to conflicting data
- No neoadjuvant therapy
- Adjuvant therapy analogous to the recommendations for colon cancer (► Chap. 3)
- For ampullary cancer survival benefit with adjuvant chemotherapy with 5 FU/leukovorin or gemcitabine (ESPAC-3) after R0 resection

Palliative Therapy

- Surgical gastroenterostomy: as a bypass procedure in symptomatic patients with inoperable tumors
- Endoscopic biliary stent/prosthesis insertion or surgical palliative biliodigestive anastomosis: in the case of obstructive jaundice
- Palliative chemotherapy: analogous to colon cancer (► Chap. 3), consider palliative radiochemotherapy if necessary

Prognosis

- 5-year survival rate: approx. 30%
- For N0, M0, R0 = 50–70% 5-year survival

1.7.3 Guidelines

Guideline program oncology (German Cancer Society, German Cancer Aid, AWMF): S3 guideline colorectal carcinoma, long version 2.1, 2019, AWMF registration number: 021-007OL, ► http://leitlinienprogrammonkologie.de/Leitlinien.7.0.html

Oncology guideline program (German Cancer Society, German Cancer Aid, AWMF): Diagnostics and therapy of squamous cell carcinomas and adenocarcinomas of the esophagus, long version 2.0, 2018, AWMF registration number: 021/023OL, ► http://leitlinienprogrammonkologie.de/Leitlinien.7.0.html

References

Becker K, Langer R, Reim D, Novotny A, Zum Meyer Buschenfelde C, Engel J, Friess H, Hofler H (2011) Significance of histopathological tumor regression after neoadjuvant chemotherapy in gastric adenocarcinomas: a summary of 480 cases. Ann Surg 253:934–939. https://doi.org/10.1097/SLA.0b013e318216f449

Connelly CL, Lamb PJ, Paterson-Brown S (2013) Outcomes following Boerhaave's syndrome. Ann R Coll Surg Engl 95:557–560. https://doi.org/10.1308/003588413X13629960049199

Siewert JR, Lordick F, Stein HJ (2010) Ösophaguskarzinom. In: Siewert JR, Rothmund M, Schumpelick V (eds) Praxis der Viszeralchirurgie Onkologische Chirurgie, vol 3. Springer, Heidelberg, pp S713–S734

Vaezi MF, Pandolfino JE, Vela MF (2013) ACG clinical guideline: diagnosis and management of achalasia. Am J Gastroenterol 108:1238–1249; quiz 1250. https://doi.org/10.1038/ajg.2013.196

von Lanz T, Wachsmuth W (2004) Praktische Anatomie. Bauch. Springer, Berlin

Small Intestine and Appendix

Didier Mutter

Contents

F. Billmann, T. Keck (eds.), *Essentials of Visceral Surgery*,
https://doi.org/10.1007/978-3-662-66735-4_2

2.1 Anatomy of the Small Intestine

Key Points

- Longest part of the gastrointestinal tract
- Difficult endoluminal access
- Surgical exploration: one of the diagnostic modalities
- New diagnostic techniques available: non-invasive assessment by double balloon endoscopy, imaging techniques (CT/MRI), capsule endoscopy

2.1.1 Measured Values

- Length = 270–290 cm (from pylorus to cecum)
  - Duodenum = approx. 20–25 cm
  - Jejunum = approx. 100–110 cm
  - Ileum = approx. 150–160 cm
- Diameter = 1.8–2.5 cm
- Surface:
  - Small intestine tube (cylinder) = 0.69 m^2 (for a 5 m long small intestine)
  - Functional resorptive surface = 120–900 m^2 (depending on author)

2.1.2 Limits

- Duodenum: from pylorus to duodenojejunal flexure
- Jejunum: Oral border = from duodenojejunal flexure (Treitz ligament)
- Ileum: No clear boundary between jejunum and ileum; ileum to ileocecal junction

2.1.3 Wall Structure of the Small Intestine

Four layers (from the outside to the inside):
- Serosa:
  - Consisting of visceral peritoneum
  - Coating of jejunoileum + anterior surface of duodenum
- Muscularis propria:
  - Smooth muscles
  - Fine longitudinal outer + thicker circular inner layer
  - Plexus myentericus: between the two layers
- Submucosa:
  - Fibroelastic connective tissue
  - Includes vessels + nerves (Meissner's plexus)
- Mucosa:
  - Muscularis mucosae + lamina propria + epithelial cell layer
  - Epithelial cell layer = goblet cells, Paneth cells, enterocytes and enteroendocrine cells

Surface Multiplication (► Sect. 2.1.1)
- Plicae circulares (Kerck ring folds): Transverse folds of the mucosa (prominent in the distal duodenum + jejunum) lead to an increase in surface area from 0.69 to 1 m^2
- Villi: surface multiplication factor up to 30-fold
- Microvilli: surface multiplication factor = 30

2.1.4 Circulation

Arterial Blood Flow

- Excluding superior mesenteric artery
- Exception = Proximal duodenum through branches of the truncus coeliacus
- Division pattern of the superior mesenteric artery:
  - Specific branches for pancreas
  - Specific branches for distal duodenum
  - Specific branches for small intestine
  - Specific branches for ascending and transverse colon
- Collateral system = vascular arcades of the mesentery
- For the jejunum: long vasa recta of one or two arcades
- For the ileum: short vasa recta of 4–5 arcades (ileum: better blood circulation)

Venous Drainage

- Superior mesenteric vein
- Drainage (with V. splenica) in V. portae hepatis (behind the neck of the pancreas)

Lymphatic Drainage

- From the mucosa through the small intestine wall
- Draining of mesenteric lymph nodes
- Main drainage pathway of fats into the bloodstream
- Immunological role + role in the distribution of cells in the case of malignant intestinal neoplasms

Mesenteric Base

- Fixed to the posterior abdominal wall
- From the left view of LWK 2, oblique to the right and caudal to the right sacroiliac joint

2.1.5 Innervation

- Innervation of the small intestine = autonomic nervous system

Parasympathetic Component

- Fibres of the vagus nerve
- Function: influence on secretion, motor function + all phases of intestinal activity

Sympathetic Component

- Nerve ganglia: Collected in the plexus around the superior mesenteric artery.
- Function: vascular contractility, intestinal secretion and motor function and pain sensation

2.1.6 Small Intestine Functions

Digestion and Nutrient Absorption

- Small intestine: main role in absorption of nutrients + water + electrolytes + minerals
- Peristalsis = intestinal contractions from oral to aboral 1–2 cm/s
  - Main function: transport of the chyme through the intestine
  - Motor pattern different between digestive phase and sobriety

Endocrinological Function

- Small intestine = largest endocrine organ in the body
- Products: Hormones + Peptides
- Paracrine + autocrine functions + neurotransmitter function

Immunological Function

- Antigen processing, humoral and cellular immunity
- Lymphoid tissue: in the Peyer's plaques, the lamina propria + intraepithelial lymphocytes

2.2 Diseases of the Small Intestine

2.2.1 Clinical Presentation

Key Points

- Small intestine diseases = broad spectrum
- Most frequent small bowel disease = small bowel ileus after previous surgery
- Exploratory laparoscopy/laparotomy = often the optimal solution:
  - Free preparation of the intestine
  - Resection or bypass
  - Well accepted: Hardly any postoperative restrictions, resection mostly limited
- Imaging: key role in diagnosis + optimal decision making in treatment of small bowel disease

General

- Mostly unspecific Clinical Presentation
- Broad spectrum of clinical signs: From simple chronic pain to acute peritonitis
- Clinical picture depends on the etiological underlying disease:
  - Inflammatory bowel disease (Crohn's disease) = most common small bowel lesion
  - Neoplastic lesions
  - Small bowel obstruction (in the context of adhesions) (► Sect. 2.2.5)
  - Other rare pathologies (e.g. Meckel's diverticulum)

Inflammatory Bowel Disease

Development

- Onset: Often insidious; rarely also acute
- Medical history: Slow + protracted
- Alternatively symptomatic phases (abdominal pain + diarrhoea) and asymptomatic phases
- Progressive increase in symptomatic phases: More frequent, longer and with more pronounced symptomatology

Symptoms

- Inflammatory symptoms of the gastrointestinal tract
- Typical triad: Chronic recurrent episodes of diarrhoea + abdominal pain + weight loss
- Possible symptoms:
  - Pain in the right lower abdomen (differential diagnosis: appendicitis)
  - Hematochezia: blood in the stool
  - Urge to stool
  - Abdominal cramps and abdominal pain
  - Feeling of incomplete evacuation
  - Constipation (up to ileus)
- General Symptomatology:
  - Fever
  - Loss of Appetite
  - Weight loss
  - Fatigue
  - Night sweats
  - Menstrual irregularities
- Extraintestinal manifestations (30% of patients):
  - Manifestation: GI (gastrointestinal) symptoms, dependent or independent
  - Skin lesions: Erythema nodosum and pyoderma gangraenosum…
  - Arthritis/arthralgias
  - Uveitis and iritis
  - Hepatitis and pericholangitis
  - Aphthous stomatitis
  - Amyloidosis
  - Pancreatitis
  - Nephrotic syndrome

Complications

- Main complications = constipation + perforation
- Constipation to the point of ileus:
  - Etiology = chronic fibrosing lesions, lumen obstruction (partial to complete)
- Perforation:
  - Free (rare) vs. covered
  - Abscesses: Localized, formation in relation to the perforations…
- Fistulas:
  - Etiology = adhesions due to inflammation
  - Abnormal connection between two adjacent organs
  - From the small intestine: to the small intestine, urinary bladder, vagina, stomach, skin
  - Generalized peritonitis = rare
- Perianal lesions (fissure, fistula, stricture, abscess): For anal/rectal involvement
- Infestation of esophagus or stomach possible
- Malignant neoplasms of the small and large intestine: Crohn's disease = predisposition

Neoplastic Intestinal Diseases

- Variable onset of disease

Symptoms

- Early symptoms: mostly non-specific, over months to years
  - Dyspepsia
  - Anorexia
  - Malaise
  - Dull abdominal pain
- Pain: most frequent symptom (often due to obstruction, partly due to intussusception)
- Intestinal bleeding: most frequent symptom (haematochezia/haematemesis)
- Obstruction/Ileus: In 15–35% of patients due to tumor infiltration and adhesions.
- Palpable mass: In 10–20% of patients.
- Perforation: up to 10% of patients (especially in sarcomas/lymphomas)

GIST (Gastrointestinal Stromal Tumors)/ Carcinoid Tumors

(► Chapter 14)

- Special separate tumor entity
- Malignant carcinoid syndrome = rare (10% of cases)

  - Hemodynamic manifestations: Flushing, asthma
  - Cardiac manifestations: Cardiac lesions
  - Intestinal manifestations: Diarrhea, hepatomegaly
- Specific markers:
  - Elevated urine markers: 5-hydroxyindolacetic acid (5-HIAA, 24 h measurement)
  - Chromogranin A in serum (marker of neuroendocrine tumors)
- Metastases: Clinical presentation = as in other neoplastic diseases

2.2.2 Imaging

- Modalities:
  - Radiological imaging
  - Endoscopic imaging
- Indications:
  - Atypical symptoms
  - Complications (e.g. bleeding, obstruction)

Radiological Imaging

Conventional Abdominal Radiograph

- Obsolete, no longer primarily indicated (also due to radiation exposure)
- Allows exclusion of ileus; no information about etiology
- Ileus sign:
  - Dilated loops of small intestine (with/without colonic dilatation)
  - Multiple air-liquid levels
- Localization of the ileal height (proximal vs. distal)

CT Examination with Contrast Medium

- Gold standard for v. a. small bowel disease/ileus
- Pros:
  - Localization of the affected segments
  - Identification of the etiology (extra- or intraluminal lesion)
  - Identification of complications: Ileus, intestinal ischemia (pneumatosis intestinalis, "portal venous gas"), intestinal necrosis
- Staging examination (TNM) in the case of a malignant tumour
- Key examination for extraluminal lesions

Colon Contrast Enema

- Obsolete due to lack of meaningfulness
- Contraindicated due to risk of perforation and when surgery is indicated

CT Enterography/MRI Enterography

- High sensitivity and specificity in the diagnosis of small intestinal diseases (especially chronic inflammatory bowel diseases)
- Principle:
  - Small bowel distension (by oral intake of 1–2 L preparation 1 h before examination)
  - i.v. contrast medium

Abdominal Sonography

- Not much use in small bowel Diagnosiss
- Exception: intestinal ultrasound with contrast medium (chronic inflammatory bowel diseases)

Endoscopic Imaging

Colonoscopy/Esophagogastroduodenoscopy (EGD)

- Very useful for CIBD (chronic inflammatory bowel disease):
  - Visualization of aphtous ulcerations
  - Cobblestone mucosa pattern
  - Discontinuity of the segments concerned
- In the setting of atypical/malignant lesions: Ideal for biopsy confirmation
- For the treatment of proximal/distal bleeding

Double Balloon Endoscopy

- Access to most of the small intestine possible
- Biopsy of a lesion possible (especially after radiological imaging)

Capsule Endoscopy

- Currently standard method of examination of the small intestinal mucosa

- Application only after exclusion of a stenosis/obstruction (CT)
- Special software for image analysis (automated analysis of anomalies)
- New generation of capsules: Integrated biopsy system

2.2.3 Crohn's Disease

Pathophysiology

- Benign lesion of the small intestine (mostly small intestine and colon)
- Chronic transmural inflammation of the intestinal tract (affected segments: all from mouth to anus possible)
- Unknown etiology
- Pathogenesis: two hypotheses:
  - Primary dysregulation of the mucosal immune system: excessive immunological response against normal microflora; as consequences:
  - Alteration in intestinal microflora or disrupted epithelial barrier function: pathologic response of the normal mucosal immune system
- Triggering/Favoring Factors:
  - Infections (Mycobacterium paratuberculosis)
  - Immunological reactions (humoral and cellular)
  - Genetic defects (IBD1 locus)
  - Environmental factors
  - Dietary factors
  - Smoking

Diagnosis

- Clinical suspicion
- Laboratory chemistry: orienting, serological markers: perinuclear antineutrophil cytoplasmic antibodies (p-ANCA) and anti-Saccharomyces cerevisiae antibodies (ASCA)
  - Atypical p-ANCA: in patients with IBD, especially ulcerative colitis
  - Atypical p-ANCA + ASCA for the differential diagnosis of ulcerative colitis (p-ANCA +) vs. Crohn's disease (ASCA +)
  - Atypical p-ANCA + ASCA prognostic for the development of IBD
- Imaging: to confirm the diagnosis by
  - CT: typical = transmural bowel wall thickening; visualization of extraintestinal complications
  - Endoscopy: typical = aphtous ulcerations with granulations; surrounding mucosa normal; biopsy: granulomas with Langerhans giant cells; systematic exploration of the ileum

Differential Diagnosis (= Other Inflammatory Bowel Diseases)

- Infectious intestinal diseases (Yersinia, Campylobacter, Salmonella, Shigella, Tuberculosis, Amoebiasis)
- Acute appendicitis
- For CIBD: Spontaneous symptom relief
- If symptoms during surgery: no resection, no biopsy (except emergency indications: abscess, perforation)

2.2.4 Small Intestinal Neoplasms

Epidemiology

- Rare + insidious tumors = diagnosis difficult
- Necessity high level of suspicion

Small bowel = 80% of GI tract, 90% of mucosal surface; small bowel tumors = rare (1–2% of GI malignancies)

- Often late diagnosis (advanced stage) = poor prognosis

Diagnosis

- Diagnosis through combined imaging modalities
- Flexible endoscopy: For lesions in the duodenum + terminal ileum
- Double balloon endoscopy: For the middle part of the small intestine
- Capsule endoscopy: contraindicated for malignant lesions with strictures
- CT:
  - For the detection of extraluminal gastrointestinal stromal tumors (GIST)

- For staging malignant tumors (mesenteric lymph nodes, liver involvement, abdominal wall infiltration)
- Very sensitive (90% diagnostic certainty)

- Somatostatin receptor scintigraphy: higher sensitivity in the localization and extension balance of these tumors

- Intestinal MRI is increasingly used
- Despite imaging modalities, diagnosis mostly during elective or emergency surgery (e.g. carcinoid tumors)

Histological Classification

- GIST = most frequent tumour in the small intestine (mostly asymptomatic)
- Adenomas = most frequent benign tumor in autopsy series
- Benign tumors = majority of small bowel neoplasms (mostly asymptomatic + incidental findings)

Adenomas

- 15% of all tumours of the small intestine
- Incidence in ileum, jejunum, duodenum = 50%, 30%, 20%
- Symptoms (if symptomatic, but usually autopsy findings): obstruction, bleeding
- Classification:
  - True adenomas
  - Villous adenomas: Mostly in the duodenum, possibly associated with FAP (familial adenomatous polyposis); possible malignancy
  - Brunner's gland adenomas: hyperplastic lesions in the proximal duodenum; can cause peptic ulcer; nonmalignant = endoscopic treatment

Hamartomas

- Part of the Peutz-Jeghers syndrome
- Heritable dominant pattern with high penetrance
- Mucocutaneous melanotic pigmentation + gastrointestinal polyps
- Small lesions (1–2 mm), brown-black, in the circumoral region of the face, oral mucosa, forearms, palm, plantar, fingers and perianal region
- Complete jejunum + ileum affected; more rarely rectum, colon, stomach
- Clinical Presentation: abdominal colic (intermittent intussusception); bleeding rare

Hemangiomas

- Submucosal vascular proliferation
  - Mostly in the jejunum
- 3–4% of benign tumours of the small intestine; multiple in 60% of cases
- Possibly part of Osler-Weber-Rendu disease or Turner syndrome
- Symptoms: Often bleeding
- Treatment: Limited resection sufficient

Gastrointestinal Stromal Tumors (GIST)

- Most frequent mesenchymal tumors of the GI tract
- Pathogenesis:
  - GIST cell: development of precursor cell of Cajal cell (myenteric plexus)
  - Activating mutation of KIT protein kinase receptor (CD117) or platelet-derived growth factor receptor α (PDGFRA)
  - Expression of CD117 and CD34
- Benign/malignant GIST = 3–4/1
- Localization: Throughout the GI tract; more common: stomach, small intestine
- Symptoms:
  - Intramural growth: obstruction (ileus)
  - Extramural growth: larger mass, bleeding
- Risk of recurrence: mitotic index >2/50 "high-power fields" = increased local recurrence/metastasis risk
- Malignant GIST:
  - 20% of malignant tumours of the small intestine
  - More frequent in the jejunum and ileum
  - Mostly >5 cm diameter at diagnosis
  - Origin = Muscularis propria: extramural growth
  - Symptoms = obstruction, hemorrhage, perforation (due to hemorrhagic necrosis)
  - Metastasis: Hematogenous: Liver, lung, bone; lymphatic = rare

- Prognosis dependent on:
  - Tumor size
  - Mitotic index
  - Invasion of the lamina propria

Adenocarcinomas

- 50% of malignant tumours of the small intestine
- Localization: Mostly duodenum + proximal jejunum
- Risk factors:
  - FAP
  - "Hereditary non-polyposis colorectal cancer" (HNPCC)
  - Peutz-Jeghers syndrome
  - Crohn's disease
  - Gluten Intolerance Enteropathies
  - Biliary diversions
  - Smoking
  - Alcohol consumption (>80 g/dL ethanol)
  - Consumption of red meat or food preserved in salt
- Prognosis dependent on:
  - Disease stage
  - Time of diagnosis: Usually late

Lymphomas

- Manifestation: Primary lesion or part of a systemic disease
- Lesion often in the ileum
- Often associated with celiac disease of immunodeficiency status
- Lesions usually large (>5 cm) with infiltration of the intestinal wall
- Symptoms:
  - Pain
  - Weight loss
  - Nausea, vomiting
  - Changes in bowel habits
- Complications:
  - Perforation: Frequent (25% of cases)
  - Fever = sign of systemic involvement

Small Intestine NET (Carcinoid Tumors)

Terminology: Small bowel NET = international consensus, instead of carcinoid tumor of the small bowel (Small Bowel NET, SBNET)

- Pathophysiology:
  - Carcinoid = part of the neuroendocrine tumors (NET)
  - Tumor cells (= multipotent cells) originate from enterochromaffin cells (Lieberkühn crypts of the small intestine)
  - Tumor cells can produce substances (depending on the cells' site of origin): Serotonin, P-substance etc.
  - Size growth = very slow
  - After serosa invasion: severe desmoplastic reaction, mesenteric fibrosis, intestinal kinking and intermittent obstruction
- Tumor location (in decreasing frequency):
  - Appendix (most frequent localization) 45%
  - Small intestine (second most common location, especially the last 60 cm of the ileum): Ileum 28%
  - Rectum 16%
  - Carcinoids mostly multicentric in the small intestine
  - Often coexistence with another malignancy of a different type (colon adenocarcinoma) or with multiple endocrine neoplasia type 1 (MEN1)
- Malignancy:
  - Carcinoids of the ileum/jejunum = higher malignancy than carcinoids of the appendix
  - Malignancy potential associated with: Tumor location, tumor size, invasion, growth type.
  - Carcinoids <1 cm: 2% are metastatic
  - Carcinoids of 1, 2 or >2 cm: metastases in 50%, 80% and 90% of cases
- Forecast:
  - Carcinoid = best prognosis of all malignant tumors of the small intestine
  - 5-year survival = 65% (in patients with regional disease), 35% (in patients with distant metastasis)
- Clinical Presentation:
  - 70–80% of patients = asymptomatic; carcinoid = incidental finding
  - Obstruction: In connection with intussusception due to tumor

- Carcinoid syndrome:
  - Only a small percentage of patients
  - Clinical Presentation: Episodic attacks of cutaneous flushing, bronchospasm, diarrhea, and vasomotor collapse
- Treatment:
  - Extended metastasis: palliative resection (because of slow-growing tumors)
  - NET of the midgut (high recurrence rate): Long follow-up, at least 7 years

Metastatic Lesions

- More common than primary tumors
- Mostly from intra-abdominal primary tumors
- Small bowel involvement:
  - Through direct extension
  - Due to peritoneal metastasis
- Metastases from extra-abdominal tumors rare (breast cancer, bronchial cancer, skin melanomas)

2.2.5 Other Diseases of the Small Intestine

Diverticula and Meckel's Diverticula

- Diverticulum of the small intestine = frequent occurrence
- Rarely symptomatic = usually no indication for surgery
- True diverticulum (congenital): Diverticulum consisting of all wall layers

Duodenum Diverticulum

- Second most frequent diverticular localization after colon
- Mostly periampullary (2-cm radius around the ampulla Vateri)
- Mostly originating from medial duodenal wall
- Mostly asymptomatic; diagnosis during endoscopy or imaging
- Complications:
  - Occlusion of the choledochal duct/pancreatic duct
  - Bleeding
  - Perforation
  - Blind Loop Syndrome
- Treatment:
  - Asymptomatic/random findings: No treatment
  - Surgical treatment: necessary in less than 5% of cases

Jejunum and Ileum Diverticula

- Rare, usually false diverticula
- Mostly multiple, protruding from mesenteric side of intestine
- Symptomatology (mostly chronic):
  - Unclear abdominal pain
  - Malabsorption
  - Functional pseudoobstruction
  - Low-grade bleeding
- Complications (rare):
  - Diverticulitis
  - Perforation
  - Abscess
  - Bleeding
  - Obstruction/Ileus
- Treatment:
  - If asymptomatic/random findings: No treatment
  - In case of complication: resection + primary anastomosis

Meckel's Diverticulum

- Most frequent congenital small intestine anomaly
- Localized antimesenteric side of the ileum, 45–60 cm proximal to the ileocecal valve
- Mostly incidental finding
- Pathophysiology
  - Origin = incomplete occlusion of the omphalomesenteric duct
  - Cells of the omphaloenteric duct = pluripotent; Meckel's diverticulum often with heterotopic tissue: gastric, colonic, pancreatic mucosa
- Clinical Presentation:
  - Bleeding (most common form of presentation)
  - Obstruction/Ileus
  - Volvulus or intussusception
  - Incarceration
  - Diverticulitis
- Treatment (symptomatic Meckel's diverticulum) = surgery (usually laparoscopic):

- Meckel's diverticulum resection: transverse stapler resection
- Small bowel segment resection of the diverticulum-bearing segment

Ulcerations and Fistulas

Ulcerations

- Rarely
- Most often associated with Crohn's disease, typhoid fever, tuberculosis, lymphoma, lesions of gastrinoma
- Drug-induced ulcerations: Coated KCl tablets, corticosteroids, NSAIDs (nonsteroidal anti-inflammatory drugs, ulceration usually in the ileum)
- Treatment (if necessary) = small bowel segment resection + anastomosis

Enterocutaneous Fistulas

- Etiology:
  - Mostly iatrogenic
  - Neighbour abscesses
  - Traumas
  - Rarely spontaneous (then in the context of Crohn's disease)
- Risk Factors/Predisposition:
  - Radiation in the anamnesis
  - Intestinal obstruction
  - CIBD
  - Mesenteric vascular disease
  - Intraabdominal sepsis
- Clinical Presentation:
  - Generalized peritonitis: Rare
  - Classification: In terms of localization and output volume (high vs. low output)
  - High-output fistula, if output ≥500 mL/24 h
  - Proximal fistulas: More serious problem due to higher output, electrolyte loss, malabsorption (distal segment eliminated)
- Poor prognostic factors (= no spontaneous healing):
  - High-Output
  - Severe interruption of intestinal continuity (>50% of circumference)
  - Active CIBD
  - Malignant disease
  - Radiation enteritis
  - Distal obstruction
  - Undrained abscess
  - Short fistula tract (<2.5 cm)
  - Epithelialization of the fistula tract
- Treatment:
  - Somatostatin: rapid reduction of output + shorter healing time of the fistula
  - Surgery: If no spontaneous healing

Small Bowel Obstruction/Ileus

- Most common disease of the small intestine

Etiology

- Postoperative adhesions (60%)
- Malignant diseases
- Crohn's disease
- Hernia

Classification of Obstruction/Ileus

- Partial vs. complete
- Simple vs. Strangulated (Trapped)

Clinical Presentation

- Abdominal pain: colicky, intermittent
  - High ileus: Briefly persistent + bilious vomiting
  - Distal ileus: progressive pain, persistent for days + abdominal distension
- Nausea, vomiting
- Diarrhoea or constipation

Complications

- Necrosis
- Perforation

Caution

Signs of necrosis/perforation are fever and tachycardia.

Diagnosis

- CT abdomen:
  - Sensitivity = 90–96%, Specificity = 96%
  - Very effective in evaluation of ileus + diagnosis of tissue damage

  - Ideal in assessing which patient can be treated conservatively vs. surgically
  - Effective in strangulation detection

- Effective detection of strangulation/complication by CT of the abdomen.
- Classic guiding paradigm of "never let the sun rise and set on an ileus" no longer appropriate
- CT diagnosis also enable conservative treatment

Treatment

- Highly dependent on Clinical Presentation + etiologies (◘ Table 2.1)
- Depending on the CT findings
- Basic indication for surgery: in case of persistence of pain for hours (laparotomy vs. laparoscopy)

2.2.6 Treatment Strategies

Drug Therapy

- Must always be considered

Surgery = mostly overtherapy, unnecessary bowel resection + surgical complications.

Crohn's Disease

- Medicinal + surgical treatment = palliative
- Therapeutic objective: alleviation of acute exacerbation + alleviation of complications
- Drug therapy: induction + maintenance of remission
  - Aminosalicylates
  - Corticosteroids

◘ Table 2.1 Therapeutic strategies for small bowel obstruction (ileus)

Etiology	Type	Management
Adhesions	Partial SBO	Non-operative treatment over 24–48 h
		Intraluminal contrast medium examinations
		Surgery
	Complete and symptomatic SBO	Surgery
Neoplasia	Primary	Resection
	Secondary	Resection, bypass or stoma
Crohn's disease	Initial presentation	Bowel resection
	Perforation, phlegmon	Bowel resection
	Multiple strictures	Bowel resection, stricturoplasty
Gallstone ileus		Enterotomy
Radiation enteritis		Bypass or resection
Meckel-Divertickel		Meckel's or bowel resection
Invagination	Spontaneous	Reduction
	Tumorous	Resection
Bezoare		Enterotomy, extraction Fragmentation/propulsion into the caeca
NSAID stricture		Bowel resection, stricturoplasty, balloon dilatation

SBO small bowel obstruction

- Immunosuppressive drugs
- Antibiotics
- Anti-TNF antibody

Malignant Lesions

- Adjuvant radiotherapy/chemotherapy: Best survival rates
- Curative resection only in 50% of patients
- Metastases in 1/3 of cases already at the time of surgery
- 5-year overall survival = 25%

GIST/Small Bowel NET (Carcinoid)

- GIST: Targeted therapies must always be considered:
  - Targeted therapy to specific molecules, e.g. imatinib with effect on KIT protein and PDGFRA protein
- Small bowel NET/carcinoids:
  - Long-acting somatostatin analogues (octreotide)
  - Effective against symptoms; no proven action on tumor inhibition
  - Also as palliative treatment for disseminated lesions

Surgical Treatment

General Principles

Segmental Small Bowel Resection + Anastomosis

- Treatment of choice in most cases
- Benign lesions: Limited resection (short segment of small bowel + limited division of mesentery).
- Malignant lesions: Oncologic resection (with control of vessels at their origin + lymphadenectomy + free small bowel resection margins)

Laparoscopic Resection

- Mostly for GIST

Surgical Procedure

Standard Procedure: Laparoscopic GIST Resection

- Lesion must be presentable laparoscopically
- Transillumination (diaphanoscopy) to visualize the vascular supply of the segment to be resected
- Incision of the mesentery, control of the vessels by ligatures or vessel sealing systems: ultrasound dissectors (Sonicision, Covidien), high-frequency thermal fusion devices (LigaSure, Covidien)
- Cutting through the intestine using a 60-mm linear stapler (e.g. EndoGIA, Covidien)
- Isoperistaltic side-to-side anastomosis to restore intestinal continuity: antimesenteric opening of the two intestinal segments, anastomosis using a linear stapler via this incision, closure of the intestinal incision

Caution

Short bowel syndrome = risk in small bowel resection due to resection of healthy tissue

Therefore, always weigh well the indication for resection

Bypass Procedures

- In selected cases of ileus/obstruction

Treatment of CIBD (E.g. Crohn's Disease)

Indications for Surgical Treatment

- Obstruction/Ileus
- Perforation
- Fistula or abscess
- Bleeding
- Complications affecting adjacent tissues

Strategy

- Preoperative imaging: essential for the clarification of multiple lesions
- Treat the affected bowel segment specifically
- Limit to one short bowel segment (recurrent resection of long segments = no better outcome + risk of short bowel syndrome)
- Obstruction/Ileus: Mostly partial/temporary

  - Drug therapy indicated
  - In targeted cases: Endoscopic dilatation
- If surgery is necessary: Segmental resection + primary anastomosis
- Intraoperatively: always careful exploration (macroscopy + palpation) of the entire peritoneal cavity (to exclude secondary lesions)
- In case of obstruction by strictures:
  - Stricturoplasty = longitudinal incision of the fibrotic tissue (preservation of the mucosa) + transverse closure
  - Indications for this technique:
    - Multiple stricture areas in long segments
    - For patients who have already undergone resection
    - If stenosis due to fibrosis: no acute inflammation
- In generalized peritonitis: external enterostomy indicated

Treatment of Benign Lesions

- Potentially malignant lesions: Resection like malignant lesions
- Symptomatic benign lesions: Endoscopic destruction/mucosal resection
- Segmental resection: laparotomy/laparoscopy; possibility of intraoperative identification of the lesion
- Always complete small bowel exploration to exclude other lesions
- Treatment of complications (obstruction/bleeding): Surgery

Treatment of Malignant Lesions

- Malignant tumors: obligatory oncological resection + regional lymphadenectomy
- Carcinoid tumors: treatment depends on tumor size + localization + presence of metastases:
  - Tumor <1 cm without local lymph nodes = segmental small bowel resection
  - Tumor >1 cm, multiple or regional LK metastases = oncological resection (wide bowel resection + mesentery)
  - Involvement of the terminal ileum = hemicolectomy on the right side
  - Cholecystectomy indicated: Because of lifelong somatostatin analogue treatment in most patients…
  - Metastases = surgery in the sense of debulking (symptom relief)

2.3 Vermiform Appendix

2.3.1 Anatomy of the Vermiform Appendix

Normal Anatomy

- Base:
  - Localized at convergence of the long taeniae (inferior surface) of the caeca
  - Anatomical relationship allows localization during surgery
- Tip: Most often retrocecal in the peritoneal space

Localization Variations (According to Wakeley and Testut & Latarjet)

- Retrocecal (65%)
- Pelvin (31%)
- Subcaecal (2%)
- Preileal (1%)
- Rare variations (1%)

The different localizations form the origin of the myriad of symptoms in acute appendicitis.

Circulation and Lymphatic Drainage

- A. appendicularis: branch of A. ileocolica
- Lymphatic drainage to the anterior ileocolic lymph nodes

Caution

Because of the prevention of postoperative bleeding, it is essential to control the appendicular artery during appendectomy (need to know the anatomy).

Histological Features

- Mucosa: goblet cells (distributed in mucosa): Mucus production
- Submucosa: Lymph follicle = important defence function (early stages of development)

2.4 Diseases of the Appendix

2

2.4.1 Appendicitis Vermiformis

Key Points

- One of the most common acute digestive diseases in children/adults
- Treatment (appendicitis and complications) as a therapeutic challenge, depending on:
  - Clinical Presentation
  - Biochemistry
  - Imaging
- Current standard = laparoscopic appendectomy
- Alternative treatment (for uncomplicated appendicitis) = conservative antibiotic treatment
- Complications: Abscess/perforation

Physiopathology

- Etiology of appendicitis = appendiceal stump obstruction
- Obstruction by stool, lymphoid hyperplasia, food debris (fibers), parasites, neoplasms.
- Obstruction:
  - Bacterial overgrowth + mucus accumulation
  - Intraluminal distension
  - Increase in wall pressure
    - Loss of the epithelial mucosal barrier
    - Perforation (after about 48 h after onset of symptoms) + abscess/peritonitis

Symptoms

Initial Symptoms

- Periumbilical pain = visceral pain (due to luminal distension)
- Nausea + Vomitus

Progressive Symptoms (Due to Inflammation of the Surrounding Structures)

- Localized pain in the right lower quadrant
- Possible vomiting
- Fever: parallel with leukocytosis + CRP elevation

Other possible symptoms: urological symptoms, diarrhoea, paralytic ileus, functional intestinal obstruction.

Clinical Presentation: Biochemistry

Clinical Presentation

- Local pain at McBurney point (possibly with defensive tension)
- Dunphy's sign: pain in the right lower abdomen during coughing
- Rovsing's sign: pain in the right lower abdomen on retrograde palpation of the colon
- Blumberg sign (= release pain): Pain in the right lower abdomen after release of pressure in the left lower abdomen
- Obturator sign: pain in the right lower abdomen on internal rotation of the hip = sign of pelvic appendicitis
- Iliopsoas sign: pain in the right lower abdomen with extension of the right hip = sign of retrocecal appendicitis
- With perforated appendicitis: pronounced intense pain + diffuse contracture

Biochemistry

- Mostly leukocytosis $>11.5 \times 10^3/mm^3$
- Elevated CRP

In the absence of one of these two signs appendicitis is unlikely. Here, surveillance should be continued (for prophylaxis of unnecessary surgery).

Imaging

- Necessary to ensure diagnosis (prevention of unnecessary surgery)
- Necessary in case of an uncertain diagnosis

Ultrasound (US)

- Sensitivity = approx. 85%; specificity >90%
- Signs of acute appendicitis:
  - Anteroposterior diameter of the appendix ≥7 mm
  - Thick-walled appendix
  - Noncompressible luminal structure
  - Cocard sign: Target in the transverse section of the appendix
  - Appendicolite

Computer Tomography (CT)

- Standard imaging in acute appendicitis
  - Sensitivity = 90%, specificity = 80%
  - Negative appendectomy after CT = rate < 10%
  - No increase in perforation rate

Diagnostic Laparoscopy

- In case of uncertain diagnosis
- Direct examination of the appendix + peritoneal cavity (other diseases)
- Indications: Primarily in young women with questionable US/CT findings

Differential Diagnosis

Operative Differential Diagnosis

- Invagination
- Meckel's diverticulitis

Non-Operative Differential Diagnosis

- Acute gastroenteritis
- Mesenteric lymphadenitis
- CIBD
- Constipation
- Functional pain
- Pyelonephritis
- Colitis
- Diverticulitis
- Ileus
- Tumour of the GI tract

Gynaecological Differential Diagnosis

- Tuboovarian abscess
- Torsion of the ovary
- Ruptured ovarian cyst
- Ectopic pregnancy
- Gynecological tumors (uterus, tube, ovary)

The large number of differential diagnoses (mostly non-operative) increases the importance of preoperative imaging.

Surgical Treatment Modalities

Treatment Strategy

Early Surgical Appendectomy

- In most cases of acute appendicitis

Antibiotic Treatment

- Perioperative antibiotic prophylaxis indicated: second generation cephalosporins (cover aerobic + anaerobic contamination)
- Systematic antibiotic treatment not recommended (no influence on postoperative complications)
- Non-perforated appendicitis: perioperative single dose, no postoperative antibiotics to reduce postoperative wound infection/intra-abdominal abscesses
- Perforated/gangrenous appendicitis: postoperative intravenous antibiotics until patient is afebrile (at least 5 days)

Laparoscopic Appendectomy

Minimally Invasive (Laparoscopic) Appendectomy = Currently the Gold Standard

Surgical Procedure

Laparoscopic Appendectomy

- Positioning as for open appendectomy (supine position, legs together, right arm abducted 90°, left arm along the body)
- Surgeon + assistant to the left of the patient; monitor to the right of the patient
- Standard instrumentation: Laparoscopy tray: 0° or 30° laparoscope with HD camera, lap scissors, atraumatic fenestrated graspers, monopolar and bipolar coagulation grasper, clip applicator, irrigation aspirator, Röder loops (e.g. Surgitie ligating loop, Covidien),

2

endoscopic salvage bag; possibly stacker (e.g. EndoGIA linear staplers, Covidien), suture material. Trocars: One 10- to 12-mm trocar (optics), and two 5-mm trocars (working trocar)
- 10-mm optic trocar placed subumbilically through open access; two 5-mm trocars suprapubically and laterally of the left rectus abdominis muscle under visual control
- Patient in Trendelenburg position + turned to the left side
- First step = exploration of the peritoneal space
  - Confirmation of the diagnosis + exclusion of differential diagnoses, especially Meckel's diverticulum, adnexa
- Second step = dissection:
  - Adequate presentation of the appendix (consequences of taenia of the caecum) + mobilization (adhesiolysis)
  - Elevation of the appendix + transection of the mesenteriolum (bipolar forceps, bipolar scissors) until adequate visualization of the appendix base
  - Control of the appendicular artery:
  - Monopolar/bipolar coagulation, vessel sealing devices (e.g., LigaSure, Covidien), stapler, suture of the artery (no technique comparatively better)
- Third step: Setting down the appendix
  - Prior to this, the base is treated with 2–3 Röder loops (e.g. Surgitie Ligating Loop, Covidien)
  - Setting down of the appendix; in case of very inflamed/necrotic stump: stapler (staple suture device) with possibly distal part of the caecum (gangrenous appendicitis, pronounced inflammation of caecal base, abscess, perforation, peritonitis)
- Fourth step: extraction of the appendix

Using a salvage bag to prevent contamination of the abdominal wall

Controversy with Normal Appearing Appendix at Laparoscopy

- Leave appendix vs. appendectomy
- Always complete exploration of the abdominal cavity to exclude differential diagnoses (e.g. Meckel's diverticulum, Crohn's disease, mesenteric lymphadenopathies, pelvic disease, abscesses, ovarian torsion, hernias)
- Current position: After exclusion of differential diagnoses = appendectomy
- Arguments for appendectomy (expert opinion):
  - Infection of the mucosa often inapparent in early phase
  - Risk for re-operation > Risk for removal of a normal appendix

- Since 1894 standard = open appendectomy (McBurney incision)
- For about 20 years standard = minimally invasive appendectomy (also for complicated appendicitis)

Advantages of the Minimally Invasive Procedure

- Less postoperative pain, shorter hospital stay, rapid recovery, low complication rate, lower readmission rate, better quality of life
- For perforated appendicitis: fewer wound infections
- Diagnostic appendectomy: Useful in cases of uncertain diagnosis
- Conversion laparoscopic open: Very rare

Resection Technique

Retrospective study (Mutter and Marescaux 2013): Consecutive series with 262 patients:

- Resection technique
  - Endoscopic ligation: 207 cases (79%)
  - Stapler appendectomy: 55 cases (21%)
- Indication for Stapler appendectomy given by the surgeon:
  - Severe inflammation: 38 cases (69%)
  - Questionable viability of the appendage base 14 cases (25.5%)
  - Necrosis of the appendix base 3 cases (5.5%)

Evidence-Based Approach

- Inverting the appendiceal stump into the caecum: No evidence of benefit
- Need for bipolar coagulation of the mucosa of the appendiceal stump (prevention of abscess by secretion); risk of local necrosis by monopolar electric current and possible postoperative fistula
- Irrigation: no evidence of benefit; risk of spreading germs (Douglas abscess); "suction only strategy" recommended
- Fascia of the 10 mm trocar must be adapted

Open Appendectomy

McBurney Incision

- McBurney incision = conventional approach
- Allows easy access to the appendix
- Limitations:
  - Complete abdominal exploration impossible
  - Impossible adnexal exploration
  - Mostly oversized incision (does not correspond to the theoretical ideal incision)

Median Laparotomy

- Indications:
  - If McBurney is insufficient for adequate exploration or if the appendix is very inflamed
  - In exceptional cases of serious intra-abdominal complications (need for preoperative imaging)
  - Some of these cases can be treated with medication, interventions or conservatively

Surgical Procedure

Open Appendectomy

- McBurney incision: oblique incision in the right lower quadrant of the abdomen
- Distraction of muscles (prevention of postoperative hernias)
- Opening of the peritoneum
- Localization of the appendix (follow taenia of the caecum) + advancement in front of the abdominal wall; minimization of the risk of rupture by careful manipulation of the inflamed tissue
- Severing of the mesenteriolum between clamps + ligation
- Skeletonization of the appendix base + ligation using absorbable sutures
- Deposition of the appendix after clamping
- Abdominal wall closure; no drainage recommended

Drug Therapy

- Indicated in two situations:
  - Uncomplicated appendicitis—only (CT evidence)
  - Severe complications of appendicitis supportive

Uncomplicated Appendicitis

- Surgical therapy = still standard for complicated appendicitis
- Evidence-based:
  - Effectiveness in the treatment of uncomplicated appendicitis: antibiotic = operative
  - Need for adequate CT diagnosis: markers of uncomplicated appendicitis
  - Duration of antibiosis (e.g. amoxicillin + clavulanic acid) = 14–21 days
  - Antibiotic therapy of uncomplicated appendicitis: supported by studies (Vons et al. 2011; Spirt 2010; Varadhan et al. 2012)

Severe Complications (Depicted by Imaging)

- Perforation: 23–73% of cases
- Perforation with abscess: 10–13% of cases
- Aim of drug therapy = to prevent major/difficult surgical procedures

Treatment Strategy

- Abscesses >5 cm: Interventionally guided drainage
- Abscesses <5 cm: Antibiotic treatment (treatment of the acute phase) + appendectomy after 6–8 weeks

2

Caution
Periappendicular abscess:
- Surgery: increased risk of bleeding, wound infection, fistula, adhesions
- Perioperative appendiceal abscess: non-operative treatment (reduction of complications)

2.4.2 Malignant Diseases

- Primary tumors of the appendix = Rare
- Usually only diagnosed postoperatively (in cases of appendicitis) in the pathological examination
- Most common: mucinous tumors and carcinoid tumors of the appendix

Mucocele of the Appendix

Pathophysiology
- Appendiceal lumen obstruction with intraluminal accumulation of mucus: appendiceal distension and mucocele
- Histological classification (Histology appendiceal mucosa):
  - Benign epithelium with retention cyst
  - Hyperplasia/low-grade atypia = low-grade mucinous appendiceal neoplasia
  - Malignant = mucinous adenocarcinoma

Epidemiology
- Simple/hyperplastic mucoceles (acellular mucus) = 5–25% of cases
- Mucinous cystadenoma (63–84% of cases): Appendix neoplasia with dysplastic epithelium (analogous to colonic polyps)
- Mucinous adenocarcinoma (11–20% of cases): High-grade cell dysplasia and invasion of muscularis mucosae + stromal invasion

Clinical Presentation
- Mostly unspecific
- Most frequently: Clinical Presentation of acute appendicitis (▶ Sect. 2.4)
- Possibly palpable tumor
- Asymptomatic patients = 25–50%

Diagnosis

Tumor Marker (Preoperative)
- CEA ("carcinoembryonic antigen"): possible indication of malignancy

Sonography
- Encapsulated cystic lesion in the lower right quadrant
- Liquid content with different echogenicity (mucus density)
- Multiple echogenic layers in the dilated appendix = pathognomonic

CT Abdomen
- Cystic mass with thin low-density wall, direct communication to the caecum
- Linear/spotted calcifications of the wall = typical for mucocele of the appendix
- No calcifications of the wall in appendiceal abscesses

Colonoscopy
- Soft erythematous mass with central ulceration (= protrusion of the appendicular ostium)
- To exclude synchronous neoplastic lesions of the colon (in up to 20% of cases)

Treatment
- Surgical therapy (strategy analogous to conventional appendectomy)
- Extent of resection: Depending on histology + extent of disease

Retention Cysts
- Resulting in: chronic obstruction of the appendiceal lumen
- Mucosa: Flat cuboidal epithelium
- Surgical extent = Simple appendectomy sufficient

Appendix Mucoceles
- Appendiceal mucoceles <2 cm without intraoperative rupture = benign
- Appendiceal mucoceles >2 cm = neoplastic
- Operation Extent:

- Appendectomy: resect appendiceal mesentery (for histological examination of lymph nodes) + prevent rupture (in case of manipulation/extraction)
- Right hemicolectomy only in case of infiltration of the residual limb

Ruptured Mucocele (= Pseudomyxoma Peritonei/Mucinous Carcinomatosis)

- Rupture = displacement of epithelial cells + mucus in the peritoneal space
- Clinical Presentation:
  - Appendicitis signs
  - Increased abdominal girth
  - Ovarian mass
  - Inguinal hernia
- Treatment: CRS (cytoreductive surgery) + HIPEC (hyperthermic intraperitoneal chemotherapy)

Forecast

Prognostic Factors

- Extent of the peritoneal tumor conglomerate
- Histological grade of the tumor

Course of the Disease

- In most patients: Dissemination of tumor cells in the abdomen at the time of diagnosis
- Most of these neoplasms are noninvasive
- Metastases = rare; locoregional recurrence = frequent (ileus)

Survival

- Without treatment: Very poor prognosis (no chance of cure + very limited survival)
- With aggressive CRS + HIPEC: 5-year survival = 50–96% in selected patient groups (if no distant metastases + complete cytoreduction)
- CRS + HIPEC must be performed early in the disease history

Carcinoid Tumors: Neuroendocrine Tumors of the Appendix

- Carcinoid tumors of the appendix = part of the carcinoids of the midgut (common embryological origin)
- Terminology: carcinoids of the appendix = well-differentiated neuroendocrine tumors (NET) of the appendix
- Histology: NET = enterochromaffin cells (expression of S-100)
- NET = malignant tumours with benign behaviour pattern

Epidemiology

- Appendix-NET = 5% of all intestinal carcinoids
- Mostly in patients around 40 years of age
- Appendiceal carcinoids <1 cm + not localized in appendiceal base = 90%
  - Appendectomy = sufficient treatment
  - Mostly retrospective postoperative diagnosis

Diagnosis

- Depending on the presence of a Clinical Presentation

Non-functional NET

- Slow growing
- Mostly years until first symptoms and diagnosis
- Mostly diagnosis in the context of surgery (pathology)

Functional NET

- Carcinoid syndrome: hormonal production = symptoms + dosable products
- Marker:
  - 5-HIAA (degradation product of serotonin) test in urine
  - Chromogranin A
  - Serotonin

Environment Diagnosis

- As with other NET: possibility of other gastrointestinal genitourinary tumors
- Colonoscopy: to exclude other colon tumors
- Other screening examination depending on age and other risk factors

Treatment (According to Recommendations of the American National Cancer Institute and ENETS)

- ◘ Figure 2.1
- NET <1 cm, not in appendix base
  - Appendectomy
- NET >2 cm
  - Hemicolectomy right + ileocecal lymphadenectomy (risk of metastases)
- 1 cm < NET < 2 cm
  - Treatment controversial
  - Hemicolectomy on the right:
    - When infiltration of the mesoappendix
    - If R1 at the resection margin
    - If N+ (lymph node metastases)
    - In case of high proliferation activity (high Ki67 index), high mitotic index, angioinvasion
    - If mixed histology (goblet cell carcinoid)

Goblet Cell Carcinoid or Adenocarcinoid

- Rare variant with mixed endocrine and exocrine properties
- Associated with poor prognosis

Aftercare

- Monitoring in patients with elevated chromogranin A (indicator for extended resection)

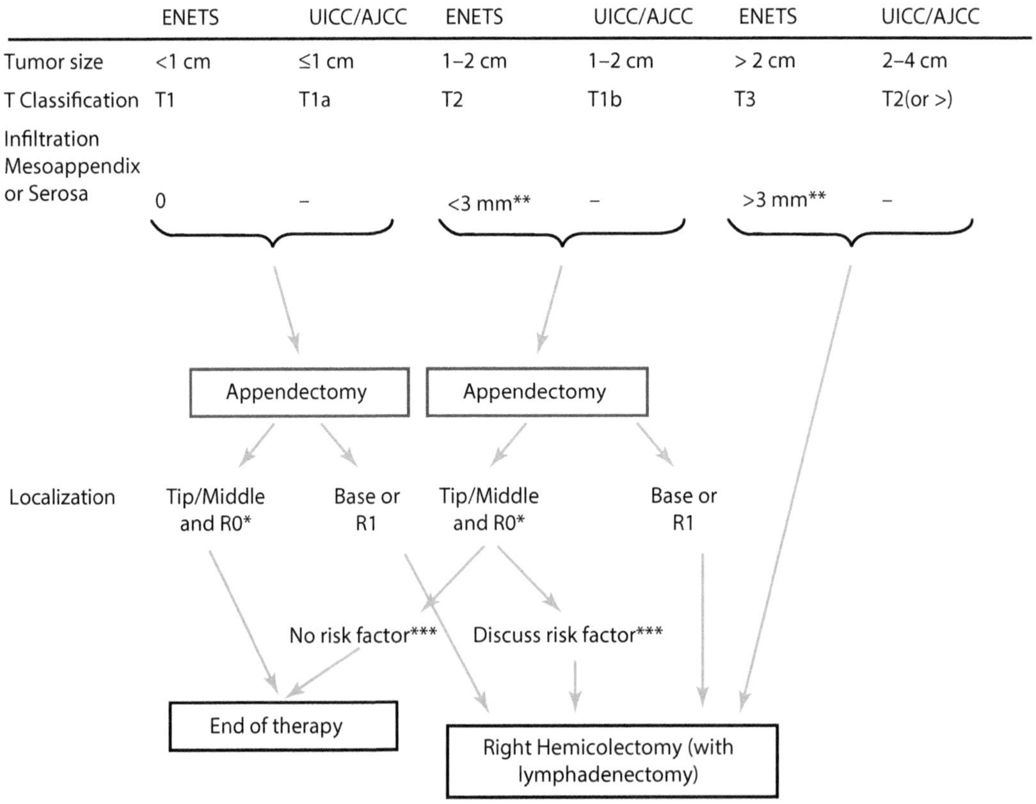

◘ **Fig. 2.1** Treatment algorithm of NETs of the vermiform appendix according to the recommendations of the American National Cancer Institute and the ENETS* R0 = tumor-free resection margins** very limited evidence*** risk factors are: V1 (histologic vascular invasion)—L1 (histologic lymphatic vascular invasion)—G2 grading—>3 mm infiltration or infiltration of the mesoappendix

- Survival:
  - Excellent for locoregional tumors
  - Tumours with distant metastases: 10-year survival = 30%

Noncarcinoid Tumors of the Appendix

- Appendix = possible location of all intestinal tumors
- Rare tumor entities

Classification According to World Health Organisation (WHO) (Table 2.2)

- Epithelial tumors
- Non-epithelial tumors

Table 2.2 Histological WHO classification of appendiceal tumours

Epithelial tumors	Non-epithelial tumors
Adenoma Tubular Villös Tubulovillous Serrated	Neuroma Lipoma Leiomyoma Gastrointestinal stromal tumor Leiomyosarcoma Kaposi's sarcoma Other
Carcinoma Adenocarcinoma Mucinous adenocarcinoma Signet ring cell carcinoma Small cell carcinoma Non-differentiated carcinoma	Malignant lymphoma
Carcinoid (well differentiated neuroendocrine neoplasia)	Secondary tumors
Tubular carcinoid	Hyperplastic (metaplastic) polyp
Goblet cell carcinoid (mucinous carcinoid)	
Mixed carcinoid adenocarcinoma	
Other	

Overview: Appendix Adenocarcinoma

- Rare: 0.08% of all carcinomas
- Mucinous appendiceal adenocarcinoma = most frequent subtype (better prognosis after resection)

Clinical Presentation

- Appendicitis in the elderly patient
- Mucocele

Treatment

- Hemicolectomy right = standard procedure
- Drug treatment/chemotherapy for specific diseases (lymphomas etc.)

References

Spirt MJ (2010) Complicated intra-abdominal infections: a focus on appendicitis and diverticulitis. Postgrad Med 122:39–51

Varadhan KK, Neal KR, Lobo DN (2012) Safety and efficacy of antibiotics compared with appendicectomy for treatment of uncomplicated acute appendicitis: meta-analysis of randomised controlled trials. BMJ 5:344

Vons C, Barry C, Maitre S, Pautrat K, Leconte M, Costaglioli B, Karoui M, Alves A, Dousset B, Valleur P, Falissard B, Franco D (2011) Amoxicillin plus clavulanic acid versus appendectomy for treatment of acute uncomplicated appendicitis: an open-label, non-inferiority, randomized controlled trial. Lancet 377:1573–1579

Colon

Oliver Thomusch

Contents

F. Billmann, T. Keck (eds.), *Essentials of Visceral Surgery*,
https://doi.org/10.1007/978-3-662-66735-4_3

3

3.1 Anatomy and Physiology

3.1.1 Definition and Limits

- Definition
  - Colon = Intestinum crassum, part of the gastrointestinal tract
  - Distally from the small intestine, proximal from the rectum
- Limits
  - Proximal = ileocecal valve (= Bauhin); border between terminal ileum and colon
  - Distal = indistinct; transition zone between sigmoid colon and rectum = transition of the taenia into closed longitudinal muscles of the rectum

3.1.2 Tasks

- Transport of chyme
- Thickening of chyme
  - Active Na^+ resorption (with diffusion of H_2O)
  - Absorption capacity = up to 5 L/day (9 L in total in the whole gastrointestinal tract)
  - Active secretion of K^+, Cl^-, HCO_3^-
- Further development of chyme
  - Breakdown of the cellulose content by bacterial colonisation of the colon (10^{10} bacteria/g faeces)
  - Resorption of 40–50% of the fibres

3.1.3 Location and Classification

- Five colonic segments from proximal to distal:
  - Caecum (= appendix, coecum) with appendix vermiformis (= appendix)
  - Ascending colon
  - Transverse colon
  - Descending colon
  - Colon sigmoideum (= sigma)
- Position of the colon in relation to the peritoenum
  - Caecum (distal part) + appendix: Intraperitoneal
  - Caecum (proximal part): Secondary retroperitoneal
  - Ascending colon: Secondary retroperitoneal
  - Transverse colon: Intraperitoneal
  - Descending colon: Secondary retroperitoneal
  - Sigmoid colon: Intraperitoneal

3.1.4 Measured Values

- Colon length = 1/4 of the length of the intestine (in adults 140–160 cm)
- Lumen of the colon varies in size: in adults
  - Caecum = approx. 6.5 cm (maximum width approx. 9 cm)
  - Colon ascendens = approx. 5.5 cm
  - Transverse colon approx. 5 cm
  - Descending colon = approx. 4 cm
  - Sigmoid colon = approx. 5.5 cm

3.1.5 Characteristic Features of the Colon

- Taeniae coli
  - 0.5–1 cm wide light bands = shirred outer longitudinal muscles of the colon
  - Beginning at cecum-appendix junction to sigmoid colon
  - Three Taenia: libera, mesocolica, omentalis
- Haustra coli
  - Puffed sleeve-like protrusions of the colon between plicae semilunares coli
- Plicae semilunares coli
  - Crescent-shaped mucosal folds of the colon
- Appendices epiploicae
  - Small sac-like protrusions of the colonic serosa filled with fatty tissue from tela subserosa
  - Located near the Taeniae libera and mesocolica

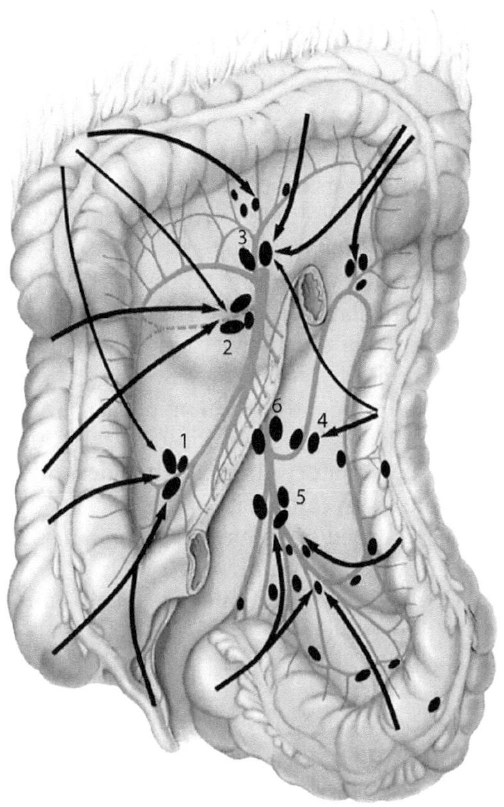

Fig. 3.1 Lymphatic drainage of the colon. *1* Ileocolic artery, *2* Right colic artery, *3* Middle colic artery, *4* Left colic artery, *5* Sigmoid arteries, *6* Inferior mesenteric artery

3.1.6 Blood Supply and Drainage

Arteries

- Superior mesenteric artery (ileocolic artery + right colic artery + middle colic artery): Caecum + appendix + ascending colon + transverse colon
- Inferior mesenteric artery (left colic artery + sigmoid artery): left half of transverse colon + descending colon + sigmoid colon
- Riolan anastomosis = anastomoses between two watershed areas: Between middle colic artery and left colic artery (Ramus ascendens), supply area superior and inferior mesenteric arteries

Veins

- Veins parallel to the arteries = portal vein/Henle loop

Lymphatic Drainage (Fig. 3.1)

- Along the associated arteries
- Paracolic at the small blood supply vessels (arcades)
- Intermediate: Along the main vessels
- Central: In the area of the aorta

Caution
Lymphatics along the marginal arteries = LN (lymph node) metastases to proximal and distal possible: safety distance to the proximal and distal resection border = 10 cm

3.2 Benign Diseases of the Colon

3.2.1 Diverticulosis and Diverticulitis

Key Points

- Acquired benign disease of the colon; incidence increasing with age
- Complications: Diverticulitis, hemorrhage, abscess, perforation, stenosis…
- Therapy: primarily conservative; surgery: in case of complications/recurrent diverticulitis

Definitions

Colon Diverticulum

- Acquired protrusion of the intestinal wall
- Diverticulum: Protrusion of the entire intestinal wall
- Pseudodiverticulum: Protrusion of the mucosa + submucosa through muscle-weak gaps of the colon wall

Diverticular Disease

- Occurrence of symptoms/complications in the context of diverticulosis

Diverticulitis (= Pathological)

- Peridiverticulitis: inflammatory process originating by the colonic diverticulum
- Pericolitis: spread to the intestinal wall (= focal pericolitis)

Epidemiology

- Prevalence of diverticulosis:
  - Increases with age
  - Under 40 years = rare
  - 60 years = approx. 30%
  - 85 years = approx. 65%
- Men:Women = 1:1
- Diverticular disease: clinical symptomatic = 10–25% of diverticular carriers (complications in 5%)
- Diverticulitis: incidence = 80–126/100,000 population/year

Etiology/Pathogenesis

- Multifactorial
- Increased intraluminal pressure
- Weakness of the intestinal wall: mostly passage of the vessels

Sigmoid colon = high pressure zone = increased intraluminal pressure; 90% of diverticula in the sigmoid.

Risk Factors

- Higher prevalence at older ages
- Genetic predisposition (e.g. Marfan syndrome, Ehlers-Danlos syndrome, polycystic kidney disease)
- Dietary fiber deficiency
- Higher body weight (BMI >30 kg/m^2)
- Recurrence rate after acute diverticulitis: depending on severity (between 2% and 35%) (= guideline)
- Complicated diverticulitis:
  - Relevant mortality (0–13%)
  - Special risk under immunosuppression (8–24%)

Increased prevalence of colorectal cancer in diverticulosis is not proven.

Complications

- Diverticulitis (see above)
  - Development due to stool retention = bacterial growth in the diverticulum = inflammation
  - Initial lesion before abscess, perforation
- Diverticular bleeding
  - In 5% of diverticula carriers (= hematochezia)
  - Independently of inflammation
  - Risk = age, nonsteroidal anti-inflammatory drugs, right-sided diverticula (Asian patients)
- Abscess and/or fistula formation
  - Severe complications
- Covered perforation/open perforation with peritonitis
- Stenosis

Symptoms

- Diverticulosis = asymptomatic
- Diverticulitis:
  - Left lower abdominal pain (abrupt onset, rapidly progressive)
  - Possibly pressure-painful roller (palpatory)
  - Fever, nausea, vomiting, dysuria
  - Change in bowel movements, possibly blood in the stool
  - Diverticular bleeding
  - Painless peranal bleeding
  - Sustained/Intermittent
  - Spontaneous healing (80% of cases)
  - High recurrence rate

Classifications

- Classification of diverticular disease according to the German S2k guideline of the AWMF (Classification of diverticular disease, CDD) (◘ Table 3.1)
- Classification according to Hinchey (for perforated sigmoid diverticulitis) (◘ Table 3.2)
- Classification according to Hansen and Stock (for sequence: diverticulosis, diverticulitis, complications) (◘ Table 3.3)

Table 3.1 Classification of diverticulitis/diverticular disease (CDD)

Type 0	**Asymptomatic diverticulosis**	
		Incidental finding; asymptomatic
		No disease
Type 1	**Acute uncomplicated diverticular disease/diverticulitis**	
Type 1a	Diverticulitis/diverticular disease without environmental reaction	Symptoms related to the diverticula
		Inflammatory signs (laboratory): optional
		Typical sectional imaging
Type 1b	Diverticulitis with phlegmonous bypass reaction	Inflammatory signs (laboratory): obligatory
		Sectional imaging: phlegmonous diverticulitis
Type 2	**Acute complicated diverticulitis** as 1b, additionally:	
Type 2a	Microabscess	Covered perforation, small abscess (≤1 cm); minimal paracolic air
Type 2b	Macroabscess	Para- or mesocolic abscess (>1 cm)
Type 2c	Free perforation	Free perforation, free air/liquid
		Generalized peritonitis
Type 2c1	Purulent peritonitis	
Type 2c2	Fecal peritonitis	
Type 3	**Chronic diverticular disease** Recurrent or persistent symptomatic diverticular disease	
Type 3a	Symptomatic uncomplicated diverticular disease (SUDD)	Typical clinical presentation
		Inflammatory signs (laboratory): optional
Type 3b	Recurrent diverticulitis without complications	Signs of inflammation (laboratory) present
		Cross-sectional imaging: typical
Type 3c	Recurrent diverticulitis with complications	Detection of stenoses, fistulas, conglomerate
Type 4	**Diverticular bleeding**	**Detection of the source of bleeding**

Table 3.2 Classification of perforated sigmoid diverticulitis according to Hinchey

Division	Definition
Hinchey I	Local pericolic abscess after perforation into the mesocolon
Hinchey II IIA IIb	Distant abscess Circumscribed, drainable distant abscess Diffuse abscess with fistula formation
Hinchey III	Purulent peritonitis
Hinchey IV	Fecal peritonitis

3

Table 3.3 Classification according to Hansen and Stock

Division	Definition
Stage 0	Asymptomatic diverticulosis
Stage 1	Diverticulitis without intestinal wall overflow, clinically unspecific complaints, inconspicuous CT findings
Stage 2a	Phlegmonous form, on CT extension into the pericolic fat tissue
Stage 2b	Spread of inflammation to adjacent organs by covered perforation, extraluminal gas inclusions in CT or abscess formation
Stage 2c	Free perforation, clinical signs of acute abdomen and evidence of free air
Stage 3	Chronic recurrent, development of intestinal wall fibrosis and luminal narrowing

Diagnosis

Medical History (Medication, Tobacco Consumption)

Clinical Examination

- Abdomen: palpation, auscultation, digital-rectal examination
- See below Symptoms
- Measurement of body temperature

Laboratory Tests

- Leucocytosis
- CRP elevation, accelerated blood sedimentation
- Urine analysis
- In sepsis: elevated procalcitonin

Diagnostic Imaging

- Ultrasound examination:
  - Bowel wall thickening
  - Dom sign: Hypo-echoic lesion, eccentric next to the intestinal wall (= inflammatory diverticulum)
  - Abscess, fatty tissue compression
- Cross-sectional imaging: CT with contrast agent = standard: confirmation of diagnosis + exclusion of complications
- Colonoscopy:
  - No colonoscopy to confirm the diagnosis of acute diverticulitis (risk of perforation!)
  - Important role in lower GI (gastrointestinal) bleeding and/or to exclude tumor
  - Colonoscopy after conservatively treated diverticulitis and planned elective sigmoid resection: (Usually after 4–6 weeks, to exclude other relevant pathologies

Caution
Colonoscopy in acute inflammatory situation = high risk of perforation.

Therapy

Prophylaxis of Diverticulitis

Primary Prophylaxis

- Regular physical activity
- High fiber diet
- Preservation of normal weight

Secondary Prophylaxis

- Insufficient data = no general recommendations possible
- Prophylaxis of recurrent diverticular disease:
  - Nutrition
  - Lifestyle
  - Physical activity
  - Medications (mesalazine, probiotics, rifaximin)

Conservative Therapy

Asymptomatic Diverticulosis

- Primary prophylaxis (see above)
- Acute uncomplicated diverticulitis without risk factors for a complicated course
  - Close clinical and laboratory control
  - Low recurrence rate
  - No indication for surgery

- Antibiotic therapy:
  - No acceleration of healing
  - No prevention of complications/recurrences
  - Exception = in the case of necessary immunosuppressive drug therapy after transplantation, collagenoses etc.

Complicated Diverticulitis

- Inpatient treatment
- If necessary, parenteral fluid substitution in case of insufficient oral fluid intake
- Oral intake of food if necessary (depending on clinical situation)
- Parenteral antibiotic therapy
- For retroperitoneal/paracolic abscesses = interventional drainage + control

Surgical Therapy

Surgery Indications

- Emergency surgery:
  - CDD Type 2c
  - Evidence of freely perforated sigmoid diverticulitis with clinical or radiological signs of peritonitis
  - Failure of conservative therapy in complicated diverticulitis (acute abdomen, sepsis)
  - Diverticular hemorrhage with circulatory effect or persistent Hb effect that cannot be controlled by interventions
- Elective surgery in the inflammation-free interval (>3–4 weeks):
  - Recurrent diverticulitis with structural changes and complications CDD type 3c (fistula formation, stenosis, unclear dignity)
  - After successfully treated complicated diverticulitis CDD type 2b (macroperforation, abscess)
  - Clinically uncomplicated symptomatic diverticular disease CDD type 3a or chronic recurrent diverticulitis CDD type 3b
  - Recurrent, localized, clinically relevant diverticular bleeding
  - Diverticular hemorrhage: endoscopic hemostasis or angiography with embolization not possible
- Surgery is not indicated:
  - Asymptomatic diverticulitis CDD type 0
  - Acute uncomplicated diverticulitis CDD type 1
  - In the interval after successful conservative therapy of complicated sigmoid diverticulitis with microabscess CDD type 2a
  - Self-limiting or interventional successfully treated diverticular bleeding

Surgical Strategy

- Objective = removal of the diverticulum (diverticulitis)-bearing intestinal segment
- Laparoscopic (or laparoscopic-assisted) vs. open resection: Laparoscopic = fewer local complications, wound infections, intra-abdominal abscesses, postoperative ileus and fascial dehiscence
- Standard procedure = sigmoid resection + primary continuity restoration (if necessary with protective ileostoma) also in case of perforated sigmoid diverticulitis
- Laparoscopic peritoneal lavage + drainage, without resection: if necessary also for Hinchey III
- Sigmoid resection with primary anastomosis superior to Hartmann's procedure in the haemodynamically stable and immunocompetent patient under 85 years of age (Lambrichts et al. (2019) Lancet 4(8), 599–610)

Caution

Continuity restoration after Hartmann resection (discontinuity resection with rectal blind closure and terminal stoma) occurs in only about 50% of patients and is associated with substantial morbidity (44%) and lethality (5%).

- Technical aspects:
  - Proximal resection margin: In any case proximal to the chronically or acutely inflammatory altered wall sections in the healthy intestine

- Distal resection margin: In the upper rectum (better blood circulation) distal of the high pressure zone
- Stapler vs. manual suture anastomosis = equivalent

- Preservation of the inferior mesenteric artery recommended = avoidance of damage to the sacral plexus (= tubular sigmoid resection preferred)
- In septic/instable patients with difficult mobilization of the left flexure = Hartmann's procedure

3.2.2 Colonic Polyps

Definition

- Growths of different genesis into the lumen of the colon

Epidemiology

- Accumulation with increasing age
- Men > Women
- Localization: >50% in the rectum

Classification (◘ Table 3.4)

- Histological classification = behaviour/precancerous lesions

Symptoms

- Mostly incidental finding (= asymptomatic)
- Peranal mucus discharge: With large polyps
- Bleeding
- Complications:
  - Degeneration (adenoma-carcinoma sequence)
  - Obstruction
  - Invagination
  - Prolapse

Diagnosis

- Digital-rectal examination
- Rectoscopy/complete colonoscopy with biopsy/ablation
- Colon contrast imaging, CT colonography (rare, obsolete)

Therapy

Endoscopic Therapy

- If possible, always endoscopic
- Ablation of the polyp (thermal snare, forceps) in sano, goal = clean-colon
- Endoscopic mucosal resection (EMR)
- Submucosal resection/dissection (SMR/SMD)

FAP (Familial Adenomatous Polyposis)

- First colonoscopy obligatory at the age of 10 years, then annually
- If adenomas are detected = proctocolectomy indicated between onset of puberty up to the age of 20 years
- Followed by annual pouchoscopy
- Human genetic counselling (diagnosis in the family)

◘ Table 3.4 Classification of colonic polyps

Designation	Definition
Adenoma	Epithelial neoplasia (precancerous lesion) with a tendency to degeneration
Hyperplastic polyp	Small benign mucosal change, low tendency to degeneration
Inflammatory polyp	Small benign mucosal change, without degenerative tendency (associated with chronic inflammatory bowel disease)
Familial adenomatous polyposis (FAP)	Obligate precancerous lesion; mutation of the APC gene (autosomal dominant); risk of degeneration = 100%
Hamartoma	Atypical differentiation of germinal tissue (mutation) = polyposis with a tendency to degeneration (e.g. Peutz-Jeghers syndrome; Cowden syndrome)
Serrated polyp	Epithelial neoplasia; adenoma with high malignant potency

Guideline: Polypectomy

Implementation

- Documentation of the localization
- Polyp >5 mm: complete resection by loop ablation
- Polyp ≤5 mm: complete resection with forceps or snare
- Endoscopic mucosal resection
- Endoscopic full-thickness resection
- Histology obligatory:
- Statement on the completeness of the removal
  - In case of carcinoma detection necessary: pT (in case of sessile polyps the sm invasion measurement in µm), grading, L-, R-classification (local complete removal in depth and to the side).
  - pT1 carcinomas: "low risk" = G1, G2, L0/ "high risk" = G3, G4, L1

Postpolypectomy Strategy

- High-risk pT1 carcinoma (even if R0 ablation) = oncological resection
- Low-risk pT1 carcinoma incompletely ablated = complete endoscopic/local surgical removal
- If R0 situation not achievable or doubt about pT1 situation = oncological surgical resection

Follow-up

- Low-risk pT1 carcinoma after complete endoscopic R0 ablation = endoscopy after 6 months, complete colonoscopy after 3 years
- After removal of small, single, non-neoplastic polyps = no need for follow-up = control colonoscopy after 10 years
- Complete ablation of neoplastic polyps
- Time of control colonoscopy depending on number, size and histology
- In case of 1–2 adenomas <1 cm without higher-grade intraepithelial neoplasia after 5–10 years

Surgical Therapy

- For large polyp with a large base
- For non-ablatable polyp
- In case of carcinoma detection, after polypectomy
- Technique:
  - Exploration, colotomy, ablation
  - Colonic segment resection
  - Transanal full wall excision

If carcinoma is detected in the histology, oncological resection of the colon segment bearing the polyp is essential (▶ Sect. 3.3).

Follow-Up Care After Colonoscopic Ablation

- Depending on the histology
- Control colonoscopy:
- After ablation of 1–2 adenomas with low-grade intraepithelial neoplasia: after 5–10 years
- After ablation of >3 adenomas or villous parts or high-grade neoplasia: After 3 years
- Sessile adenomas or questionable in-toto removal: After 2–6 months

3.2.3 Ulcerative Colitis

Key Points

- Chronic inflammatory bowel disease confined to the colon and rectum, continuous affection of the mucosa
- Risk of formation of DALM ("dysplasia associated lesion or mass") → colon carcinoma
- Cure through restorative proctocolectomy

Definition

- Inflammatory bowel disease
- Mucosa + submucosa of the colon and rectum affected
- Continuous spreading of the lesions = ulcerations
- Autoimmunity in the pathogenetic background = genetic predisposition + specific triggers (stress, infection)

Epidemiology

- Incidence: 3.0–3.9 per 100,000 population
- Prevalence: 160–250 per 100,000 population
- Age peak at 16–25 years
- Women > Men

Etiology

Etiopathogenesis

- Not fully clarified
- Autoimmune pathogenesis: genetic predisposition + specific triggers (stress, infection)
- Positive family history, currently more than 160 known gene loci
- Other factors: diet, psychosomatic causes, nicotine, intestinal microbiome

Course

- Onset of inflammation: In the rectum
- Spread in oral direction, restricted exclusively to rectal and colonic mucosa
- Acute phase: red edematous mucosa, contact bleeding, microscopy: granulocytic crypt abscesses
- Chronic phase: mucosa destruction with loss of fold relief = pseudopolyps; microscopy: lymphocytic histiocytic infiltration

Clinical Presentation

Intestinal Manifestations

- Bloody-mucous diarrhea = leading symptom
- Abdominal discomfort: Pain, tenesmus
- Systemic signs of infection (e.g. reduced general condition, fever)

Extraintestinal Manifestations (15–20%)

- Erythema nodosum
- Aphtae, pyoderma gangraenosum
- Episcleritis, uveitis
- Peripheral and axial arthritis (ankylosing spondylitis)
- Primary sclerosing cholangitis (PSC), increased risk for development of chronic sclerosing cholangitis (CSC)

Course

- Acute-fulminant (5%): Sudden onset of illness (diarrhea, septic temperatures, septic shock); complications: Toxic megacolon; lethality approx. 30%
- Chronic-Continuous (10%): Without complete remission
- Chronic-recurrent (85%): Recurrent exacerbations; periods of complete remissions

Complications

- Massive bleeding
- Toxic megacolon
- Growth disorder
- Backwash ileitis (in up to 10% of patients spread to the ileum DD Crohn's disease)

Caution

Risk of colon cancer development due to ulcerative colitis!

Diagnosis

Anamnesis

- Type and onset of symptoms, food intolerances, medications, etc.
- Stool anamnesis

Complete Physical Examination

- Digital-rectal examination (blood detection)
- Extraintestinal manifestations (especially skin)

Lab

- Inflammatory status (leukocytosis, blood sedimentation rate, CRP, α_2-globuline)
- Hemoglobin, iron balance (exclusion of bleeding)
- Kidney function

- Transaminases, cholestasis parameters (bilirubin, alkaline phosphatase, γ-glutamyltransferase) in primary sclerosing cholangitis
- p-ANCA (antineutrophil cytoplasmic antibodies): 60–70% of cases
- Calprotectin/Lactoferrin in stool: progression parameter in any inflammatory bowel disease)
- Exclusion of intestinal infection: e.g. Clostridium difficile, CMV (cytomegalovirus), travel history
- Stool diagnosis

Imaging

- Colon double contrast enema:
  - Loss of the mucosal relief = "bicycle tube"
  - Pseudopolyps
- Sonography: Thickened colonic mucosa
- Hydro-MRI

Endoscopy

- Rectoscopy, ileocolonoscopy
- Biopsies of all intestinal sections
- Danger of perforation in case of inflammation

Endoscopic Classification

- Proctitis (limited to rectum)
- Left-sided colitis (to left flexure)
- Extensive colitis

Differential Diagnosis

- Crohn's disease
- Diverticulitis
- Infectious colitis
- Ischemic colitis
- Drug-toxic colitis
- Colon Cancer
- Irritable Bowel Syndrome

Therapy

Conservative-Medical Therapy

Long-term remission maintenance therapy should be given to all patients after successful relapse therapy

Uncomplicated Ulcerative Colitis

Proctitis

- Mesalazine ≥1000 mg/day as suppository
- Plus topical steroids (budenoside-rectal foam) or additional oral administration of mesalazine, if necessary

Left-Sided Colitis

- Rectal mesalazine as an enema or foam (≥1 g/day) in combination with oral mesalazine-releasing preparations (≥3 g/day)
- If necessary, systemic steroid therapy 0.5–1 mg/kg body weight/day prednisolone equivalent

Cancer Prevention

- Significantly increased risk of cancer = colonoscopy annually in patients with ulcerative colitis (after 8 years of disease)
- Risk reduction: Aminosalicylate long-term therapy
- In case of high-grade IEN (intraepithelial neoplasia) = proctocolectomy

Complicated/Severe Ulcerative Colitis

- Inpatient treatment, interdisciplinary
- Thrombosis prophylaxis
- Parenteral fluid and electrolyte balance
- No motility inhibiting drugs
- Systemic steroid therapy, e.g. 1 mg/kg body weight/day prednisolone equivalent
- In case of contraindication for system. Steroid therapy, Infliximab, Ciclosporin A or Tacrolimus can be used
- In case of insufficient clinical efficacy of steroids, these can be supplemented with TNF antibodies, tofacitinib, or with ciclosporin A or tacrolimus. In the case of infliximab, combination therapy with a thiopurine should preferably be used
- Surgical proctocolectomy
- Definition of severe colitis = criteria of Truelove and Witts:
  - More than six bloody diarrhea per day

3

  - Fever
  - Tachycardia
  - Anemia
  - BSR >30 mm/h
- Always interdisciplinary therapy

Time-Adapted Approach

- Time points for response to therapy, onset of remission, time point for discontinuation of medication in remission (Table 3.5)

Infliximab and ciclosporin are comparable as salvage therapy in acute severe steroid-insensitive ulcerative colitis.

Caution
- Before anti-TNF-α therapy: exclude latent tuberculosis!
- Before immunosuppressive therapy in chronic inflammatory bowel disease patients with a negative VZV (varicella-zoster virus) history (chickenpox/herpes zoster) or negative VZV serology, perform vaccination:
  - HPV (human papillomavirus) vaccination in girls and young women
  - Pneumococcal vaccination

Surgical Therapy

Surgery Indications

- Free or covered perforation
- Therapy refractory bleeding
- Drug-therapy refractory relapse
- Conservative-therapy refractory course
- Colon stenosis (of unclear dignity)
- Suspicion or detection of carcinoma, DALM

Important: Intraepithelial neoplasia (IEN) (WHO criteria) → continence-preserving proctocolectomy
- Histopathologically graded (low/high grade)
- In flat, non-inflamed mucosa
- Secondary assessment by reference pathologists
- DALM (inflammatory bowel disease-associated): Dysplasia-associated lesion or mass
- ALM: "adenoma like mass"

Standard Surgery: Restorative Proctocolectomy

- Laparoscopic or conventional open surgery
- If necessary, staged surgery: e.g. 3-stage procedure
  - Subtotal colectomy with terminal ileostomy
  - Residual proctocolectomy (with ileoanal pouch anastomosis) + double barrel ileostomy

Table 3.5 Time-adapted approach, time points for response to therapy, onset of remission, time point for discontinuation of medication in remission

Drug	Response after	Remission after	Time of weaning
5-aminosalicylic acid	2–4 weeks	8–12 weeks	After 2 years
Budenoside	2 weeks	8–10 weeks	(After 6–12 months)
Systemic steroids	1 week	4 weeks	No permanent therapy
Anti-TNF-α	1st–2nd gift	8 weeks	After 2 years
Azathioprine, 6-mercaptopurine, methotrexate	8 weeks	12–16 weeks	After >3.5 years
Calcineurin inhibitors	5–7 days	3 months?	After 6–12 months

TNF tumour necrosis factor

- Reversal of Ileostomy
- In case of ileoanal pouch = leave not longer than 2 cm rectal mucosa, if necessary secondary transanal mucosectomy

- Contraindications:
  - Severe sphincter insufficiency (check sphincter function, e.g. enema)
  - Perianal fistula
  - Age >60 years (relative CI)

Surgical Procedure

Restorative Proctocolectomy

- Transabdominal total colon and rectum resection (comparable to FAP Procedure—▶ Sect. 3.3.3)
- Peranal exposure of the rectal stump (Parks retractor)
- Injection of the mucosa above the dentate line
- Dissection the mucosa cranially
- Transanal/transabdominal transection of the rectal wall (with/without preservation of a rectal cuff)
- Mobilization of the ileum = tension-free anastomosis
- Reservoir formation: Formation of a 15-cm ileum J-pouch with stapling suture device (GIA 90 mm), via antimesenteric incision in the ileum loop
- Peranal anastomosis: machine/hand anastomosis
- Hand anastomosis: pull-through of the reservoir through rectal cuff + pouch-anal anastomosis (single stitch suture, all-layer)
- Protective double barrel loop ileostomy

Follow-Up

- Ileostomy reversal (after 2–3 months): Only after checking the reservoir tightness (pouchoscopy + CM imaging) + continence check (e.g. enema).
- Pouchoscopy: annually = exclusion of cancer or pouchitis

Alternative Procedure

- In case of cancer: surgery according to oncological criteria
- Turnbull procedure (creation of ileostoma and colostoma) for toxic megacolon
  - Double barrel ileostomy
  - Two colonic fistulas (transverse colon + sigmoid colon)
  - Lethality = 2–5% vs. 30% for subtotal colectomy
- Subtotal colectomy
  - Emergency surgery
  - Blind closure of the rectum (Hartmann operation)
  - Interval proctocolectomy
  - High lethality

Preventive Care (Cancer Prophylaxis)

- Indication
  - Ulcerative pancolitis that has been present for >8 years
  - Left-sided colitis persisting for more than 15 years
  - Synchronous primary sclerosing cholangitis (PSC)
  - If the rectum is left in place or if there is a terminal ileostomy with rectal stump
- Complete colonoscopy with step biopsies
  - At least four biopsies every 10 cm
  - Annually
- Primary prevention of colorectal carcinoma (CRC) = aminosalicylates

3.2.4 Chronic Constipation

In Short

- Rule out laxative abuse
- Neuronal pathologies: usually very early manifestation
- Rule out rectocele

Definition

- Subjectively unsatisfactory (<3 bowel evacuation per week or ≥2 leading symptoms of constipation: heavy straining,

lumpy or hard stool, subjectively incomplete defecation, subjective obstruction, manual maneuvers to facilitate defecation)
- For at least 3 months

3

Epidemiology

- Western countries: incidence = approx. 15%
- Women > Men
- Age-associated: Increases with age

Etiology

- Low-fiber diet: association, but no causal relationship
- Reduced fluid intake
- Lack of exercise
- Neuromuscular factors: enteric neuropathy: Cajal cells, myopathy: intestinal smooth muscle
- Diseases that can lead to secondary constipation (◘ Table 3.6)
- Medications with constipation potency (◘ Table 3.7)

◘ Table 3.6 Diseases that can lead to secondary constipation

Endocrinopathies	Diabetes mellitus Hypothyroidism Hyperparathyroidism MEN 1 and MEN 2
Neurological diseases	Parkinson's disease Multiple sclerosis Apoplexy Paraplegic Syndrome Paraneoplastic intestinal Neuropathies
Psychiatric diseases	Depression Somatization disorder
Other diseases	Ovarian carcinoid Scleroderma Amyloidosis Myotonic dystrophy Obstructive/Stenosing Intestinal disorders

MEN Multiple endocrine neoplasia

Diagnosis

Anamnesis

- Defecation disorder
- Medication

◘ Table 3.7 Drugs with constipation potency

Drug group	Drugs
Analgesics	Opiates
Antacids	Aluminium hydroxide, calcium carbonate
Antidepressants (anticholinergics)	Tricyclics (imipramine, clomipramine, amitriptyline, dibenzepine), tetracyclics (maprotiline, mianserine)
Antiepileptic drugs	Carbamazepine
Antihypertensives	β-blockers (e.g. atenolol), calcium antagonists (e.g. verapamil), clonidine
Anti-Parkinson's medication	Anticholinergics (e.g., biperiden), amantadine, bromocriptine
Antiemetics	5-HT3 antagonists (e.g. ondansetron)
Antitussives	Preparations containing codeine
Chemotherapeutics	Vincristine, vinblastine
Diuretics	Thiazides, sulfonamides
Iron supplements	Iron(II) and iron(III) salts
H_2 blocker	Cimetidine, Famotidine, Ranitidine
Lipid-lowering agent	Ion exchangers (e.g. colestipol, colestyramine)
Neuroleptics	Phenothiazines (e.g. chlorpromazine), thioxanthenes, butyrophenones, dibenzodiazepine (clozapine)
X-ray contrast agent	Barium salts
Spasmolytics	Butylscopolamine, trospium chloride

Physical Examination

- Rectal digital examination
- Gynaecological examination if necessary

Further Diagnosis

- Abdominal Ultrasound
- Colonoscopy after the age of 55
- Anorectal manometry
- MRI Defecography
- Colonic transit time

Therapy

Step-By-Step Therapy (Fig. 3.2)

- First stage: General recommendations = high-fibre diet, if necessary addition of psyllium husks, wheat bran
- Second stage:
  - Suppositories and clysms, plentiful fluid intake, adequate exercise, refraining from suppressing the urge to defecate
  - First choice: macrogol (osmotic laxative), bisacodyl, narium picosulfate (stimulate colonic motility and water secretion)
  - Second choice: sugars e.g. lactulose, anthraquinones
- Third Stage:
  - Prucalopride: e.g. Resolor®: prokinetic serotonin (5 HT4) receptor agonist = promotion of intestinal motility
  - Lubiprostone: e.g. Amitiza®: direct chloride channel activator = increase water and chloride secretion
  - Linaclotide: e.g. Constella®. Agonist = guanylate cyclase agonist = increase water and chloride secretion
- Fourth stage: Combinations of stages 1–3 (after special diagnosis)
- Fifth Stage: Sacral nerve stimulation

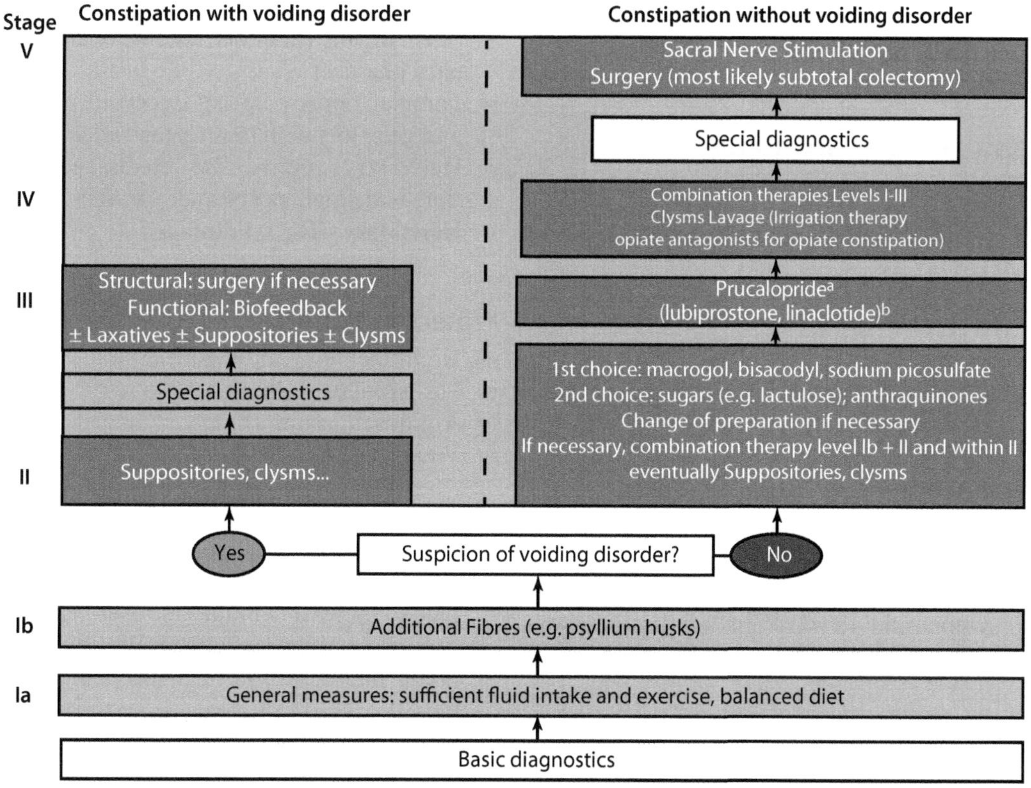

Fig. 3.2 Therapeutic algorithm for chronic constipation. 1st choice Approved for constipation in women if laxatives are ineffective or intolerant. 2nd choice Available through international pharmacies, linaclotide approved for obstipation-predominant IBS

Surgery

- Rarely indicated, after careful consideration most likely subtotal colectomy (80–90% improvement)
- Estimation of the potential effect: Temporary ileostoma or permanent ileostoma on patient's request
- Alternative: Antegrade irrigation via appendix or caecal stoma

3.2.5 Guidelines

AWMF guideline: S2k guideline diverticular disease/diverticulitis, register number 021/20. Currently under revision, planned completion 31.07.2021

AWMF guideline colorectal cancer January 2019, registration number 021/007OL.

S3 guideline ulcerative colitis 8/19, AWMF registration number 021/009

3.3 Colon Cancer and Hereditary CRC Syndromes

3.3.1 Colon Carcinoma

In Short

- Adenoma-carcinoma sequence: screening colonoscopy
- Standard procedure: Surgery with adjuvant chemotherapy (from T3/N+)

Definition

- Epithelial malignancy of the colon (between the caecum and rectosigmoid junction)
- Upper limit (level) of rectum (rigid rectoscopy) = 16 cm from ano (in Europe)

Epidemiology

- Second most common tumor in western industrialized nations
- Incidence in Germany = 80/100,000 inhabitants per year
- Men = Women
- Multiple synchronous colorectal carcinomas = 2–5%
- From 50 years of age: doubling of incidence and mortality per decade of life

Etiology and Pathogenesis

- Interaction of genetic factors and environmental influences

Risk Categories

- Sporadic: approximately 70%, acquired somatic mutation associated with:
  - Higher age (>40 years)
  - Tobacco consumption, alcohol consumption
- Risk-increasing diseases: Colorectal adenomas, chronic inflammatory bowel diseases (► Sect. 3.2.3 Ulcerative colitis), ureterosigmoideostomy, carcinomas of other organs (mamma, uterus, ovary, urinary bladder)
- Familial: approx. 20–30%, polymorphisms and gene loci with lower penetrance
- Hereditary: approx. 5%, hereditary mutation with high penetrance (► Sect. 3.3.2 Hereditary CRC syndromes)

Protective Factors

- High-fiber, low-fat, low-meat diet
- Fast stool passage
- Aminosalicylates
- Vitamin C, folic acid

Pathogenesis

- Adenoma-carcinoma sequence (90%): Due to increasing mutations over years
- De novo carcinomas (10%): Without adenoma manifestation (e.g. ulcerative colitis)
- Hereditary forms: Germline mutations already existing = carcinoma at a young age

Classification

TNM Classification (2017)

- T (tumor)
  - Tx Primary tumor not assessable
  - T0 No evidence of primary tumor
  - Tis carcinoma in situ: intraepithelial or invasion of the lamina propria
  - T1 Invasion of the submucosa
  - T2 Invasion of the muscularis propria
  - T3 invasion of the subserosa, or pericolic fat tissue
  - T4a Perforation of the visceral peritoneum
  - T4b Invasion of adjacent organs
- N (lymph nodes)
  - N0 No regional lymph node metastases
  - N1a 1 affected lymph node
  - N1b 2–3 affected lymph nodes
  - N1c Tumour nodule in the pericolic fat tissue
  - N2a 4–6 affected lymph nodes
  - N2b More than 6 affected lymph nodes
- M (metastases)
  - M0 No distant metastases
  - M1a Metastases in another organ
  - M1b Metastases in more than one other organ

UICC Staging of Colorectal Cancer

UICC stage	T (tumor)	N (lymph nodes)	M (metastases)
0	Tis	N0	M0
I	T1, T2	N0	M0
IIA	T3	N0	M0
IIB	T4a	N0	M0
IIC	T4b	N0	M0
III	Each T	N1, N2	M0
IIIA	T1, T2	N1a	M0
	T1	N2a	M0
IIIB	T3, T4a	N1	M0
	T2, T3	N2a	M0
	T1, T2	N2b	M0
IIIC	T4a	N2a	M0
	T3, T4b	N2b	M0
	T4b	N1, N2	M0
IVA	Each T	Each N	M1a
IVB	Each T	Each N	M1b

Histological Grading

- G1: Well differentiated
- G2: Moderately differentiated
- G3: Poorly differentiated (e.g. mucinous)
- G4: Undifferentiated (e.g. small cell, signet ring cell)
- V0/V1: Vein intrusion present/absent
- L0/L1: Intrusion into lymphatic vessels present/absent
- Pn0/Pn1: Perineural sheath infiltration present/absent

Symptoms

- Mostly uncharacteristic features
- Blood in the stool
- Change in bowel habits
- B-symptoms (fever, night sweats, weight loss)
- Performance drop, fatigue
- Tumor Anemia
- Rare abdominal pain

Complications

- Ileus
- Tumor perforation
- Fistulas
- Relevant bleeding

Diagnosis

Standard Investigations

- Anamnesis
  - Stool habits, body weight, blood in the stool, pain

3

– Family history: for risk assessment of hereditary colorectal cancer (Tables 3.8, 3.9, and 3.10)
- Clinical examination of the abdomen
  – Digital rectal examination
  – FOBT (Fecal Occult Blood Test = Haemoccult®)

Table 3.8 Amsterdam I criteria[a]

1	CRC was diagnosed in at least 3 relatives
2	One of you should be a first degree relative of the other two
3	At least 2 consecutive generations are affected
4	At least 1 CRC was diagnosed before the age of 50 years
5	Familial adenomatous polyposis (FAP) was excluded
6	CRC are verified by histopathological examination

CRC colorectal carcinoma
[a] Families must meet all criteria

Table 3.9 Amsterdam II criteria[a] (risk assessment of hereditary colon carcinoma)

1	Lynch syndrome-associated carcinoma has been diagnosed in at least 3 relatives[b]
2	One of you should be a first degree relative of the other two
3	At least 2 consecutive generations are affected
4	At least 1 tumor was diagnosed before the age of 50 years
5	Familial adenomatous polyposis (FAP) was excluded
6	Tumors are verified by histopathological examination

[a] Families must meet all criteria
[b] Colorectal tumor or tumor of the endometrium, small intestine, ureter, or renal pelvis

- Lab
  – Blood count, electrolytes, kidney function, coagulation status
- Complete colonoscopy

Guideline-Based Preoperative Diagnostic of Tumor Staging

- Digital-rectal examination
- Complete colonoscopy + biopsy
- Tumor not passable = colonoscopy 3–6 months postoperatively or intraoperatively
- Pneumocolon CT if necessary
- Abdominal ultrasound (especially liver)
- Chest X-ray in 2 planes

Table 3.10 Revised Bethesda guidelines (risk assessment of hereditary colon carcinoma[a])

1	CRC before the age of 50
2	Presence of synchronous, metachronous CRC (or Lynch syndrome)-associated tumors[b], regardless of age
3	CRC with MSI-H histology[c] diagnosed in patients <60 years of age
4	CRC diagnosed in patients with one or more first degree relatives with Lynch syndrome-associated tumor, one of whose carcinomas was diagnosed before age 50 years
5	CRC diagnosed in a patient with 2 or more first or second degree relatives with Lynch syndrome-associated tumor, regardless of age

[a] MSI investigation required if only one criterion is met
[b] Endometrial, gastric, ovarian, pancreatic, biliary, small bowel, brain tumors (usually glioblastoma in Turcot syndrome), seborrheic gland adenomas, and keratoankanthomas in Muir-Torre syndrome, hepatobiliary carcinomas, transitional cell carcinomas of the renal pelvis or ureter
[c] Presence of tumor-infiltrating lymph nodes, Crohn's disease-like lymphocytic infiltration, mucinous/seal-ring differentiation, or medullary growth pattern

- CEA (carcinoembryonic antigen) determination
- Useful in individual cases: spiral CT or MRI abdomen, spiral Chest CT

Colorectal Cancer Screening (in the Asymptomatic Population)

- Colonoscopy = standard procedure
  - From the age of 50
  - If the findings are unremarkable = repetition after 10 years
- Alternative: Sigmoidoscopy every 5 years + yearly FOBT (Guajak procedure)
- FOBT = consisting of 3 test letters with 2 order fields each for 3 consecutive stools
- Positive FOBT test = colonoscopy check!

Caution

In first degree relatives of patients with CRC or colorectal adenomas, a complete colonoscopy should be performed before the age of 50 years approximately 10 years before the age of onset of the cancer in the index patient, latest at the age of 50 years.

Guideline: Polypectomy

- ► Section 3.2.2

Therapy

Treatment Strategy

- Colon cancer = indication for surgery
- Always aim for R0 resection
  - Contraindication to surgery:
  - General inoperability of the patient
  - Inoperability of the tumor (R0 not achievable): Diffuse peritoneal carcinomatosis with distant metastases, infiltration of the great vessels

Surgical Therapy

Principles of Surgical Therapy

- Oncological resection principles
- Laparoscopic vs. open: equivalent if oncologic principles are adhered to
- Extent of resection (Fig. 3.3) depending on resection of the supplying vessels and the lymphatic drainage areas
- Right Hemicolectomy:
  - Indication: cancer of the caecum, ascending colon; for cancer of the right flexure = extended right hemicolectomy
  - Complications: Injury to the branches of the superior mesenteric artery, injury to the right ureter, injury to the duodenum, tearing of the pancreatic head veins (loop of Henle)
  - CME = complete mesocolic resection
- Left Hemicolectomy:
  - Indication: cancer of the descending colon, of the proximal sigmoid; in case of cancer of the left flexure = extended left hemicolectomy
  - Complications: Injury to the spleen, hemorrhage from splenocolic ligament, injury to the left ureter
- Colon transversum resection
  - Indication: Cancer of the middle of the transverse colon; for tumors close to the flexure = hemicolectomy
  - Complications: Insufficient anastomotic perfusion = anastomotic leakage
- Colon sigmoideum resection
  - Indication: Cancers of the middle/distal sigmoid colon
  - Complications: Injury to the left ureter, inadequate anastomotic perfusion = anastomotic leakage

Surgical Procedure
Right Hemicolectomy

- Longitudinal laparotomy vs. upper abdominal transverse laparotomy vs. laparoscopic approach
- Complete mesocolic excision (CME)
- Exploration, marking (e.g. vessel loops) of the colon at the level of the resection margins (proximal margin = 10–20 cm of the Bauhin valve)
- Mobilization of the caecum and ascending colon; exposure of the right ureter; detachment of the colon/mesocolon from Gerota's fascia

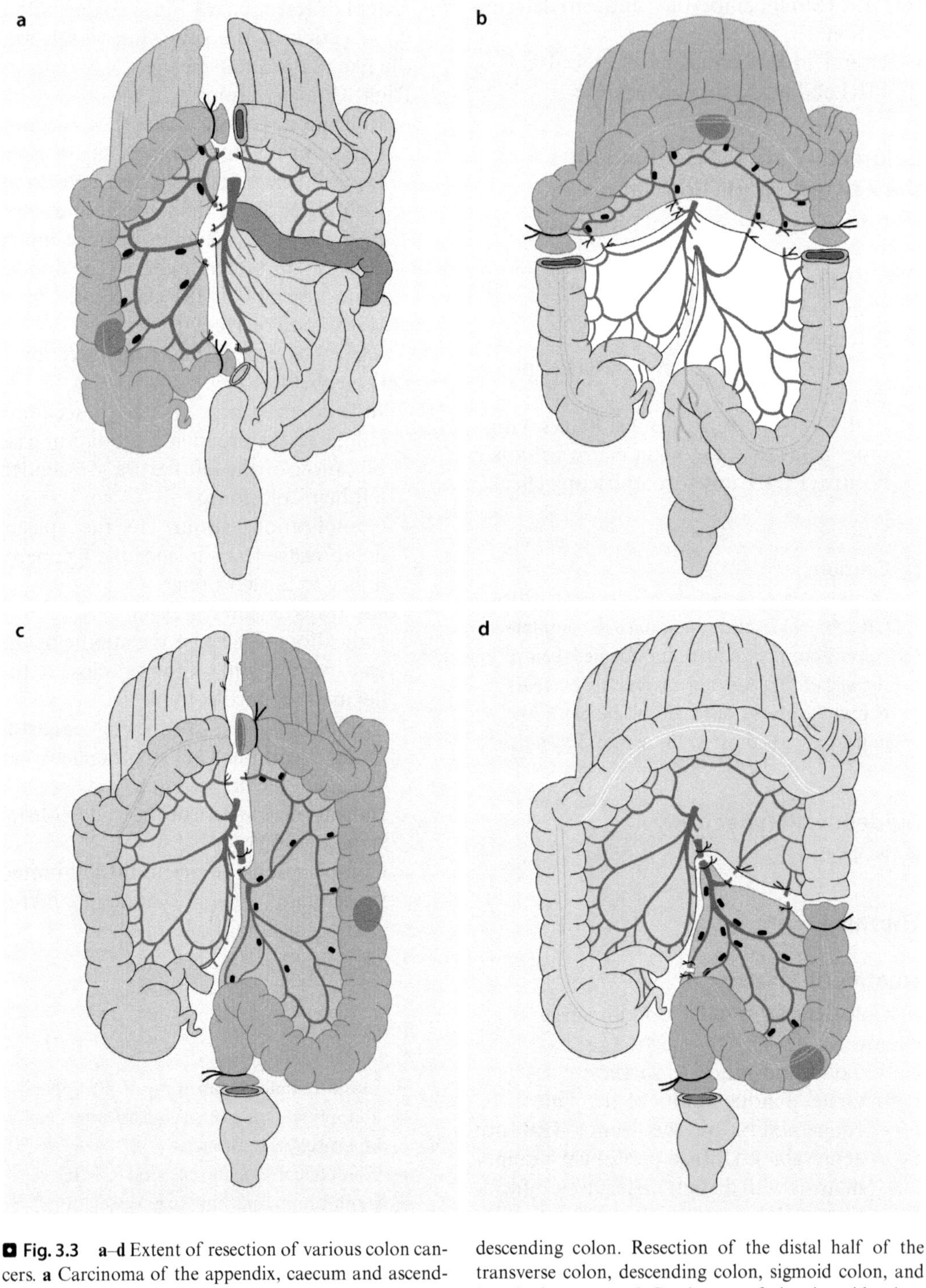

Fig. 3.3 **a–d** Extent of resection of various colon cancers. **a** Carcinoma of the appendix, caecum and ascending colon. Right hemicolectomy and lymphadenectomy. **b** Carcinoma of the transverse colon. Resection of the transverse colon including the flexurae coli dextra and sinistra and lymphadenectomy. **c** Carcinoma of the descending colon. Resection of the distal half of the transverse colon, descending colon, sigmoid colon, and lymphadenectomy. **d** Carcinoma of the sigmoid colon. Resection of the distal descending colon, sigmoid colon, proximal rectum, and lymphadenectomy

- Mobilization of the right flexure (transection of the hepatocolic and duodenocolic ligaments)
- Transection of gastrocolic ligament for distal resection border
- Transection of the great omentum at the level of the distal resection margin; omentum remains en bloc on the specimen
- Transection of the mesentery (with mesenteric vessels) between ligatures
- Ligation of the ileocolic vessels close to superior mesenteric vein and colic arteries and the right branch of the colic artery and vein close to Henle's loop (CME)
- Remove the bowel at the level of the resection margins
- Side-to-side ileotransversostomy
- Closure of the mesenteric gap

Surgical Procedure
Left Hemicolectomy

- Longitudinal laparotomy vs. laparoscopic approach
- Complete mesocolic excision (CME)
- Exploration, marking of the colon at the level of the resection margins (proximal: depending on tumor location; distal: above the peritoneal fold)
- Incision of the white line (Toldt) and mobilization of the descending colon + sigmoid; exposure of the left ureter
- Dissection of the left mesocolon from Gerota's fascia medially
- Transection of the great omentum at the level of the proximal resection margin; omentum remains en bloc on the specimen
- Mobilization of the left colonic flexure (transection of the splenocolic and phrenocolic ligaments)
- Severing the mesentery between ligatures
- Transection of the inferior mesenteric vein at the inferior border of the pancreas (lateral to lig. Treitz), transection of the inferior mesenteric artery centrally
- Pay attention to the course of the parasympathetic nerves
- Remove the bowel at the level of the resection margins
- Transversorectostomy (usually circular end to end anastomosis)
- Closure of the mesenteric gap

Surgical Procedure
Colon Transversum Resection

- Longitudinal laparotomy vs. upper abdominal transverse laparotomy vs. laparoscopic approach
- Complete mesocolic excision (CME)
- Exploration, marking of the colon at the level of the resection margins
- Transection of the gastrocolic ligament
- Mobilization of the right colonic flexure and the ascending colon
- Mobilization of the left colonic flexure
- Radicular resection of the A. and V. colica media
- Transection of the transverse mesocolon at the lower border of the pancreas; including lymphadenectomy
- Transection of the mesentery between ligatures
- Remove the bowel at the level of the resection margins
- Ascendodescendostomy as end-end anastomosis
- Closure of the mesenteric gap

Surgical Procedure
Oncological Colon Sigmoideum Resection

- Median lower abdominal laparotomy vs. laparoscopic approach
- Complete mesocolic excision (CME)
- Exploration, marking of the colon at the level of the resection margins (proximal: transition descending colon—sigmoid; distal: rectosigmoid transition)

3

- Incision of the white line (Toldt) and mobilization of the descending colon + sigmoid; exposure of the left ureter
- Dissection/Mobilization of the mesosigmoid from Gerota fascia medially
- Exposure and resection of the inferior mesenteric artery (preservation/non-preservation of the left colic artery); check of the blood supply of the proximal end of the intestine
- Transection of the inferior mesenteric vein at the inferior border of the pancreas
- Medial incision of the mesenteric peritoneum at the insertion along the aorta and blunt detachment from the retroperitoneum; Attention: protection of the autonomic nerves
- Resection of the superior rectal artery
- Transection of the mesosigma between ligatures
- Mobilization of the proximal rectum
- Incision of the pelvic floor peritoneum
- Exposure of the rectum, dorsally in the Waldeyer space, then ventrally and laterally (paraproctia).
- Transection of the upper mesorectum up to the level of the distal resection border (No **Coning** = thinning of the distal mesorectum)
- Resection of tumor bearing colon segment
- Circular end-to-end descendorectostomy (usually mechanically with transanal CEEA ("circular end-to-end anastomosis") stapler)

Postoperative Complications

- Suture insufficiency = anastomotic insufficiency
  - With peritonitis: relaparotomy, lavage, Hartmann resection or resection + anastomosis, creation of protective ileostoma
- Abscess: drainage (possibly CT-guided), irrigation, if necessary creation of protective ileostoma
- Fecal fistula without peritonitis (infraperitoneal): stoma creation + Endo-VAC-application until cleaning of the cavity, waiting for spontaneous healing.
- Postoperative bleeding
- Mechanical ileus due to adhesive small bowel obstruction = relaparotomy + adhesiolysis
- Hernia
- Cancer Recurrence

Principles for Specific Situations

- Multivisceral resection:
  - In case of adherence of the tumor to adjacent organs = en bloc multivisceral resection
- **Caution:** Biopsies should be strictly avoided = risk of tumor cell dissemination (spillage)
- Carcinoma in FAP: Restorative proctocolectomy with small bowel pouch + lymph node dissection according to the location of the carcinoma
- Carcinoma in HNPCC:
  - Proceed in the same way as for sporadic CRC
  - If necessary subtotal colectomy + prophylactic hysterectomy + salpingoovarectomy at the time of abdominal surgery
- Carcinoma in ulcerative colitis: restorative proctocolectomy + systematic oncologic lymphadenectomy with CME

Principles in Metastatic Colon Cancer

- Liver metastases
  - If R0 resection for liver and all other lesions possible = liver resection
  - Neoadjuvant systemic chemotherapy if necessary
- Pulmonary metastases
  - If R0 resection possible = resection
  - For synchronous liver and lung metastases → resection of liver metastases first
- Peritoneal carcinomatosis
  - If R0 (CC-0) resection possible = cytoreductive surgery (CRS) + peritonectomy + hyperthermic intraperitoneal chemotherapy (HIPEC) indicated

Adjuvant Chemotherapy

Caution

- Prerequisite is the oncological R0 resection!
- Indication based on histology with TNM classification (pN0 classification possible if at least 12 regional lymph nodes in specimen) (see above)

Indications

- Stage III (UICC)
- Stage II (UICC) (with microsatellites instability) or with risk factors:
  - pT4 tumor, tumor perforation/rupture
  - Emergency Operation
  - Number of examined lymph nodes too low
- Adjuvant chemotherapy may be considered after R0 resection of synchronous or metachronous liver metastases

Contraindications

- Poor general condition
- Uncontrolled infection
- Liver cirrhosis Child B/Child C
- Severe coronary heart diseases (CHD); heart failure: NYHA (New York Heart Association) III/IV
- Preterminal/terminal renal failure
- Limited bone marrow insufficiency

Standard Chemotherapy = FOLFOX (5-FU/Folinic Acid/Oxaliplatin)

- Protocol Examples:
  - FOLFOX4: folinic acid, 5-FU (5-fluorouracil), oxaliplatin every 2 weeks for 12 cycles
  - Guideline states that patients over 70 years of age should not receive oxaliplatin-containing therapy
  - In case of contraindication to oxaliplatin-containing regimens = monotherapy with fluoropyrimidines: oral 5-FU prodrug capecitabine, 8 cycles of 3 weeks each
  - In R0-resected stage III colon cancer, additional administration of cetuximab does not add benefit to FOLFOX even in KRAS wild type

No age restriction for adjuvant chemotherapy (general contraindications to be considered) = patients ≥75 years of age in stage III have survival benefit from adjuvant chemotherapy; oxaliplatin provides little additional benefit.

Palliative Chemotherapy

- Stage IV: Indicated for primary irresectability, independently of metastasis-related symptoms
- For example, FOLFOX, FOLFIRI, bevacizumab, cetuximab…
- Regorafenib (small molecule multikinase inhibitor) = survival benefit in metastatic colorectal cancer after failure of all standard therapies

Oncologic Follow-up

- Stage I: Not indicated
- Stage II and III: Follow-up indicated after R0 resection
- Principles of oncologic follow-up: ◘ Table 3.11

Prognosis

- Cumulative 5-year survival rate = 60%
- 5-year survival rate by UICC stage:
  - UICC I = approx. 70–100%
  - UICC II = approx. 60–91%
  - UICC III = approx. 44–60%
  - UICC IV = approx. 3–7% (without therapy)

3.3.2 HNPCC (Hereditary Non-polyposis Colorectal Cancer): Lynch Syndrome

Key Points

- Hereditary disease associated with colorectal cancer
- Also associated with other cancers (including endometrial cancer)
- Defect in mismatch repair genes

Table 3.11 Programmed follow-up for colon cancer UICC II and III (S3 Guidelines Colorectal Carcinoma)

Investigation	Months										
	3	6	9	12	15	18	21	24	36	48	60
Medical history, physical examination, CEA		x		x		x		x	x	x	x
Colonoscopy		x[a]		x[b]					x[b]		
Abdominal Sonography[c]		x		x		x		x	x	x	x
Sigmoidoscopy (rectoscopy)[d]		x		x		x		x			
Spiral CT[e]	x										
Chest X-ray (no consensus)											

[a] If a complete preoperative colonoscopy has not been performed
[b] If the findings are unremarkable (no adenoma, no carcinoma) next colonoscopy after 5 years
[c] A meta-analysis showed an advantage for an imaging procedure to detect liver metastases in follow-up. For this reason, application of the simplest and less expensive procedure
[d] Only for rectal cancer without adjuvant or neoadjuvant radiochemotherapy
[e] Only for rectal cancer 3 months after completion of tumor-specific therapy (surgery or radiation/chemotherapy) as initial findings

Definition

- HNPCC = Lynch syndrome
- Most frequent form of hereditary colorectal cancer
- Autosomal-dominant inheritance, no 100% penetrance

Epidemiology

- Approx. 1–3% of all CRC patients
- 2% of all endometrial cancers
- Most common form of hereditary CRC
- Lynch syndrome: Compared to sporadic CRC
  - Younger patient age
  - Better prognosis
  - Much lower metastatic tendency: synchronous CRC 18%, metachronous CRC 30% after 10 years, 50% after 15 years, right-sided CRC 60%
  - Lifetime risk of CRC (up to 75 years) (Table 3.12)

Etiology

- HNPCC: "hereditary non-polyposis colorectal cancer" (introduced in 1985)
- Bethesda/Amsterdam criteria for the diagnosis of HNPCC
- Lynch syndrome: mutation identified
- Mismatch repair (MMR) gene: mutation (MSH2, MLH1, MSH6, PMS2)
- Malignancies in LS (Lynch syndrome) patients: Due to somatic mutation of the second gene = microsatellite instability (MSI)
- Lynch I: CRC only

Table 3.12 Cumulative lifetime risks in patients with Lynch syndrome

Cancer	Lynch syndrome (%)	General population (%)
CRC male	54–74	5
CRC female	30–52	5
Endometrium	28–60	2
Ovary	6–7	1
Stomach	6–9	<1
Small intestine	3–4	<1
Pancreas	<1–4	1
Hepatobiliary	1	Rarely
Urinary tract	3–8	Rarely
Brain	2–3	<1
Seborrhoeic skin tumour/keratoankanthoma	1–9	Rarely

- Lynch II: CRC + cancer of the genitourinary tract
- Muir-Torre syndrome: Lynch syndrome + sebaceous gland cancers or keratoacanthomas

Diagnosis

Anamnesis

- Amsterdam criteria I + II (Tables 3.8 and 3.9)
- Bethesda criteria (Table 3.10)

Test for Mismatch Repair Defect

- If Bethesda criteria met
- By PCR, much cheaper = immunohistochemistry
- Histology
- In biopsy of CRC, MSI can be identified with almost 100% sensitivity and specificity
- Increased incidence of mucinous carcinomas, signet ring carcinomas, medullary carcinomas

Caution

A significant proportion of loss of MLH1 expression is the result of promoter methylation (BRAF V600 mutation) and not an MMR defect

Prevention

- Monitoring of Lynch syndrome mutation carriers (Table 3.13)
- Complete colonoscopy: annually from the age of 25, in any case 5 years before the lowest age of onset of the disease in the family
- Females at risk: From the age of 25 annual gynaecological examination + transvaginal US
- If there is a positive family history of gastric cancer: annual EGD from the age of 25
- Upper abdominal Ultrasound annually

Surgical Therapy

Despite regular monitoring, the relative risk of developing a tumor is 5.8 times higher compared to a mutation-negative cohort.

Table 3.13 Recommendations for surveillance of Lynch syndrome mutation carriers by the German S3 guideline (compared with the recommendations of the Mallorca group (European branch of InSIGHT, ► http://www.mallorca-group.eu), EGAPP (► https://www.egappreviews.org/recommendations/Lynch.htm), and NCCN (► https://www.nccn.org)

	Colonoscopy interval (years)	Lower age limit	Gastroscopy interval (years)	Lower age limit	Abdominal ultrasound interval (years)	Lower age limit	Gynecology Interval (years)	Lower age limit	Other
S3 guideline	1	25[a]	1[b]	25	1	25	1	25	Genetic counseling at the age of 18
Mallorca Group	1–2	20–25	1–2[b]	30–35	1	30–35	1–2, TVU, aspiration biopsy…	30–35	Urinalysis and cytology if there is a family history of urinary tract cancer.
EGAPP	1–2	20–25					1–2, TVU, endometrial biopsy…	30–35	Genetic counselling
NCCN	1–2	20–25[c]					1–2, TVU or endometrial aspirate	30–35	

TVU transvaginal ultrasound
[a] Same age or at least 5 years younger than the youngest age at diagnosis in the family
[b] When cancer runs in the family
[c] Same age or 10 years younger than youngest age at diagnosis in the family

- Oncological resection: According to the standard rules for CRC
- Extended resection: e.g. subtotal colectomy + ileosigmoidostomy = justified in individual cases
- If necessary prophylactic hysterectomy + salpingo-oophorectomy at the time of abdominal surgery

3.3.3 Other Hereditary CRC Syndromes

Familial Adenomatous Polyposis (FAP)

Definition

- Obligate precancerous lesion
- Risk of cancer = almost 100% from the age of 15 onwards
- About 1% of all CRC
- Other extracolic manifestations

Etiology

- Mutation APC gene
- Autosomal dominant inheritance (75% of cases)
- New mutation (25% of cases)

Tumour Spectrum

- Duodenal and papillary adenomas
- Gastric Adenomas
- Abdominal and extraabdominal desmoid tumors
- Thyroid cancers
- Malignant CNS tumours (mostly medulloblastomas)
- Hepatoblastomas
- Osteomas, epidermoid cysts, pigmentary abnormalities of the retina

Prevention

- From the age of 10, after human genetic counselling predictive genetic diagnosis
- If mutation confirmed:
  - Rectosigmoidoscopy annually from the age of 10 at the latest
  - If adenomas are detected = complete colonoscopy
  - Until proctocolectomy annual repetition of complete colonoscopy
- Esophagogastroscopy (EGD) with inspection of the papilla region: At the latest from the age of 30 every 3 years, if necessary annually in case of changes
- Extracolic manifestations: Annual ultrasound of the abdomen, from the age of 10 onwards annual ultrasound of the thyroid gland

Therapy

- Sphincter-preserving proctocolectomy (▶ Sect. 3.2.3)

Follow-Up

- Pouchoscopy yearly
- If preserved rectal stump = rectoscopy every 4 months

Hamartomatous Polyposis Syndromes

Definition

- Peutz-Jeghers Syndrome
- Juvenile polyposis coli
- Cowden syndrome: PTEN ("phosphatase and tensin homolog") gene

Prophylaxis

- No general recommendations due to sparse evidence available

Diagnosis and Therapy

- See above (CRC)
- No general recommendations due to sparse evidence available

3.3.4 Guidelines

S3 Guideline Colorectal Carcinoma 1/2019, AWMF Register Number 021/007/OL

Schmiegel W, Reinacher-Schick A, Arnold D, Graeven U, Heinemann V, Porschen R, Riemann J, Rödel C, Sauer R, Wieser M, Schmitt W, Schmoll HJ, Seufferlein T, Kopp I, Pox C (2008) S3 guideline colorectal carcinoma. Z Gastroenterol 46:1–73

Reference

Lambrichts DPV, Vennix S, Musters GD, Mulder IM, Swank HA, Hoofwijk AGM, Belgers EHJ, Stockmann HBAC, Eijsbouts QAJ, Gerhards MF, van Wagensveld BA, van Geloven AAW, Crolla RMPH, Nienhuijs SW, Govaert MJPM, di Saverio S, D'Hoore AJL, Consten ECJ, van Grevenstein WMU, Pierik REGJM, Kruyt PM, van der Hoeven JAB, Steup WH, Catena F, Konsten JLM, Vermeulen J, van Dieren S, Bemelman WA, Lange JF, LADIES trial collaborators (2019) Hartmann's procedure versus sigmoidectomy with primary anastomosis for perforated diverticulitis with purulent or faecal peritonitis (LADIES): a multicentre, parallel-group, randomised, open-label, superiority trial. Lancet Gastroenterol Hepatol 4(8):599–610

Suggested Reading

Alberts SR, Sargent DJ, Nair S, Mahoney MR, Mooney M, Thibodeau SN, Smyrk TC, Sinicrope FA, Chan E, Gill S, Kahlenberg MS, Shields AF, Quesenberry JT, Webb TA, Farr GH, Pockaj BA, Grothey A, Goldberg RM (2012) Effect of oxaliplatin, fluorouacil and leucovorin with or without cetuximab on survival among patients with resected stage III colon cancer. JAMA 307:1383–1393

Chabok A, Påhlman L, Hjern F, Haapaniemi S, Smedh K, AVOD Study Group (2012) Randomized clinical trial of antibiotics in acute uncomplicated diverticultis. Br J Surg 99:532–539

Chang KH, Burke JP, Coffey JC (2013) Infliximab versus cyclosporine as rescue therapy in acute severe steroid-refractory ulcerative colitis: a systematic review and meta-analysis. Int J Color Dis 28:287–293

Ehehalt R, Krammer HJ (2014) Aktuelle Diagnostik und Therapie der Colitis ulcerosa. Coloproctology 36:409–420

Frei P, Rogler G (2014) Topische Therapie bei chronisch-entzündlichen Darmerkrankungen. Coloproctology 36:353–358

Grothey A, Van Cutsem E, Sobrero A, Siena S, Falcone A, Ychou M, Humblet Y, Bouché O, Mineur L, Barone C, Adenis A, Tabernero J, Yoshino T, Lenz HJ, Goldberg RM, Sargent DJ, Chon F, Cupit L, Wagner A, Laurent D, CORRECT Study Group (2013) Regorafenib monotherapy for previously treated metastatic colorectal cancer (CORRECT); an international, multicenter, randomized, placebo-controlled, phase 3 trial. Lancet 381:303–312

Kremer K, Lierse W (1992a) Chirurgische Operationslehre, Band Darm. Georg Thieme, Stuttgart

Kremer K, Lierse W (1992b) Chirurgische Operationslehre, Band Darm. Thieme, Stuttgart

Kucharzik T, Koletzko S, Kannengießer K, Dignaß A (2020) Ulcerative colitis-diagnostic and therapeutic algorithms. Dtsch Arztebl Int 117:564–574. https://doi.org/10.3238/arztebl.2020.0564

Leifeld L, Germer CT, Böhm S, Dumoulin FL, Häuser W, Kreis M, Labenz J, Lembcke B, Post S, Reinshagen M, Ritz JP, Sauerbruch T, Wedel T, von Rahden B, Kruis W (2014) S2k Leitlinie Divertikelkrankheit/Divertikulitis, AWMF Registriernummer 021/20. Z Gastroenterol 52:663–710

Lock JF, Galata C, Reißfelder C, Ritz JP, Schiedeck T, Germer CT (2020) The indications for and timing of surgery for diverticular disease. Dtsch Arztebl Int 117:591–596. https://doi.org/10.3238/arztebl.2020.0591

Pehl C (2014) Chronische Obstipation. Definition, Diagnostik und Therapie nach der S2k-Leitlinie. Coloproctology 36:495–505

Rauber A, Kopsch F (1987) Lehrbuch und Atlas der Anatomie des Menschen, Band 2: Innere Organe. Thieme, Stuttgart

Rogers AC, Collins D, O'Sullivan GC, Winter DC (2012) Winter laparoscopic lavage for perforated diverticulitis: a population analysis. Dis Colon Rectum 55:932–938

Sanoff HK, Carpenter WR, Stürmer T, Goldberg RM, Martin CF, Fine JP, McCleary NJ, Meyerhardt JA, Niland J, Kahn KL, Schymura MJ, Schrag D (2012) Effect of adjuvant chemotherapy on survival of patients with stage III colon cancer diagnosed after age 75 years. J Clin Oncol 30:2624–2634

Schneider R, Schneider C, Kloor M, Fürst A, Möslein G (2012) Lynch syndrome: clinical, pathological, and genetic insights. Langenbecks Arch Surg 397:513–525

Standring S (2009) Gray's anatomy. The anatomical basis of clinical practice, vol 40. Churchill Livingstone, Elsevier, London

Steinke V, Engel C, Büttner R, Schackert HK, Schmiegel WH, Propping P (2013) Erblicher Darmkrebs ohne Polyposis. Dtsch Arztbl Int 110:32–38

Vennix S, Musters GD, Mulder IM, Swank HA, Consten EC, Belgers EH, van Geloven AA, Gerhards MF, Govaert MJ, van Grevenstein WM, Hoofwijk AG, Kruyt PM, Nienhuijs SW, Boermeester MA, Vermeulen J, van Dieren S, Lange JF, Bemelman WA, Ladies Trial Colloborators (2015) Laparoscopic peritoneal lavage or sigmoidectomy for perforated diverticulitis with purulent peritonitis: a multicentre, parallel-group, randomised, open-label trial. Lancet 386:1269–1277. https://doi.org/10.1016/S0140-6736(15)61168-0

von Lanz T, Wachsmuth W (2004) Praktische Anatomie. Bauch. Springer, Berlin

Wittekind (2017) TNM – Klassifikation maligner Tumoren, 8. Aufl. VCH, S 98–100. Wiley-VCH, Weinheim. ISBN 978-3-527-34280-8

Rectum

Jens Wannenmacher and Stefan Willis

Contents

F. Billmann, T. Keck (eds.), *Essentials of Visceral Surgery*,
https://doi.org/10.1007/978-3-662-66735-4_4

4.1 Anatomy and Physiology

S. Willis

4.1.1 Definition, Location and Structure

Definition

- Part of the large intestine between sigmoid colon and anus

Location

- In the pelvis with close relationship to neighbouring organs—therefore special features in diagnosis and therapy

Limits

- Boundary between colon and rectum defined differently: in Germany at 16 cm and in the USA at 12 cm (from anocutaneous line (a.a.) measured with rigid rectoscope (caution literature comparison)
- According to the Union for International Cancer Control (UICC) division into 3 parts:
  - Upper third 12–16 cm a.a. (= intraperitoneal portion)
  - Middle third 6–12 cm a.a.
  - Lower third <6 cm a.a.

4.1.2 Anatomy and Embryology

Topographic Anatomy

- Curved course along the sacrum and the coccygeal bone to the levator funnel
- Dorsal retroperitoneal position up to the promontory, ventral variable peritoneal envelope (excavatio rectouterina in females or rectovesicalis in males)
- Extraperitoneal envelopment of the rectum by the mesorectum with the lymphovascular pathways
- Circumferential boundary of the mesorectum by the visceral pelvic fascia, which turns into the parietal pelvic fascia at the level of the pelvic floor, in between avascular separating layer
- Denonvillier's fascia = ventral part of the parietal pelvic fascia (covering of vagina or seminal vesicle and prostate together with associated vessels and nerves)
- Waldeyer's fascia = dorsal part of the parietal pelvic fascia (covering the presacral venous plexus and the vegetative hypogastric and pelvic nerves)
- Inferior part of the rectum without mesorectal and fascial envelope

Blood Supply and Drainage

- Arterial Supply:
  - From cranial = superior rectal artery (end section of the inferior mesenteric artery, course: dorsal in the mesorectum)
  - From caudal: inferior rectal artery (from A. iliaca interna), occasionally inconstant middle rectal artery
- Venous drainage:
  - 2/3 oral: drainage in superior rectal vein to inferior mesenteric vein and portal vein
  - 1/3 aboral: drainage in middle rectal veins + inferior rectal veins to internal iliac vein and inferior vena cava
- Lymphatic drainage: bidirectional
  - Cranial along the superior rectal artery to paraaortal nodes and vessels
  - Distally along the internal iliac artery
  - No lymphatic vessel arcades near the intestinal wall

Caution
Caudal portion = intramural lymphatic drainage (due to missing mesorectum)

Innervation

- Through autonomic nerves:
  - Sympathetic innervation:
    - inferior mesenteric trunc ventral to the aorta at the level of the outlet of the inferior mesenteric artery, becomes the superior hypogastric

plexus presacral at the level of the promontory, than divides into right and left hypogastric nerves, which course dorsal to the mesorectum

Damage of the sympathetic portion leads to retrograde ejaculation.

- Parasympathetic innervation:
  - pelvic splanchnic nerves unite with the sympathetic hypogastric nerves at the level of the seminal vesicles and form the inferior hypogastric plexus (= pelvic plexus).
  - Further course along the lateral border of the prostate gland

Damage of the parasympathetic part leads to erectile dysfunction or disturbance of lubrication and bladder emptying disorder.

4.1.3 Physiology

- Direct continuity with sigmoid colon, but different function

Special Functions of the Rectum

- Defecation: action of defecation
- Continence: ability to retain stool; controlled voiding
- anorectal continence apparatus

4.2 Benign Diseases

S. Willis

4.2.1 Benign Neoplasms/ Malformations

Polyps/Adenomas (Chap. 3)

- Mostly asymptomatic
- Symptoms:
  - Mostly incidental findings during screening endoscopy
  - Bleeding
  - Mucus production
  - Passage obstruction
  - Histology obligatory

Caution
Adenoma = facultative precancerous lesion

- Therapy:
  - Endoscopic ablation with snare, EMR (endoscopic mucosal resection) or submucosal dissection
  - Surgical therapy by means of transanal resection or TEM (transanal endoscopic microsurgery) possible
  - Avoid peacemeal resections (histology, topographic assignment for R1 resection)

Schwannomas, Leiomyomas, Angiomyomas

- Very rare
- Diagnosis occasionally by CT- or EUS (endoscopic ultrasound)-guided puncture
- Therapy: Enucleation in healthy tissue is sufficient

Hirschsprung's Disease

- Congenital intestinal aganglionosis
- Pathophysiology:
  - Aganglionic segment starting from linea dentata, reaching to different degrees proximally, dilated intestine above it
  - Mostly disease of childhood
- Diagnosis: by deep rectal biopsy
- Therapy: Resection of the aganglionic segment and the adjacent dysfunctional dilated section

Infiltrating Endometriosis

- Unclear pathogenesis, mostly young women
- Symptoms:
  - Unspecific, cyclically occurring complaints
  - Pelvic pain, rectal bleeding, constipation, diarrhoea

- Therapy:
  - Primarily conservative/symptomatic therapy
  - Recurrence rate: up to 60%
  - Resection required in individual cases
  - Interdisciplinary approach at specialised centres

4.2.2 Rectal Prolapse

Key Points

- Etiology unclear
- Mainly older, female patients affected
- Diagnosis by inspection
- Often simultaneous constipation + incontinence
- Choice of procedure dependent on: size of the prolapse + comorbidity of the patient
- Perineal procedures: Lower morbidity but worse long-term outcomes
- Abdominal procedures: Better results, but higher risk

Definition, Classification, Differential Diagnosis, Epidemiology

Definition

- Protrusion of the entire rectal wall outwards through the anal sphincter apparatus

Classification

- Grade 1: Internal, partial prolapse (intussusception)
- Grade 2: Internal prolapse extending to the anocutaneous line
- Grade 3: External solid wall prolapse

First-degree prolapse can also be detected in a high percentage of healthy individuals; findings requiring treatment only when symptoms occur.

Differential Diagnoses

- Anal prolapse (▶ Sect. 5.2.1 Haemorrhoids)
- Mucosal prolapse alone

Epidemiology

- Age peak: children around 3 years and older women
- Incidence = 1% in the over-65s
- Combination with bladder, vagina and/or uterus prolapse = frequent

Etiology and Pathogenesis

- Variable expression of morphological/functional changes:
  - Abnormally deep rectovesicale/rectovaginale space ("Cul de sac")
  - Atone pelvic floor and sphincter muscles
  - Diastasis of the pelvic diaphragm (levator ani muscle)
  - Mobile mesorectum with lack of lateral + dorsal fixation
  - Pudendal nerve neuralgia
- Causal pathogenesis vs. secondary phenomenon = unclear
- Often associated with:
  - Functional disorders (e.g. excessive pressing during defecation)
  - Structural changes (e.g. hysterectomy, post anal atresia in children)

Symptoms and Diagnosis

Symptoms

- Common concomitant symptomatology:
  - Symptoms of constipation (up to 65%)
  - Symptoms of incontinence (up to 90%)
- Rectal prolapse = clinical diagnosis

Diagnosis

- Inspection
- Rectal digital examination = crucial!
  - Spontaneously reducible in the initial stage
  - If more severe: Manual reduction required
- Dynamic pelvic floor MRI: Helpful for evaluation of the ventral compartments and detection of an enterocele
- Rectoscopy/colonoscopy: to exclude endoluminal concomitant diseases
- Anal manometry not required

Therapy

- Therapy goals
  - Permanent removal of the prolapse
  - Restoration of adequate function
- Strategy: Choice of procedure depends on:
  - Prolapse size
  - Comorbidity of patients

Non-surgical Therapy

- Preoperative exhaustion of conservative options (stool regulation, pelvic floor exercises, biofeedback if necessary)
- Possible combination of all procedures with:
  - Sacral nerve neuromodulation/stimulation (SNS, stable good continence improvement)
  - Sphincteroplasty/levatoroplasty (poor long-term results)

Surgical Therapy

- Therapy principles
  - Resection, fixation or plication of the redundant bowel
  - Abdominal or perineal/transanal procedure
- Strategy
  - No significant risks = laparoscopic resection rectopexy (= best functional long-term result)
  - In moderate prolapse without constipation: Current preference for laparoscopic ventral rectopexy
  - In case of high risk for abdominal surgery: perineal procedures

No clear recommendations based on evidence-based randomized trials.

Perineal and Transanal Procedures

- Wrapping procedure of the anus
  - Techniques: Thiersch ring, subcutaneous placement of foreign material.
  - Results: unsatisfactory + partly considerable complication rates = obsolete
- Rehn-Delorme operation/procedure
  - Principle:
    - Transanal mucosal resection + suprasphincteric plication of the prolapsed rectum
    - Possible in analgosedation
  - Results:
    - Low morbidity and mortality, mean recurrence rate approx. 20% after 2 years
    - In many cases improvement of continence
- Altemeier Rectal resection
  - Principle:
    - Perineal rectum resection with reanastomosis ± pouching at the level of the dentate line
    - Circular resection of the prolapse possible using staple suture devices Transtar®
  - Results:
    - Recurrence rate lower than after Rehn-Delorme (5–15%), immanent risk of anastomotic insufficiency with pelvic sepsis (4%)
    - Significant improvement in constipation, frequent worsening of continence (urge incontinence, stool smearing)

Surgical Procedure
Rehn-Delorme Procedure

- preoperative colonic irrigation
- General anaesthesia, spinal anaesthesia
- Lithotomy position (Lloyd-Davis position), single-shot antibiotics with metronidazole i.v.
- Sphincter dilation, maximum eventration of the prolapse with 2 clamps
- Injection of the submucosa with diluted adrenaline saline solution (better separation of the layers)
- Incision of the mucosa 1 cm orally of the dentate line and circular dissection and resection of the mucosa cylinder of the entire prolapse.
- Accordion-like folding and reduction of the intestinal tube by 4–5 mattress sutures
- Reanastomosis of the mucosa

Abdominal Procedures

- Rectopexy without resection
  - Principle:
    - Dorsal suture rectopexy

- Laparoscopic ventral mesh rectopexy (d'Hoore), posterior mesh fixation (Ripstein / Wells) largely abandoned
- Avoidance of lateral mobilization leads to improved postoperative function
- Use of foreign materials (alloplastic meshes) with risk of erosion, fistula and stenosis formation
- Results:
  - Recurrence rates around 10%
  - Significant variation in functional outcomes
  - Loop formation and kinking of the redundant sigmoid: marked increase in constipation
  - Resection rectopexy
- Principle:
  - Stable stretching and fixation of the rectum + removal of the redundant sigmoid + usually suture rectopexy at the promontory
  - Due to anastomosis, alloplastic material is usually not used
- Results:
  - Recurrence rate = 2–8%
  - Improvement of constipation in more than 50% of patients
  - Improvement of continence in 60–90% of patients

Today's standard = laparoscopic procedure (additional advantages)

Surgical Procedure
Laparoscopic (Resection) Rectopexy

- General anesthesia, lithotomy position (Lloyd-Davis), perioperative antibiosis
- Trocar placement (see laparoscopic sigmoid resection)
- Lateral mobilization of the sigmoid, visualization of the left ureter
- Entering the vessel-free dorsal layer at the level of the promontory, preparation down to the pelvic floor
- Incision of the peritoneum at the anterior fold, anterior dissection up to the upper third of the vagina or up to the seminal vesicles
- **Caution:** Do not cut the lateral ligaments!
- If resection: Tubular transection of the mesosigmoid with preservation of the superior rectal artery, transection of the rectum above the promontory with a stapler, Pfannenstiel incision, resection of the bowel at the descendosigmoid junction, double-stapling anastomosis
- Fixation of the rectum to the presacral fascia at the level of the promontory by non-absorbable simple interrupted sutures close to the midline (**caution:** injury to the presacral venous plexus or pelvic nerves)
- reconstruction of the anterior rectovaginal peritoneum by continuous suture

4.3 Malignant Diseases

S. Willis and J. Wannenmacher

Key Points: Rectal Cancer

- Most common malignancy of the rectum
- Locoregional risk of recurrence: Higher than for colon cancer (due to lymphatic spread pathways, narrowness of the pelvis)
- Operative standard = en bloc resection of the tumor with regional vascularization. Systematic pathoanatomical examination on perirectal tumor spread
- Continence-preserving surgery (approx. 85% of rectal carcinomas): Through better understanding of continence mechanisms + optimized surgical technique.
- Current Standards:
  - Tumors of the upper third of the rectum: Proximal partial mesorectal excision + reconstruction by end-to-end descendorectostomy

- Tumors of the middle and distal third of the rectum: Total mesorectal excision obligatory + side-to-end anastomosis/colonic pouch-anal anastomosis
- Local excision (transanal or by TEM): for limited to small and histologically favorable uT1 tumors
- For extraperitoneally located T3/4 tumors: Neoadjuvant therapy approaches > postoperative radiochemotherapy

4.3.1 Histological Tumour Entities

- Rectal carcinoma = most frequent malignancy of the rectum
- GIST (Chap. 14)
  - Mesenchymal submucosal tumor
  - High malignancy potential at >5 cm and/or >5 mitoses per 50 HPF (high power field = microscopy field)
  - Aim for complete surgical removal
  - if necessary, follow-up treatment with Imatinib
- Neuroendocrine carcinoma/carcinoid
  - Rectum = most frequent localization in the intestine
  - Increasing incidence
  - Malignancy potential: depending on the degree of differentiation (G1–G3)
  - Tumours <2 cm mostly benign: local resection sufficient
  - Oncological radical resection for tumours >2 cm + proven malignancy
  - Simultaneous cholecystectomy if planned therapy with somatostatin analogues
- Lymphomas, sarcomas = rarities

4.3.2 Rectal Cancer

Definition

- All epithelial malignancies from the linea dentata to 16 cm ab ano measured with the rigid rectoscope

Forms/Classification

- By growth:
  - Exophytic polypous
  - Endophytic ulcerative
  - Diffusely infiltrating
- By histological cell type:
  - Mostly adenocarcinomas
  - Rare adenosquamous carcinomas
- By differentiation:
  - Low grade
  - High grade

Epidemiology and Etiology

- s. Colon cancer
- More than 50% involve the rectum

Tumor Spread

- Continuous
  - Intramural
  - Direct organ infiltration
- Discontinuous
  - Tumor satellites in the mesorectum outside lymph nodes
  - At a distance of up to 4 cm from the tumor
- Lymphogenous
  - Mesorectal and para-aortic lymph nodes
  - Rarely iliac lymph nodes
- Hematogenous
  - Into the liver via portal vein
  - Into the lungs (rare) in distal tumors via the vena cava

Classification

Classification According to Mason (Clinical Staging)

- After palpation
  - CS I Mucosa displaceable
  - CS II Intestinal wall displaceable
  - CS III Intestinal wall partially fixed
  - CS IV Intestinal wall fixed
  - CS V Disseminated disease

TNM Classification (2017)

- T (tumor)
  - T0 No infiltration
  - T1 Infiltration of the submucosal layer

- T2 Infiltration of the muscularis propria
- T3 Infiltration of the subserosa
- T4a Infiltration of the visceral peritoneum
- T4b Infiltration of other organs/structures
- N (lymph nodes)
  - N0 No metastases in the lymph nodes
  - N1 Metastases in 1–3 regional lymph nodes
  - N2a Metastases in 4–6 regional lymph nodes
  - N2b Metastases in >6 regional lymph nodes
- M (metastases)
  - M0 No distant metastases
  - M1 distant metastases

4

Derivation of UICC Stages from TNM Classification

Stage I	T1, T2	N0	M0
Stage II	T3, T4	N0	M0
Stage III	Each T	N1, N2	M0
Stage IV	Each T	Each N	M1

Symptoms

- Section 3.3 Colon cancer

Diagnosis

Rectal Digital Examination

- Assessment of the tumor location
- Infiltration depth and sphincter function

Rigid Rectoscopy

- Biopsy
- Exact localization (distance from anocutaneous line)

Colonoscopy

- Exclusion of second tumor

Endorectal Ultrasound

- Infiltration depth
- Crucial for the evaluation of T1 tumors
- Limited for the assessment of lymph node involvement

MRI Pelvis

- Distance to circumferential resection margin (CRM)
- Infiltration depth
- Crucial for local staging of T2 to T4 tumors
- Limited for evaluation Lymph node involvement

Thoracic CT, Abdominal CT

- Exclusion of distant metastases; sonography abdomen and Chest X-ray alternatively possible, but less sensitive

PET-CT

- Not required for primary diagnosis
- Helpful in recurrence diagnosis

Therapy

Indication

- Therapeutic procedure according to guidelines depending on preoperative staging (◘ Table 4.1)
- Increasing trend towards neoadjuvant therapy depending on the distance of the tumor from the mesorectal fascia, currently evaluation in trials: distance to CRM <1 mm: neoadjuvant therapy; distance to CRM ≥1 mm: primary resection.
- Optimal procedure for cancer in the upper third of the rectum = unclear = neoadjuvant therapy and surgery vs. treatment as in sigmoid cancer (primary surgery ± adjuvant chemotherapy)
- Increased morbidity in emergency surgery for ileus:
  - In case of ileus: relief by insertion of a double-barrel transverse colostomy or endoscopic insertion of a fully covered metal stent, followed by definitive therapy according to the guidelines

Table 4.1 Therapy strategy depending on preoperative staging

Tumor stage	Therapy
T1 "low risk"	Local excision
T1 "high risk", T2 N0 M0	Primary resection
T3/4 N0 M0 Tx N+ M0	Neoadjuvant therapy, followed by resection + adjuvant chemotherapy
Tx Nx M1	Radical resection of tumor and metastases ± adjuvant chemotherapy Primary tumor resection followed by additive chemotherapy and metastasectomy or vice versa Palliative therapy

Neoadjuvant Therapy

- Neoadjuvant radiotherapy: Significant reduction of local recurrence rate in locally advanced tumor stages from 27 to 11%.
- Adjuvant radiotherapy: positive effect after optimal surgery smallerwhen compared with neoadjuvant, but still present

Long-Term Radiochemotherapy (Preferred in Germany and USA)

- Target:
  - Downstaging + Downsizing
  - Increase in the rate of sphincter-preserving surgery
- Implementation:
  - Conventional fractionated radiotherapy with 45–50 Gy (28 single doses of 1.8 Gy each) + concomitant chemotherapy with 5-FU and folinic acid (5-fluorouracil) or capecitabine over a period of 6 weeks
  - Operation 6–8 weeks later
  - In recent meta-analyses, higher remission rates after 10–12 weeks (but contradictory RCT from France)
  - Postoperative: Adjuvant chemotherapy

Short-Term Therapy (Preferred in the Netherlands, Poland and Scandinavia)

- No tumor reduction
- In the lower third of the rectum: less effective than long-term radiochemotherapy
- Implementation:
  - Exclusively radiotherapy with 25 Gy distributed over 5 individual doses
  - Operation in the immediate aftermath
  - Comparable results with regard to the oncological outcome—in recent studies, delayed surgery with subsequent tumor reduction is also possible
- **Problems of Neoadjuvant Therapy as a Whole:**
  - Preoperative overstaging in 18% of UICC-II/-III classified patients, especially correct detection of lymph node status (see above)
  - Long-term side effects possible: sphincter weakness, potency disorders, secondary cancers
  - No significant effect on survival rate, therefore generally not indicated in the metastatic stage
  - Neoadjuvant chemotherapy without radiotherapy or intensified neoadjuvant chemotherapy with prior or subsequent radiotherapy (= "total neoadjuvant therapy"): Currently the subject of trials (RAPIDO)
  - Complete remission after neoadjuvant therapy: radical surgery generally indicated due to remaining vital tumor cells, "watch and wait" = individually possible, preferably only in studies

Adjuvant Therapy

Modalities

- As adjuvant chemotherapy after long-term neoadjuvant therapy (see above)
- As combined radiochemotherapy after R0 resection and not-performed neoadjuvant therapy in stages II and III
- After R1 resection, tumor perforation or intraoperative tumor rupture also indicated in stage I

Results

- Lower local recurrence rate and higher morbidity than after neoadjuvant therapy
- Benefit of adjuvant chemotherapy in the context of long-term neoadjuvant therapy = controversial
- No benefit from intensification of chemotherapy

Additive/Palliative Therapy

Principles

- Individual approach depending on tumor location, extent of metastasis and general condition of the patient
- Distant metastasis = prognostic in non-stenosing/non-bleeding tumor with extensive metastasis
- Benefit of primary tumor resection before chemotherapy = unclear

Strategy

- In stenosing cancer and multimorbid patients:
  - Use of a double-barrel stoma or insertion of a flexible metal stent
  - With or without subsequent chemotherapy
- In patients in good general condition and potentially resectable metastases = curative approach:
  - Primary resection of the primary tumor, if necessary additive chemotherapy and subsequent resection of the metastases
  - Alternatively primary resection of the metastases with subsequent resection of the primary tumor
  - Depending on the localization, thermoablation instead of or in combination with resection of metastases
  - Additive chemotherapy not longer than max. 5 cycles; also in case of complete radiological response: Metastasectomy obligatory (in 30% still vital tumor cells detectable).
  - Up to 30% long-term survival after R0 resection of primary tumor and metastases
  - Benefit of additional "pseudoadjuvant" chemotherapy after R0 resection of primary tumor and metastases = not proven
  - Benefit of "pseudoneoadjuvant" chemotherapy before resection of primary resectable metastases = controversial
- Palliative chemotherapy with as few side effects as possible (e.g. 5-FU, capecitabine), additive chemotherapy with as good a response as possible (e.g. FOLFOX/FOLFIRI ± EGFR/VEGF antibodies)

Operative Therapy Principles

Local Limited Procedures

- Indication:
  - For malignant, non-invasive polyps
  - For carcinomas with early infiltration of the submucosa, maximum T1 sm 1–2, maximum size 3 cm without other negative predictors (G1–2, R0, L0, V0, Pn0).
- Disadvantages:
  - No assessment of lymph node status possible, but under these conditions low risk of metastasis (approx. 2%)
  - Increased risk of local recurrence compared to anterior resection (approx. 10%)
- Principle:
  - Surgical rectal full wall excision
  - Endoscopic resection (endoscopic mucosal resection, submucosal dissection)
  - Avoid peacemeal resection
- Surgical procedure:
  - Transanal full wall excision (lower third of the rectum)
  - Transanal endoscopic microsurgery: TEM/TEO = transanal endoscopic surgery, TAMIS ("transanal minimally invasive surgery"); middle and upper third of the rectum

In multimorbid patients, locally limited rectal resection is permissible as an individual therapy after appropriate patient information, even in the case of locally advanced tumours (exception).

Surgical Procedure
Local Limited Rectal Resection
- Bowel preparation helpful
- General or locoregional anaesthesia
- Positioning with tumor at floor level
- Safety distance 1 cm
- Transanal resection: exposition of tumor using anal spreader, placement of holding sutures, pulling the tumor caudally, excision with electrocautery, transverse suture closure
- Transanal microsurgery/endoscopy: insertion of the instrumentation, marking of the resection line with electrocautery, dissection of the rectal wall with electric knife, transverse suture closure
- Rapid opening of the suture in case of suspicion of pararectal infection

Rectal Resection
- Principles of resection:
  - Removal of the rectum + en bloc removal of the locoregional lymphatic drainage area
  - Preparation along the anatomical enveloping fasciae (see above)
  - For tumors in the upper third: Anterior rectal resection with partial mesorectal excision (PME)
  - For tumors in the middle and lower third: low anterior rectal resection with total mesorectal excision (TME)
  - Radicular ligation of the inferior mesenteric artery and vein, no prognostic difference between truncal ligation and preservation of the left colic artery
  - Protection of the autonomic nerves (see above) essential
  - Maintain sufficient distal clearance margin:
    - Anterior resection with PME: 5 cm
    - Low anterior resection with TME for high-grade tumors: 2–3 cm
    - Low anterior resection with TME for low-grade tumors: 1 cm
    - After neoadjuvant therapy and negative frozen section: At least 0.5 cm
  - En bloc resection of tumor-adherent organs (multivisceral resection)
  - Laparoscopic surgery is oncologically equivalent in suitable patients (less favourable results possibly in low-located rectal carcinoma (ALACART, ACOSOC Trial)—value of robot-assisted procedures in lower conversion rate in men with narrow pelvis (ROLARR Trial))
- Principles of Reconstruction:
  - Reconstruction depending on the extent of resection:
    - PME: End-to-end anastomosis (residual rectal pouch available)
    - TME: colon-J-pouch-anal anastomosis, alternatively in case of narrow pelvis or voluminous mesentery coloplasty-pouch-anal anastomosis or side-to-end anastomosis (= reduction of stool frequency and imperative urge to defecate)
  - Anastomosis:
    - Double-stapling technology
    - For very distally located tumors: intersphincteric resection with coloanal hand suture
    - Ta TME (transanal TME) developed as a transanal adjunct to TME in obese men with low-seated tumors—possible advantages in clarity but higher incidence in urethral lesions.
    - Protective stoma after low anterior resection
  - Background:
    - Insufficiency rate increases distally (up to 30%), therefore optional after PME
    - Does not prevent the insufficiency, but significantly reduced inflammatory reaction in the pelvis
    - Double-barrel ileostomy with less prolapse and lower complication rate than reverse transversostomy
    - Double-barrel transversostoma with less postoperative fluid loss (preferred in elderly patients with renal insufficiency)

4

Preoperative bowel irrigation and marking of the stoma position (lying, standing and sitting) are important.

Surgical Procedure
Open Low Anterior Rectal Resection

- General anesthesia, lithotomy (Lloyd-Davis) positioning, peridural catheter
- Median laparotomy, exploration of the abdomen
- Lateral mobilization of the descending colon, exposure of the left ureter
- Mobilization of the left colonic flexure from lateral to medial
- transection of the inferior mesenteric artery approx. 1 cm preaortic, transection of the inferior mesenteric vein at the lower edge of the pancreas
- Radicular transection of the mesentery, transection of the colon at the descendosigmoidal junction
- Start of TME dorsally, sharp dissection between mesorectum and Waldeyer's fascia, sparing the hypogastric nerves down to the pelvic floor
- Anterior dissection along the Denonvillier's fascia, protection of seminal vesicles and prostate or vagina
- Transection of lateral bridges along the hypogastric nerves, circular preparation of the rectum at the pelvic floor
- "Rectal washout", transection of rectum with a linear stapler
- Colon J-pouch: limb length 5–6 cm, coloplasty pouch: 6–8 cm incision ventrally between the taeniae coli with transverse closure, side-to-end anastomosis: stump with 2–3 cm length
- Transanal double stapling anastomosis, protective stomy
- Eventually placement of a suprapubic bladder catheter in men

Surgical Procedure
Laparoscopic Low Anterior Rectal Resection

- Lithotomy (Lloyd-Davis) positioning, vacuum mattress, shoulder supports
- Pneumoperitoneum, insertion of the trocars
- Preliminary transection of the vessels, mobilization of the descending colon and the left flexure from medial to lateral (**caution:** vegetative nerves and pancreatic tail)
- TME as for open resection
- Distal transection with angled stacker, several magazines may be required
- Retrieval of the specimen through widening of the incision in the left lower abdomen or suprasymphyseal Pfannenstiel incision
- Reconstruction and anastomosis as for open resection

Abdominoperineal Rectal Extirpation

- Indication:
  - For tumors infiltrating the sphincter/anal canal
  - If the distal clearance margin is not sufficient (see above)
- Principles:
  - For deep-seated T1/2 tumors: classical abdominoperineal extirpation leaving the lateral levator muscles intact
  - In advanced tumor stages: Cylindrical rectal extirpation including the levator musculature, coverage by pedicled myocutaneous flap (VRAM, bilateral gluteal shift flap)
- Results:
  - Higher local recurrence rate than after sphincter-preserving surgery
  - Conventional and laparoscopic procedure = oncologically equivalent

Surgical Procedure
Abdominoperineal Rectal Extirpation

- Insertion of a transurethral bladder catheter
- Abdominal part:
  - Mobilization of the left colonic flexure not required

- TME as in anterior resection with sphincter preservation in classical extirpation, preparation only up to the levator attachment in cylindrical extirpation
- Creation of a terminal descendostoma, prevention of a parastomal hernia by mesh augmentation or extraperitoneal drainage
- Insertion of an omental patch into the sacral cavity

- Perineal part:
  - Preparation for classical extirpation in lithotomy (Lloyd-Davis) position, for cylindrical extirpation: knee-chest position if necessary (better overview for large tumors)
  - Suture (closure) and circular dissection of anus
  - Transection of the ischiorectal fat
  - Transection of the anococcygeal ligament or coccygeal resection
  - Transection or resection of the levator ani muscle
  - Ventral release of the specimen (**caution**: urethral injury)
  - Layered wound closure or flap plastic reconstruction

Prognosis

Prognostic Factors

- Depth of infiltration into the intestinal wall
- Presence of lymph node and distant metastases
- Tumor cell differentiation

5-Year Survival Rates

- 5-year survival rate = on average 40–60% (most frequent finding = stage III)
- 5-year survival rates by UICC stage:
  - Stage I = approx. 80–100%
  - Stage II = approx. 60–80
  - Stage III = approx. 30–60
  - Stage IV = approx. 0–57%
- 5-year survival rate in stage IV dependent on:
  - Lymph node status
  - Number and size of metastases
  - CEA level (tumor marker >200 μg/L unfavorable)
  - Disease-free interval (<12 months unfavorable)

Follow-up

Targets

- Early detection of potentially curable local recurrences (up to 25%)
- Early detection of distant metastases (up to 25%)
- Early detection of metachronous second tumors (up to 10%)

Time Intervals

- Every 6 months:
  - Anamnesis
  - Physical examination
  - CEA determination
  - Abdominal Ultrasound
- After 1 and 5 years:
  - Colonoscopy
  - Exception: If no preoperative complete colonoscopy due to e.g. stenosis: colonoscopy within the first 6 months postoperatively
- On a yearly basis:
  - Thoracic X-ray = optional

Special Features

- Stage I after radical resection (very low risk): Colonoscopy only recommended
- After local resection (due to increased risk of local recurrence): Endoscopic controls after 6, 24 and 60 months recommended
- CT, MRI and PET-CT = suitable for detecting recurrences; not recommended in routine follow-up due to insufficient evidence
- No age limit for follow-up
- No follow-up after palliative therapy

4

4.3.3 Guidelines

Guideline program oncology (German Cancer Society, German Cancer Aid, AWMF): S3 guideline colorectal carcinoma, long version 2.1, 2019, AWMF registration number: 021-007OL, ► https://www.leitlinienprogramm-onkologie.de/fileadmin/user_upload/Downloads/Leitlinien/Kolorektales_Karzinom/Version_2/LL_KRK_Langversion_2.1.pdf

Further Reading

Alkatout I, Egberts JH, Mettler L et al (2015) Interdisziplinäre Diagnostik und Therapie der tief infiltrierenden Endometriose. Zentralbl Chir 140:630–638. https://doi.org/10.1055/s-0034-1383272

Braun J, Kasperk M, Saklak M, Ulmer F, Willis S (2011) Gutartige Erkrankungen von Dickdarm und Rektum. In: Siewert JR, Rothmund M, Schumpelick V (Hrsg) Praxis der Viszeralchirurgie, Gastroenterologische Chirurgie, 3 Aufl. Springer, Heidelberg, pp S527–S584

Church JM, Raudkivi PJ, Hill GL (1987) The surgical anatomy of the rectum—a review with particular relevance to the hazards of rectal mobilisation. Int J Color Dis 2(3):158–166

Fleshman J, Branda M, Sargent DJ et al (2015) Effect of laparoscopic-assisted resection vs open resection of stage II or III rectal cancer on pathologic outcomes: the ACOSOG Z6051 randomized clinical trial. JAMA 314(13):1346–1355. https://doi.org/10.1001/jama.2015.10529

Fritzmann J, Weitz J (2013) Rektumkarzinom—Teil 1: Präoperative Diagnostik. Allgemein Viszeralchirurgie 7:59–69

Horisberger K, Kienle P (2013) Rektumkarzinom—Teil 2: Operationstechnik. Allgemein Viszeralchirurgie 7:163–181

Jayne D, Pigazzi A, Marshall H et al (2017) Effect of robotic-assisted vs conventional laparoscopic surgery on risk of conversion to open laparotomy among patients undergoing resection for rectal cancer: the ROLARR randomized clinical trial. JAMA 318(16):1569–1580. https://doi.org/10.1001/jama.2017.7219

Lefevre JH, Mineur L, Kotti S et al (2016) Effect of interval (7 or 11 weeks) between neoadjuvant radiochemotherapy and surgery on complete pathologic response in rectal cancer: a multicenter, randomized, controlled trial (GRECCAR-6). J Clin Oncol 34(31):3773–3780

Lindsey I, Guy RJ, Warren BF, Mortensen NJ (2000) Anatomy of Denonvilliers' fascia and pelvic nerves, impotence, and implications for the colorectal surgeon. Br J Surg 87(10):1288–1299

Luo C, Plank AW, Merrie AE, Plank LD, Bissett IP, Saramanayake CB (2010) Systematic review on ventral rectopexy for rectal prolapse and intussusception. Dis Colon Rectum 12:504–512

Matzel KE, Heuer S, Zhang W (2008) Rektumprolaps. Chirurg 79:444–451

Pox CP (2014) Rektumkarzinom Teil 3: multimodale Therapie und Nachsorge. Allgemein Viszeralchirurgie 8:287–295

Ramage JK (2008) Consensus guidelines for the management of patients with digestive neuroendocrine tumours: well-differentiated colon and rectum tumour/carcinoma. Neuroendocrinology 87:31–39

Standring S (2009) Gray's anatomy. The anatomical basis of clinical practice. 40 Aufl. Churchill Livingstone, Elsevier, London

Stevenson AR, Solomon MJ, Lumley JW et al (2015) Effect of laparoscopic-assisted resection vs open resection on pathological outcomes in rectal cancer: the ALaCaRT randomized clinical trial. JAMA 314(13):1356–1363. https://doi.org/10.1001/jama.2015.12009

Ulrich A (2019) Chirurgir des Rektumkarzinoms UpDate 2019. Dtsch Arztebl 116(23–24):4

Willis S, Schumpelick V (2010) Rektumkarzinom. In: Siewert JR, Rothmund M, Schumpelick V (Hrsg) Praxis der Viszeralchirurgie Onkologische Chirurgie, 3 Aufl. Springer, Heidelberg, pp S713–S734

Wittekind C (2017) TNM—Klassifikation maligner Tumoren, 8 Aufl. WILEY-VCH, Weinheim, pp S98–S100. isbn:978-3-527-34280-8

Suggested Reading

Bahadoer RR, Dijkstra EA, van Etten B et al (2021) Short-course radiotherapy followed by chemotherapy before total mesorectal excision (TME) versus preoperative chemoradiotherapy, TME, and optional adjuvant chemotherapy in locally advanced rectal cancer (RAPIDO): a randomised, open-label, phase 3 trial. Lancet Oncol 22:29–42

Kreis ME, Ruppert R, Ptok H, Strassburg J, Brosi P, Lewin A, Schön MR, Sauer J, Junginger T, Merkel S, Hermanek P, OCUM Study Group (2016) Use of preoperative magnetic resonance Imaging to select patients with rectal cancer for neoadjuvant chemoradiation—interim analysis of the German OCUM Trial (NCT01325649). J Gastrointest Surg 20(1):25–32

Anorectum

Jens Wannenmacher and Stefan Willis

Contents

F. Billmann, T. Keck (eds.), *Essentials of Visceral Surgery*,
https://doi.org/10.1007/978-3-662-66735-4_5

Key Points

- Complex anatomy and physiology of the anorectum: variety of proctological diseases
- Treatments as different as etiologies
- Defecation/Stool Continence: Complex Interaction of the Large Intestine Rectum Pelvic Floor: Different Therapeutic Approaches Required for Fecal Incontinence/Outlet Obstipation

5.1 Anatomy and Physiology

5.1.1 Anatomy

- Anatomy of anal canal: approx. 0.5 cm distal to the linea anocutanea to dentate line (pectinate line)
- Length = approx. 3–4 cm
- 10–25 crypts (excretory ducts of the proctodeal glands) at the level of the dentate line
- Hemorrhoidal plexus (Corpus cavernosum recti): subepithelial venous plexus at the upper edge of the anal canal
- Epithelial lining: Tripartite
  - Distal to the linea anocutanea: keratinizing squamous epithelium
  - Anal canal: Non-keratinizing squamous epithelium (anoderm)
  - Proximal to the dentate line: transitional cell area (cylindrical epithelium)
- Musculature: Smooth + striated
  - Internal anal sphincter: smooth muscle; continuation of the ring muscle of the rectum; innervation: autonomous via stretch receptors in rectal wall
  - External anal sphincter: transversely striated muscle; encloses the internal sphincter like a cylinder; pars subcutanea, superficialis, profunda; innervation: somatic = pudendal plexus
  - Puborectal muscle (M. puborectalis): transversely striated muscle; cranial of the external sphincter, corresponds to the lowest part of the levator ani muscle; embraces the rectum from the dorsal side (= in the form of a loop); innervation: somatic = pudendal plexus
- Blood supply: inferior rectal artery, middle rectal artery

5.1.2 Physiology

- Continence:
  - Internal anal sphincter: Involuntary continuous contraction (resting pressure)
  - External anal sphincter: voluntary contraction on demand (pinch pressure); contraction prevents relaxation of the internal sphincter (= voluntary inhibition reflex)
  - Puborectal muscle: voluntary contraction = maintenance and reduction of the anorectal angle
  - Hemorrhoidal plexus: venous outflow of the “haemorrhoids”; contraction of the internal anal sphincter = partial throttling of the outflow; erectile tissue function = intraluminal sealing of the anal canal = fine continence
  - Rectum: variable reservoir function (compliance); retrograde stool transport possible through segmental contractions
- Defecation:
  - Stool-filled ampoule = stimulation of the stretch receptors
  - Stimulation = contraction of the detrusor recti
  - Relaxation of the internal anal sphincter ani: rectoanal inhibition reflex
  - By abdominal pressure + voluntary relaxation of the external anal sphincter and puborectal muscles (enlargement of the anorectal angle) = defecation.

5.2 Benign Diseases

5.2.1 Hemorrhoidal Disease

Key Points

- Typical localisation: 3 (left lateral), 7 (right posterior) and 11 (right anterior) o'clock in lithotomy (Lloyd-Davis) position
- Hemorrhoids = physiological: important role in fine continence
- Hemorrhoidal disease = at the appearance of symptoms
- first and second degree hemorrhoids = conservative/interventional therapy
- third and fourth degree hemorrhoids = surgical therapy

Definition

- Normal anal cushions (pads): Usually at 3 o'clock, 7 o'clock and 11 o'clock in Lloyd-Davis position
- By placing these pads next to each other = precise closure of the anal canal = fine continence; anal cushions contribute about 15% of resting anal pressure
- Haemorrhoidal disease = in the case of hypertrophy and/or the appearance of symptoms =

Classification

- First-degree hemorrhoid:
  - Only proctologically visible protrusion
- Second-degree hemorrhoid:
  - Cushion prolapse during pressing
  - Spontaneous reduction
- Third-degree hemorrhoid:
  - Cushion prolapse during pressing
  - Manual reduction necessary (no spontaneous reduction)
- Fourth-degree hemorrhoid:
  - Cushion permanently prolapsed
  - Irreducible or reducible, with immediate reprolapse
  - Subdivision possible into:
    - Grade 4a: reducible under anaesthesia
    - Grade 4b: Not reducible under anaesthesia
  - Anal prolapse: fourth degree circular hemorrhoids ± mucosal prolapse, radial folding (does not correspond to the circular folding seen in rectal prolapse; ► Sect. 4.2)

Epidemiology

- No exact data on prevalence and incidence
- One of the most common diseases in western industrialised countries (70% of people suffer from hemorrhoids at least once in their lives)
- Men: Women = 2: 1
- Frequency peak: 45–65 years

Etiology

- Main Causes:
  - Genetic factors
  - defecation disorder
  - Stool consistency
- Mechanism:
  - Disturbed venous outflow = swelling of the hemorrhoidal plexus = in the course hypertrophy of the tissue
  - Hypertrophy of the tissue = among other things loosening of the ligamentous connections = lack of retraction of the cushions after defecation
- Causal factors (among others):
  - Increased intra-abdominal pressure (e.g. heavy pushing, pregnancy)
  - Chronic sphincter hypertrophy
  - Increased resting tone with inadequate relaxation
  - Fecal impaction in chronic constipation
  - Also chronic diarrhea tendency: No sufficient stretching and relaxation of the anal canal = traumatization of the still bulging anal cushion.

Symptoms

- Transanal bleeding = cardinal symptom:
  - Mostly bright red blood during or after defecation
  - Often bleeding from the congested vessels of the covering mucosa, not from hemorrhoid itself

  - Extensive bleeding can lead to hemorrhagic shock
- Pain:
  - Not typical, as not located in the sensitively supplied area of the anal canal
  - Painful in incarcerated haemorrhoidal prolapse and thrombus formation
- Other symptoms:
  - Smearing and oozing due to disturbance of fine continence
  - Irritative-toxic anal eczema with pruritus ani: Resulting from oozing

5

Diagnosis

- Anamnesis
- Inspection, rectal digital examination
- Procto/rectoscopy
- Colonoscopy (exclusion of other diseases, especially colorectal carcinoma)

Differential Diagnosis

- Sentinel Pile (marisc): flap-like folds of skin on the external anal ring which do not fill up during pressing
- Anal vein thrombosis (► Sect. 5.2.2)
- Fissures (► Sect. 5.2.3)
- Rectal prolapse (► Sect. 4.2 Benign diseases of the rectum)
- Anal fibromas: benign fibromas lined with squamous epithelium; length up to 4 cm (fibroma pendulans)
- Malignant and benign tumors

Therapy

Basic Therapy

- Change of defecation behaviour + adjustment of diet = avoidance of strong pressing and especially post pressing (= high-fibre diet)
- Drug therapy (hemorrhoidalia): Only symptomatic, no long-term therapy with ointments containing cortisone
- Treatment of secondary changes (e.g. irritative-toxic anal eczema with e.g. zinc paste)

Conservative and Interventional/ Semioperative Therapy

- For hemorrhoids grade 1 and 2

Sclerotherapy (Blond or Blanchard or Bensaude procedures)

- Blond: submucosal injection of e.g. polidocanol or quinine into the hemorrhoidal tissue
- Blanchard or Bensaude: Injection of e.g. phenol-almond solution into the area of the afferent hemorrhoidal arteries.
- Principle: Fixation of the convolutes above the linea dentata by inflammation and scarring
- Complications:
  - Bleeding
  - Allergic reactions
  - Rectal Necrosis

Infrared Coagulation

- Principle: Infrared rays = superficial tissue necrosis above the linea dentata = scarring + fixation of hemorrhoids

Rubber Ring Ligation (According to Barron)

- Principle: Ligation of the convolutes via an applicator = necrosis of the tissue with scarring
- Complications:
  - Post-operative bleeding up to 14 days after intervention (**caution:** anticoagulated patients!)
  - Severe pain with application below the linea dentata
  - Allergic reactions
  - Rectal Necrosis
  - Abscesses
  - Urinary retention

Doppler-Guided Hemorrhoidal Artery Ligation (HAL)

- Principle: Localization + ligation of the haemorrhoidal arteries via a special proctoscope with built-in Doppler transducer = shirring + scarring

Recto-Anal Repair

- Principle: localization + ligation of the hemorrhoidal arteries + additional continuous shirring of the haemorrhoidal convolutes

- Successful even without (expensive) Doppler support

Surgical Therapy

- For hemorrhoids ≥ grade 3 = surgical therapy

Milligan-Morgan Hemorrhoidectomy

- = gold standard

> **Surgical Procedure**
> **Milligan Morgan Operation**
> - General anesthesia, spinal anesthesia, saddle block
> - Lithotomy position, single-shot antibiotics with metronidazole i.v.
> - Sphincter dilatation, insertion of the spreader
> - Start with the largest hemorrhoid
> - Placement of 2 sharp clamps on anocutaneous line and hemorrhoid
> - Injection of the anocutaneous tissue with e.g. diluted adrenaline saline solution (better separation from the internal sphincter)
> - Arch-shaped incision of the perianal skin and wedge-shaped incision of the anoderm on both sides in the direction of the vascular pedicle
> - If present, co-resection of the sentinel piles (mariscs)
> - Dissection of the hemorrhoid with scissors or diathermy
> - Resection of the base of hemorrhoid and suture with absorbable suture
> - Same procedure at the other two positions
> - Hemostasis, if necessary insertion of a tamponade
> - Ensure that the anoderm bridges are wide enough

Ferguson Hemorrhoidectomy

- Principle: Resection as in Milligan-Morgan-OP, additionally continuous closure of the anoderm defect except for a small drainage field
- Pros:
  - Less pain
  - Better bleeding control
  - Anatomically correct reconstruction of the anal canal
- Disadvantage: Higher stenosis rate

Subanodermal Resection (Parks Procedure)

- Principle: Y-shaped incision of the anoderm, subanodermal/submucosal resection of the hemorrhoid, reconstruction of the anoderm
- Advantage: Low anoderm loss (especially if extensive findings)
- Disadvantage: Quite complex surgical technique

Stapler Hemorrhoidopexy (Longo Procedure)

- Principle: Circular resection of the rectal mucosa by means of a stapler at the point of attachment of the hemorrhoids = pexie of the haemorrhoids at their place of origin
- Pros:
  - No violation of the sensitive anoderm
  - Less postoperative pain
  - Anatomically correct reconstruction of the anal canal
  - Reduction of mucosal prolapse
- Disadvantages:
  - Significantly higher costs (stapler device)
  - No histological workup of the hemorrhoids
  - Significant stretching of the anal canal

> **Surgical Procedure**
> **Stapler Hemorrhoidopexy**
> - General anaesthesia, spinal anaesthesia or saddle block
> - Single-shot antibiosis optional
> - Sphincter dilation, insertion of the transparent speculum, fixation with single stitch sutures
> - Starting at 12 o'clock in Lloy-Davis, placement of a mucosal, purse string suture with monofilament suture 2–3 cm above the linea dentata

- Inserting the fully opened stapler, placing the pressure plate above the purse string suture, closing the same
- Pulling the two suture ends through openings on the stapler head and knotting a tab
- Under continuous pull on the sutures, closure of the stapler
- **Caution:** In female patients, check that the posterior vaginal wall is not traped in the device!
- Firing and removal of the stapler after 1 minute compression time
- Checking for blood dryness, arterial bleedings should be stitched
- Insertion of a tamponade if necessary

5

Therapy Strategy for Grade 4 Hemorrhoids

- In the acute stage: First cooling, analgesia and local therapy to reduce the oedema (if possible)
- Plastic Reconstructive Procedures (Fansler-Arnold):
  - Resection of haemorrhoids + reconstruction of the anal canal with transposition flap
  - Operatively demanding, time-consuming, high complication rate
- Combined procedures: e.g. Ferguson's procedure for the most extensive findings + hemorrhoidal artery ligation with recto-anal repair for the smaller findings
- Two-stage approach
  - For hemorrhoids that can be reduced under anesthesia: In experienced hands Longo's stapler hemorrhoidopexy possible (with increased recurrence rate)
  - For all resecting procedures: Keep anoderm loss as low as possible

Grade-Adapted Therapy

- In all stages: High-fibre diet, fluid intake, correct defecation as flanking measures.
- Grade 1: Sclerotherapy, infrared coagulation, if necessary HAL
- Grade 2: Rubber band ligation, HAL, if necessary sclerotherapy, recto-anal repair
- Grade 3: Closed/open hemorrhoidectomy, stapler haemorrhoidopexy
- Grade 4: Closed/open hemorrhoidectomy, stapler hemorrhoidopexy if necessary, two-stage procedure if necessary

Complications

- Postoperative pain (less common with stapler hemorrhoidopexy than with resecting procedures)
- Bleeding
- Urinary retention
- Sentinel piles (Mariscs)
- Recurrence
- Anal Fissure
- Fecal Incontinence
- Anal stenosis (especially with extensive resections of the anoderm = Whitehead anus)
- Recurrence (approx. 15%)
- Most severe complications (rectovaginal fistula, Fournier's gangrene, pelvic sepsis) = very rare

5.2.2 Anal Vein Thrombosis

Key Points

- Blood clots of the subcutaneous and subanodermal veins of the external anal region
- Incision and expression (in very painful patients = immediate relief from symptoms); disadvantage = high recurrence rate
- Therapy of choice for pronounced findings = total excision

Definition

- Acute thrombosis of the subanodermal and subcutaneous veins of the inferior hemorrhoidal plexus
- Singular or pearled (chambered)
- Size: Up to plum size

"External hemorrhoid" is an Incorrect denomination.

Epidemiology

- Approx. 5% of proctological patients
- Men: Women = 2: 1

Etiology

- Exact etiology is not clear
- Often, however, no cause can be identified

Triggering Factors

- Thermal influences (cold, muggy weather)
- Physical exertion (e.g. jogging, cycling)
- Intra-abdominal pressure (e.g. pressing, defecation, pregnancy)
- Nutritive factors (alcohol, hot spices)
- Mechanical factors (proctological surgery, anal intercourse)
- Diarrhea
- Enlarged hemorrhoidal cushions (connection to the succutaneous venous plexus = slowing of blood flow)

Symptoms

- Usually abrupt pain in the anal area with swelling
- Infrequent moderate dull ache, occasionally on touch only
- Other symptoms:
  - Itchy
  - Stitch
  - Burning

Diagnosis

- Analogous to the diagnosis of hemorrhoidal disease (▶ Sect. 5.2.1)

Differential Diagnosis

- Thrombosed hemorrhoids
- Mariscs
- Abscesses
- Anal Fibroids
- Melanoma(!)
- Anal (marginal) carcinoma

Therapy

Conservative Therapy

- In patients with few symptoms and chronic findings:
  - Application of antiphlogistic local therapeutics
  - Administration of systemic acting non-steroidal anti-inflammatory drugs

Surgical Therapy

- Incision, drainage, expression of the thrombus under local anesthesia:
  - Suitable for small findings
  - Mostly immediate relief from complaints
  - Disadvantage: High recurrence rate
- Complete excision under anesthesia:
  - Indicated for larger findings
  - Advantages: Low recurrence rate + histological examination possible
  - Disadvantage: Larger wound area

Complications

- Rare in open wound healing
- Recurrences: the more complete the excision, the rarer

5.2.3 Anal Fissure

Key Points

- Elongated, painful ulceration in the anal canal, usually at 6 o'clock in Lloyd-Davis position
- Acute anal fissure: anaesthetic creams, sphincter stretching, sphincter relaxing drugs
- In case of unsuccessful therapy or chronicity with formation of outpost fold and hypertrophic anal papilla: excision (Gabriel procedure)
- In case of post-operatively non-healing fissures and high tonus: if necessary lateral sphincterotomy

Definition

- Elongated ulceration of the anal canal, about 90% at 6 o'clock in Lloyd-Davis position
- Transition from acute to chronic fissure often fluent

Acute Anal Fissure

- Superficial, elongated defect of the anoderm with sharply defined edges
- Bloody or greasy wound bed

Chronic Anal Fissure

- Rough, raised rim wall
- Sclerosed internal fibers at the base of the fissure
- Cranially hypertrophied anal papilla, caudally "outpost fold" (Marisc)

Epidemiology

- Approx. 15% of proctological patients
- Men: Women = 1: 1

Etiology

Main Cause = Heavy Pressing

- Strong pressing during hard defecation → tearing of the anoderm → reactive cramping of the musculature due to pain → difficult defecation, reduced perfusion → poor healing tendency = vitious circle

Other Causes

- Anal fistula
- Manipulation
- Cryptitis
- Diarrhea
- Chronic spincter spasm
- Chronic inflammatory bowel diseases
- Hemorrhoidal disease (cofactor)

Symptoms

- Acute pain: onset with defecation, possibly lasting for hours
- Proctogenic constipation: due to fear of pain recurrence
- Light red blood accumulation
- Secretion, smearing of stool
- Dyscontinence
- Pencil thin stool

Diagnosis

- Corresponds to the diagnosis of hemorrhoidal disease (► Sect. 5.2.1)
- If impossible due to pain = injecting the fissure with a local anaesthetic
- If, despite anaesthesia, impossible and there is doubt about the diagnosis = proctological examination under anaesthesia to exclude e.g. an abscess

Differential Diagnosis

- Fissure in Crohn's disease
- Anal lues, AIDS-associated lesions
- Anal Carcinoma
- Intersphincteric abscesses
- Rhagades

Therapy

Conservative Therapy

- Primary conservative therapy for acute anal fissure
- Stool regulation, sufficient drinking quantity, creams
- Sphincter stretching:
  - Daily self-stretching of the sphincter with anal dilator
  - If necessary, subsequent insertion of an anal tampon
  - Anaesthetic creams, occasionally local anaesthesia required
  - Effective, but currently largely abandoned in favor of drug therapy
- Nitroglycerin:
  - Application of 0.2% nitroglycerine ointment = reduction of sphincter tone + improvement of blood circulation
  - 3 times daily for 8 weeks into the entire anal canal
  - Systemic side effects common (especially headache)
- Calcium antagonists:
  - 0.2% nifedepine or 2% diltiazem ointment = reduction of sphincter tone + improvement of blood flow
  - Intraanal use not required
  - Systemic side effects rare
  - Higher recurrence rate
- Botulinum toxin:

- Injection of botulinum toxin = muscle paralysis for up to 3 months = support of the healing process
- Temporary incontinence up to 5%
- High costs

Surgical Therapy

- Indication: Chronic anal fissures
- Sphincter stretching and fissurectomy (Gabriel procedure) = standard in German-speaking countries

Surgical Procedure

Gabriel Procedure

- General anesthesia, spinal anesthesia, saddle block
- Lithotomy (Lloyd Davis) position
- Cautious sphincter dilatation, insertion of the spreader
- **Caution:** Sphincter stretching (Lord technique) (8 fingers) = obsolete
- Exclusion of fistula, probing of the crypts at the level of the anal papilla
- Excision of outpost fold, fissure and hypertrophic anal papilla en bloc with protection of the sphincter with diathermy or scissors
- Targeted transection of remaining, sclerosed sphincter fibers
- Waiver of sphincterotomy
- Triangular drainage, wider towards the outside
- Insertion of a tamponade if necessary
- Lateral sphincterotomy
  - Widespread in the Anglo-American area
  - Transection of the lower two thirds of the internal sphincter at 3 o'clock Lloyd-Davis position with protection of the anoderm
  - Reduced tone as a prerequisite for fissure healing
  - Disadvantage: Considerable risk of (late) incontinence
- Eisenhammer fissurectomy:
  - With additional deep sphincterotomy in the area of the fissure

Obsolete because of the risk of formation of a keyhole defect with disturbance of fine continence

Stage-Appropriate Therapy

- High-fibre diet, fluid intake, correct defecation as accompanying measures
- Conservative:
  - Anal stretchers, anesthetic creams
  - Nitroglycerin
  - Calcium antagonists
  - Botulinum toxin
- Operative therapy:
  - Sphincter stretching and Gabriel fissurectomy
  - Eventually lateral sphincterotomy

Complications

- Systemic side effects (nitroglycerin, Botox)
- abscess-, fistula formation
- Incontinence (Botox, lateral sphincterotomy)
- Recurrence

5.2.4 Anorectal Abscess

Key Points

- Classification depends on the localization
- Origin mostly in cryptoglandular tissue
- Anorectal abscess = emergency indication
- Therapy = surgical

Definition

- Classification of the anorectal (periproctitic) abscess: According to the localization
- Classification:

- Subanodermal abscess
- Intersphincteric abscess
- Ischioanal abscess
- Supralevator/pelvic abscess

Epidemiology

- Incidence = approx. 2–3 per 10,000 inhabitants/year
- Frequency peaks between 30 and 50 years of age
- Men: Women = 3: 1

Etiology

Cryptoglandular Origin

- >90% of the cases
- obstruction of the proctodeal glands (e.g. stool) = cryptitis = secondary abscess = abscess spread along avascular planes (path of least resistance)

Rarer causes

- Inflammatory bowel diseases, especially Crohn's disease
- Rectal perforation (e.g. swallowed toothpicks, anal foreign bodies)
- Diagnosis or surgical manipulation
- Tuberculosis

Caution
Gravity abscess in e.g. appendicitis, pyelonephritis or sigmoid diverticulitis

Symptoms

- Mostly acute painful swelling, possibly reddening in the anal area
- With advanced findings: Fever, general ill feeling, sepsis…

Caution
Supralevatorial abscess: Often dull pain in the pelvis, back pain, externally inconspicuous.

Diagnosis

- Inspection:
  - Usually sufficient
  - Further invasive examinations usually not tolerated by the patient
- Supralevator abscess:
  - Exception
  - Fluctuation and circumscribed tenderness during rectal examination
- In unclear cases:
  - Rectoscopy + endosonography (if tolerated by the patient)
  - CT/MRI if necessary
  - In case of doubt = proctological examination/endosonography under anaesthesia

Differential Diagnosis

- Carbuncle
- Infected atheroma
- Acne inversa
- Anal fissure, anal vein thrombosis
- Pilonidal sinus
- Neoplasia

Therapy

Conservative Therapy

- Not purposeful
- Even with spontaneously perforated abscesses = usually no sufficient drainage

Surgical Therapy

- Therapy of the anorectal abscess = operative
- Subanodermal, ischioanal, and most intersphincteric abscesses = generous excision.
- For high intersphincteric and supralevatoric abscesses = transrectal discharge (avoidance of fistula formation)

Surgical Procedure
Abscess Excision

- General anesthesia, spinal anesthesia, saddle block
- Lithotomy (Lloyd Davids) position
- Antibiotics for extensive phlegmon or sepsis
- Procto-/rectoscopy, if necessary endosonography
- Longitudinal oval excision of the abscess with sparing of the sphincter
- If a fistula can be visualized without any problems, thread placed in fitula (seton procedure) or split (fistulotomy)

if it is deeply seated (experience of the surgeon!)
- **Caution**: Never force a fistula presentation in an acute situation (via falsa)
- Tamponade insertion
- Specimen to pathology
- Proctoscopy to exclude fistula disease after a few weeks

Complications

- Sepsis, Fournier's gangrene with delayed treatment
- Recurrence, especially if external drainage field is too small
- Sphincter damage
- Fistula formation as a late consequence

5.2.5 Anorectal Fistulas

Key Points

- Classification according to course (path)
- Anal fistula = chronic stage, anorectal abscess = acute stage of the same usually cryptoglandular disease
- Therapy = surgical
- Goodsall rule: Above a line between 9 and 3 o'clock Lloyd-Davis position the fistulas run in a straight line (inner and outer ostium on a same radial line), below in an arc (inner ostium mostly at 6 o'clock in Lloyd Davis position)

Definition and Classification

Definition

- Connection of the anal canal with the skin surface lined with granulation tissue

Classification of Anorectal Fistulas (According to Course)

- Subanodermal fistula
- Intersphincteric fistula
- Transsphincteric fistula
- Suprasphincteric fistula
- Extrasphincteric fistula

Epidemiology

- Incidence = approx. 2 per 10,000 inhabitants/year
- Frequency peak: between 30 and 50 years of age
- Men: Women = 3: 1

Etiology

- Anorectal fistula = chronic form
- Anorectal abscess = acute form of the same disease

Cryptoglandular Origin

- >90% of the cases
- Proctodeal gland obstruction (e.g. faecal) → cryptitis → secondary abscess → abscess spread along avascular plane (path of least resistance) → perianal perforation (spontaneous or surgical): Connection between anal canal and body surface (skin)

Rarer Forms of Fistula

- Atypical fistulas in Crohn's disease
- Ischiorectal fistulas
- Rectovaginal fistulas
- Superficial fistulas in acne inversa
- Congenital fistulas

Symptoms

- Putrid, occasionally feculent secretion
- Recurrent, usually spontaneously perforating abscesses
- In the case of prolonged progression: Reduction of continence performance

Diagnosis

- Rectal digital examination
- Careful atraumatic probing of the fistula tract
- If the fistula is already thread-reinforced (seton procedure), have the patient pinched = good estimation of the fistula' course possible
- Procto/rectoscopy
- Endosonography, if necessary MRI (fistula course, exclusion of fuchsbau)
- Colonoscopy: mainly for Crohn's disease

5

Differential Diagnosis

- Differentiation of fistulas of cryptoglandular origin from other forms of fistulas (see above)
- Anal Fissure
- pilonidal sinus

Therapy

Conservative Therapy

- When excising a periproctitic abscess = do not force fistula presentation, since spontaneous healing is possible
- Established fistula = indication for surgery (no spontaneous healing + high probability of recurrent abscesses)
- Malignant degeneration possible (fistula carcinoma)

Surgical Therapy

- Thread drainage (seton procedure):
  - Principle: Insertion of a non-absorbable suture/plastic vessel loop ("Vessel loop" = more comfortable for patient)
  - Therapeutic approaches: Healing of the acute inflammation, fibrosis of the fistula tract, two-stage definitive treatment.
  - In cryptoglandular fistulas: Spontaneous healing not to be expected (occasionally successful with Crohn's disease fistulas under drug therapy).
  - Permanent solution for pre-damaged sphincter (**caution:** rarely malignant degeneration)

Caution

"Cutting seton" should no longer be used due to high risk of incontinence.

- Fistula Splitting/Cleavage:
  - Subanodermal, intersphincteric or deep transsphincteric fistula = splitting over probe + open wound treatment
  - Cure rates = up to almost 100%
  - Individually different sphincter weakening after splitting (pre-damaged sphincter, narrower ventral sphincter in women, etc.)
  - In no case cut more than 1/3 of the sphincter mass.
- Fibrin Glue:
  - Principle: curettage of the fistula tract + filling with fibrin glue
  - Long-term healing rates = only 20%
  - Possible therapy option in the case of a clearly damaged sphincter, since the sphincter muscle is not affected.
- Fistula Plug:
  - Principle: Occlusion of the fistula tract with porcine submucosa/biocompatible synthetic polymer plug.
  - Cure rates = 20–28%
  - Indication: Similar to fibrin glue
- LIFT("ligation of intersphincteric fistula tract")-OP:
  - Relatively new procedure
  - Cure rates = 50–80%
  - Low incontinence rate, as the sphincter apparatus is only slightly affected by the gentle surgical technique.
  - In the case of very scarred findings, visualization of the fistula tract in the (narrow) intersphincteric space is often difficult.

Surgical Procedure

LIFT-OP

- General anesthesia, spinal anesthesia, saddle block
- Lithotomy (Lloyd Davis) position
- Perioperative antibiotic therapy optional
- Incision anocutaneous line above the (thread-armed) fistula
- Dissection of the intersphincteric space and visualization of the intersphincteric fistula tract
- Suture ligature of the duct at the junction with the internal sphincter muscle
- Severing or excision of the duct
- Curettage of the external duct, if necessary drainage field extension
- Suture ligature of the duct at the junction with the external sphincter muscle
- Adaptive suture

Plastic fistula closure by flap:

- Principle: Fistula excision, muscle suture and covering of the internal ostium by mucosa-submucosa flap, rectum full wall flap (advancement flap) or anodermal flap
- Studies on cure rate = very inhomogeneous (46–95%)
- Relatively demanding surgical technique
- Incontinence rate is low, as the sphincter apparatus is only slightly affected in this procedure

Fistula excision with primary sphincter reconstruction:

- Principle: splitting of the sphincter, complete excision of the fistula tract, reconstruction of the sphincter
- Relatively good cure rates of 60–80%
- Relatively high risk of continence disturbance, especially in case of dehiscence of the sphincter suture (4–32%)
- Sophisticated surgical technique = prerequisite = great experience of the surgeon

Stage-Appropriate Therapy

- Superficial fistula, good continence performance:
  - Fistula splitting
- High fistula or limited continence performance:
  - Plastic reconstruction
- Poor continence performance, hidden situs:
  - Consider occluding procedures (in case of high recurrence rate)
  - Consider lifelong thread drainage (rarely malignant degeneration possible)

Complications

- Septic complications
- Recurrence
- Incontinence
- Malignant degeneration with long course

5.2.6 Pilonidal Sinus

Key Points

- Frequent disease, which mostly affects young men
- Acute or chronic inflammation, mostly of the coccyx region
- **Caution:** The acute abscessing form is a surgical emergency
- Complete excision with open wound treatment is the most frequently performed operation

Definition

- Inflammation of the subcutaneous tissue, mostly of the coccyx region
- In the sinus: granulation tissue, cell detritus, hair
- Different clinical forms:
  - Asymptomatic form
  - Acute abscessed form
  - Chronic form

Epidemiology

- Frequency = 48/100,000 inhabitants (Germany, 2012)
- Frequency peaks between the tenth and 30th year of life
- Men: Women = 2.5–3: 1

Etiology

Risk Factors

- Genetic disposition possible
- Strong hairiness
- Profuse perspiration
- Deep anal fold
- Sitting activity

Pathophysiology

- Rubbing movements of the buttocks → penetration of broken hairs with their ends close to the roots into the skin → skin scales act as barbs → migration of the hair into the subcutaneous fat → foreign body granuloma → abscess possible

5

Symptoms

Asymptomatic Form

- Irritationless primary openings
- Incidental finding

Acute Abscessed Form

- Swelling
- Redness
- Pain
- eventually Perforation
- If it progresses = fever, sepsis…

Chronic Form

- Purulent secretion

Diagnosis

- As a rule, the clinical examination is sufficient

Differential Diagnosis

- Carbuncle
- Anorectal Abscess
- Anorectal Fistula

Therapy

Conservative Therapy

- Instillation of 80% phenol solution (not approved in Germany due to toxicity)
- Epilation by means of shaving (also as recurrence prophylaxis) = not useful

Surgical Therapy

- Radical en bloc excision with open wound treatment
  - Most frequently used surgical procedure
  - Recurrence rate = 2–13%
  - Disadvantage: Often healing time of several weeks with corresponding incapacity to work

Surgical Procedure
En Bloc Excision of the Pilonidal Sinus

- General anaesthesia, for very small findings local anaesthesia
- Prone position
- Antibiotics for extensive phlegmon or sepsis
- Staining of the ducts with e.g. methylene blue solution
- Whetstone-shaped excision of the complete findings with all lateral passages with diathermy, if necessary down to the sacral fascia
- Bevelling of incision edges
- Tamponade insertion
- Plastic procedures:
  - Defect coverage after excision by flap plastic of different types (e.g. Karydakis, Cleft-Lift, Limberg, see below)
  - Also referred to as "off-midline procedures" because of the lateral displacement of the wound
  - Significantly shorter healing time
  - Number of "real" recurrences comparable with open wound treatment
  - Disadvantage: Number of abscesses, dehiscences, wound healing disorders relatively high (up to 45%), if not performed in a completely infection-free area

Surgical Procedure
Karydakis Flap/Cleft-Lift Procedure

- Symmetrical, elliptical excision of the sinus
- Mobilization of a subcutaneous flap of the opposite side
- Three-layer wound closure outside the midline

Surgical Procedure
Limberg Plastic

- Rhombic excision of the sinus
- Mobilization of rhombic-shaped flap down to the gluteal fascia
- Pivoting and tension-free sewing in of the flap
  - Sparing excision of the pori, curettage of the fistula tracts
  - Only for locally limited findings
- Procedures with unclear data:
  - Fibrin instillation

- Autologous stem cells
- Laser therapy
- Not recommended:
  - Excision with marsupialization of the wound edges
  - Midline suture excision

Stage-Adapted Therapy
- Asymptomatic form:
  - Prophylactic surgery does not seem necessary
- Acute abscessing form (emergency):
  - Definitive radical excision, or
  - Abscess relief and definitive therapy with plastic covering if necessary in the infection-free interval
- Chronic form:
  - Definitive radical excision, if necessary with plastic covering
  - In the case of locally limited findings, a semi-interventional procedure can be considered

Complications
- Sepsis if delayed therapy
- Recurrence
- Long healing process (with open wound treatment)
- Abscess, wound healing disorder (with plastic covering)
- Malignant degeneration (rare)
- Cosmetically unsightly scarring

5.2.7 Fecal Incontinence

- In this chapter, only the surgical therapy methods are discussed in detail.

Key Points
- Frequent clinical picture with a high number of unreported cases
- Often multifactorial
- Therapy of fecal incontinence usually conservative at first

Definition
- Loss of intestinal contents at the wrong time or in the wrong place

Clinical Classification
- Grade I: Inability to hold air (winds) in a controlled manner
- Grade II: Inability to retain liquid stools
- Grade III: inability to retain normally formed stools

Score Classification
- Better, as quality of life is also taken into account
- For example, Cleveland Clinic Score (Table 5.1), Jorge/Wexner Score

Epidemiology
- Prevalence = up to 3% of the population (depending on the study); up to 30% of patients in nursing homes
- Prevalence increases with age
- Women more frequently affected overall

Etiology

Pathophysiology
- Mostly multifactorial
- For example, delivery lesion (defect) at a young age → atrophy of the sphincter with age → constipation tendency → prolapse formation with chronic nerve damage → combined incontinence

Table 5.1 Cleveland Clinic Incontinence Score (CCIS)[a]

	Air	Liquid stool	Formed stool	Using incontinence pads
Occasionally	1	4	7	1
>1/week	2	5	8	2
Daily	3	6	9	3

[a]Incontinence index (IC): 0 perfect continence, 1–7 good continence, 8–14 moderate incontinence, 15–20 severe incontinence, >20 complete incontinence

5

Risk Factors

- Congenital (anomaly, spina bifida, Hirschsprung's disease)
- Neurological (e.g. multiple sclerosis, Parkinson's disease)
- Autonomic nervous system (diabetes mellitus)
- Gastrointestinal diseases
- Tumors
- Procedures in the pelvis: low anterior rectal resection, irradiation
- Sphincter injuries (delivery, trauma, surgery)
- Rectal voiding disorders (overflow incontinence, prolapse)
- Increasing age

Symptoms

- Uncontrolled continence (air and stool)
- Stool smearing ("soiling")
- Often anal eczema

Diagnosis

- Anamnesis: Essential!
- Inspection
  - Eczema, stool stains on the anus?
  - Let the patient push: Prolapse?
- Palpation
  - Tonus
  - Palpable dent
  - Rectocele, prolapse?
- Procto/rectoscopy
  - Tumor exclusion
  - Changes in the anal canal, internal prolapse?
- Holding tests
  - If the clysma/enema can be held for minutes without any problems, the diagnosis must be questioned
- Endosonography: sphincter damage?
- Manometry
- Colonoscopy
  - In the presence of inflammatory bowel disease
  - To exclude tumor disease
  - In individual cases: MRI, (MR) defecography, neurological examination

Therapy

Conservative Therapy

- Use of aids (e.g. anal tampons, pads)
- Pelvic floor training
- Biofeedback Training
- Electrostimulation
- Tibial nerve stimulation
- Medicinal stool regulation
- Anal irrigation

Surgical Therapy

- Sphincter reconstruction:
  - Butt-on-put or overlapping suture of a (fresh) sphincter defect
  - Also possible for older defects
  - Result: Initially mostly good, in the course of the years = often deterioration of continence performance (especially with concomitant neurogenic disorder)
  - Disadvantages: Relatively high rate of postoperative complications (wound healing disorder, suture dehiscence) = deterioration of preoperative continence performance
- Muscle tightening ("pre-/post-anal repair", "total pelvic floor repair"):
  - Constriction of the anal canal without severing the muscle
  - Result: Initial success rates = 60–80%; in the 5-year course = approx. 25%
- Sacral nerve modulation (SNM) formerly sacral nerve stimulation (SNS):
  - Principle: Peripheral stimulation of the sacral spinal nerves; stimulation takes place far away from the target organ = iatrogenic damage to the sphincter is therefore excluded
  - Indication now also extended to higher grade sphincter defects
  - Result: Success rate = 58% over the longer term
  - 2 surgical steps: PNE (percutaneous nerve evaluation) testing and permanent sacral nerve modulation (SNM, SNS); high predictive value (90%) regarding therapy success due to test stimulation

- Postoperative: 2-week phase with external stimulation, then 2-week phase without stimulation
- Keeping a stool diary by the patient
- If symptoms improve >50% in the stimulation phase = indication for permanent stimulation

Surgical Procedure
PNE Testing and SNM

- General anaesthesia (no muscle relaxation medication), for patients insensitive to pain also local anaesthesia
- Prone position
- Single-shot antibiosis with cephalosporin
- Marking of the sacral foramina S2–S4 under fluoroscopy or using anatomical landmarks
- Puncturing the foramina at a 60-degree angle with a needle electrode
- Contraction of the sphincter after application of current to the electrode indicates correct position
- Selection of the ideal foramen (uniform contraction, low threshold, low involvement of the lower extremity)
- Insertion of the foramen electrode using the modified Seldinger technique
- Subcutaneous placement of the foramen electrode, position control, connection with stimulator

Surgical Procedure
If Indication for Permanent Stimulation

- Complete removal of the percutaneous extension
- Creation of a pacemaker pocket gluteal outside the seating area
- Attaching and connecting the generator aggregate
- Sinking of the aggregate
- Skin closure
- Dynamic Graciloplasty (gracilis muscle transposition):
  - Principle: The pedunculated, mobilized gracilis muscle is wrapped around the anal canal; permanent stimulation via neurostimulator = long-term transformation of type 2 fibers into enduring type 1 fibers
  - Result: Continence rate = 50–83%.
  - Demanding, complex operation, complication rate = 50%
- Artificial sphincter:
  - Principle: Closure sleeve around the anal canal; control pump in the scrotum or labium
  - Result: High continence rate (up to 95% for solid and liquid stools)
  - Demanding procedure with high complication rate > 50% (infections)
- Magnetic sphincter:
  - Principle: Band with several magnets, which is placed around the anal canal, similar to a bracelet; when at rest the magnets stick together = closure of the anal canal; when pressed = the magnets move apart = opening of the anal canal.
  - Relatively new procedure, conclusive studies are lacking
- Definitive stoma placement:
  - If all conservative and surgical measures fail
  - If the patient suffers psychological stress: stoma (= controlled incontinence) = significant improvement in quality of life
- Other procedures:
  - "bulking agents": ultrasound-guided instillation of silicone or similar into the intersphincteric space

Questionable indication in case of minor symptoms and limited defect

Complications

- Social isolation, depression with delayed diagnosis
- Recurrence
- Wound healing disorder
- Implant infections with consecutive removal
- Rectal perforation, rectal necrosis, sepsis…

- Allergic reactions ("bulking agents")
- Deterioration of continence performance due to surgery

5.2.8 Anorectal Voiding Dysfunction (Outlet Constipation)

5

Key Points

- Frequent clinical picture with a high number of unreported cases
- Often multifactorial
- Therapy usually conservative at first or, if clearly possible, elimination of the underlying cause
- As a rule, combination therapy is necessary after surgical removal of the cause (stool regulation, nutritional counseling, exercise, etc.)
- Difference Outlet-Obstipation vs. Slow-Transit-Obstipation

Definition

Definition

- Chronic constipation = if at least 2 of the following criteria are present in 3 months of the last 12 months (ROM III criteria):
  - Strong pressing
  - Hard stool
  - sensation of incomplete emptying
  - Subjective obstruction
  - Manual support for defecation in >25% of defecations
  - <3 stools per week

Classification

- In scores possible (e.g. Cleveland Clinic Score for chronic constipation; ◘ Table 5.2)

Epidemiology (Of All Forms of Constipation)

- Incidence: increasing with age, 30% of those over 60 years of age
- Men: Women = 1: 3

Etiology

- Pelvic floor dyssynergy
- Anismus: involuntary, spontaneous contraction
- Symptomatic rectocele
- Intussusception: invagination of excess rectum
- Compression of the rectum due to enterocele/sigmoidocele
- Anal Stenosis
- Anal Fissure
- stenosing tumor

Symptoms

- Strong pressing during defecation
- sensation of incomplete emptying
- Fractionated emptying of small amounts of stool
- Digital clearing out
- Dull pressure pain in the pelvis

Diagnosis

- Anamnesis
  - Concomitant diseases
  - In particular, keeping a stool diary
- Inspection
- Palpation
  - Sphincter tone
  - Rectocele, prolapse
  - Stenosing process
  - Dyssynergy
- Procto/rectoscopy
  - Tumor exclusion
  - Changes in the anal canal
  - Internal prolapse
- Manometry not obligatory
- Balloon Expulsion Test: Ability of the patient to evacuate a water-filled balloon inserted into the rectum.
- Colonoscopy: In case of suspected inflammatory bowel disease/tumour disease
- Hinton test: differentiation from slow transit obtipation
- (MR) Defecography:
  - (Internal) prolapse
  - Rectocele, enterocele
  - Intussusception
  - Pelvic floor dyssynergy
  - In individual cases: MRI, CT, neurological examination

Table 5.2 Cleveland clinic constipation score[a]

Bowel movement frequency	Difficulty: painful emptying	Completeness: feeling of incomplete emptying	Pain: abdominal pain	Time: minutes of toilet use per trial	Aid: type of aid	Failure: unsuccessful emptying attempts per 24 h	History: duration of constipation (years)	Points
1–2 times/day	Never	Never	Never	Less than 5	Without help	Never	0	0
2 times/week	Rarely	Rarely	Rarely	5–10	Stimulant laxatives	1–3	1–5	1
1 time/week	Sometimes	Sometimes	Sometimes	10–20	Digital aid or enema	3–6	5–10	2
Less than 1 time/week	Mostly	Mostly	Mostly	20–30		6–9	10–20	3
Less than 1 time/month	Always	Always	Always	More than 30		More than 9	More than 20	4

[a]Minimum score = 0, maximum score = 30, constipation = score > 15

Therapy

Surgical Therapy

- Depends on underlying cause
- Pelvic floor dyssynergy:
  - Biofeedback Training
  - Pelvic floor exercises under professional guidance
- Anismus (involuntary, spontaneous contraction):
  - Biofeedback Training
  - Botulinum toxin injection
- Symptomatic rectocele:
  - Posterior colporrhaphy
  - Transanal shirring with mucosal resection

> **Caution**
> Rectoceles = also frequent in healthy women, only in 10–20% of the obstipated patients the symptoms are due to it

- Intussusception (invagination of rectum excess):
  - STARR surgery ("stapled trans anal rectal resection"): Circular transanal rectal full wall resection = circular anastomosis + "straightening" of the rectum
  - Transtar® surgery: larger resection possible (► Sect. 4.2.2 Rectal prolapse)

The term ODS (obstructive defecation syndrome) is often used synonymously for the symptom triad intussusception, rectocele and voiding dysfunction.

- Compression of the rectum by enterocele/sigmoidocele:
  - Elevation of the pelvic floor + (resection) rectopexy
- Anal stenosis: surgical correction
- Anal fissure: ► Sect. 5.2.3
- Stenosing tumor: Depending on the dignity
  - Resection
  - Stoma creation, if necessary radiochemotherapy

Complications

- Depending on the chosen therapy method

5.3 Malignant Disease: Anal Carcinoma

> **Key Points**
>
> - Anal canal carcinoma and anal margin carcinoma
> - Anal canal carcinoma:
>   - Surgical therapy of anal canal carcinoma limited to very small findings/recurrences
>   - Standard = Radiochemotherapy
> - Anal marginal carcinomas (therapy analogous to skin tumors): Primary surgical treatment

5.3.1 Definition

Anal Carcinoma

- Anal canal = from anocutaneous line to anorectal junction (anoderm + transitional zone)
- Histology:
  - Unkeratinized squamous epithelium 85%
  - Remainder = adenocarcinomas

Classification: TNM Classification

- T (tumor)
  - T1 Tumor <2 cm
  - T2c Tumor >2 cm < 5 cm
  - T3 Tumor >5 cm
  - T4 Infiltration of adjacent organs
- N (lymph nodes)
  - N0 No regional lymph node metastases
  - N1 Metastases in regional lymph nodes
  - N2 Metastases unilateral inguinal or iliacal LN
  - N3 Metastases bilaterally perirectal, inguinal or iliacal LN
- M (metastases)
  - M0 No distant metastases
  - M1 distant metastases present

Anal Margin Carcinoma

- Anal margin = from linea anocutanea to 5 cm distal thereof
- Histology: keratinizing squamous epithelium

5.3.2 Epidemiology

- Incidence = 0.5–1.5/100,000 population per year
- Men: Women = 1: 1.5
- Peak incidence: 50–70 years of age

5.3.3 Aetiology

- Known risk factors:
  - Infections with human papilloma virus (HPV)
  - HIV infections
  - Immunosupression
  - Anal sex
  - Long-term therapy with corticosteroids
  - Smoking

5.3.4 Symptomatology

- Blood accumulation, mucous discharges
- Pain
- Itchy skin
- Stool irregularities
- Continence disorders
- Enlarged inguinal lymph nodes

5.3.5 Diagnosis

- Clinical examination
- Proctoscopy, rectoscopy, endosonography
- Colonoscopy: To exclude a second carcinoma
- Sonography/MRI pelvis + groin (lymph node metastases?)
- Exclusion of distant metastases
- Biopsy, in the case of small findings also excision biopsy (= simultaneously therapeutic!)

5.3.6 Differential Diagnosis

- Hemorrhoids, Mariscs
- Anal fistula, anal fissure
- Anal Fibroids
- Rectal Cancer
- Melanoma, anal marginal carcinoma, basal cell carcinoma, fistula carcinoma
- Dermatological diseases

5.3.7 Therapy

Conservative Therapy

- Combined radiochemotherapy = therapy of choice for advanced findings
  - External radiation including the inguinal lymph nodes
  - Total dose: Up to 60 Gy
  - 5-FU (fluorouracil) continuous infusion: weeks 1 and 5
  - Mitomycin as radiosensitizer
  - 5-year survival depending on stage = up to 80%

Surgical Therapy

- Anal canal carcinoma:
  - In case of findings <1 cm after exclusion of sphincter infiltration and lymph node metastases and in case of good differentiation = complete excision with safety margin possible
  - In case of recurrence/contraindication to radiotherapy = cylindrical abdominoperineal rectum extirpation, if necessary as multivisceral resection.
  - In case of stenosing tumor = protective stoma creation before planned radiotherapy
- Anal margin carcinoma:
  - Therapy of anal margin carcinoma = therapy of skin tumours
  - Radical excision with a safety margin of 1 cm
  - In case of lymph node involvement: lymph node dissection
  - Radiatiotherapy if necessary
  - Photodynamic therapy if necessary

Complications

- After radiotherapy:
  - Incontinence
  - (Refractory) Proctitis
  - Diarrhea
  - Recurrence
- Post-op:
  - Wound healing disorders
  - Bladder emptying disorders
  - Impotence

– Stoma problems (prolapse, parastomal hernia, stenosis)
– Recurrence

5.4 Guidelines

5

German Society for Neurogastroenterology, German Society for Digestive and Metabolic Diseases, DGIM, CACP, DGAV, DGK, Deutsche Reizdarmselbsthilfe e.V. (2013) S2k-Leitlinie Chronische Obstipation: Definition, Pathophysiologie, Diagnostik und Therapie. AWMF registration number 021/019, AWMF online: ► http://www.awmf.org/uploads/tx_szleitlinien/021-019l_S2k_Chronische_Obstipation_2013-06_01.pdf

German Society for Coloproctology, BCD, DGAV, CACP, DGVS, DDG (6/2020) S3 Guideline: Sinus pilonidalis. AWMF registration number 081/009, AWMF online: ► http://www.awmf.org/leitlinien/detail/ll/081-009.html

Ommer A, Herold A, Berg E, Farke S, Fürst A, Hetzer F, Köhler A, Post S, Ruppert R, Sailer M, Schiedeck T, Strittmatter B, Lenhard BH, Bader W, Gschwend JE, Krammer H, Stange E (2011) S3 guideline: cryptoglandular anal fistulas. Coloproctol 33:295–324

Ommer A, Herold A, Berg E, Farke S, Fürst A, Hetzer F, Köhler A, Post S, Ruppert R, Sailer M, Schiedeck T, Strittmatter B, Lenhard BH, Bader W, Gschwend JE, Krammer H, Stange H (2011) S3 guideline: anal abscess. Coloproctol 33:378–392

Suggested Reading

Alasari S, Kim NK (2014) Overview of anal fistula and systemic review of ligation of the intersphincteric fistula tract (LIFT). Tech Coloproctol 18:13–22

Barussaud ML, Mantoo S, Wyart V, Meurette G, Lethur PA (2013) The magnetic anal sphincter in faecal incontinence: is initial success sustained over time? Color Dis 15:1499–1503

Bock S, Wolff K, Marti L, Schmied BM, Hetzer FH (2013) Long-term outcome after transanal rectal resection in patients with obstructed defecation syndrom. Dis Colon Rectum 56:246–252

Gingert C, Hetzer FH (2014) Stuhlinkontinenz. Coloproctol 36:125–137

Hasse C, Brune M, Bachmann S, Lorenz W, Rothmund M, Sitter H (2004) Laterale, partielle Sphinkteromyotomie zur Therapie der chronischen Analfissur. Langzeitergebnisse einer epidemiologischen Kohortenstudie. Chirurg 75:160–167

Heitland W (2012) Perianale Fistel und Analfissur. Chirurg 83:1033–1039

Herold A, Joos A, Bussen D (2012) Operationen beim Hämorrhoidalleiden. Chirurg 83:1040–1048

Hirschburger M, Schwandner T, Hecker A, Kierer W, Weinel R, Padberg W (2014) Fistulectomy with primary sphincter reconstruction in the treatment of high transsphincteric anal fistulas. Int J Color Dis 29:247–252

Joos AK, Herold A (2010) Hämorrhoidalleiden. Gastroenterologe 5:326–335

Karakayali F, Karagulle E, Karabulut Z, Oksuz E, Moray G, Haberal M (2009) Unroofing and marsupialization vs. rhomboid excision and Limberg flap in pilonidal disease: a prospective, randomized, clinical trial. Dis Colon Rectum 52:496–502

Lange J, Mölle B, Girona J (2012) Chirurgische Proktologie. Springer, Heidelberg

Milligan ET, Morgan CN, Lond LE (1937) Surgical anatomy of the anal canal, and the operation treatement of haemorrhoids. Lancet 2:1119–1124

Raptis D, Schneider I, Matzel KE, Ott O, Fietkau R, Hohenberger W (2015) The differential diagnosis and inter-disciplinary treatment of anal carcinoma. Dtsch Arztebl Int 112:243–249. https://doi.org/10.3238/arztebl.2015.024

Rojanasakul A (2009) LIFT procedure: a simplified technique for fistula-in-ano. Tech Coloproctol 13:237–240

Runkel N (2011) Analfissur. Coloproctol 33:128–129

Schiedeck T (2008) Diagnostik und Therapie der Stuhlinkontinenz. Chirurg 79:379–390

Schulte N, Hofheinz RD (2013) Analkarzinom. Coloproctol 35:309–314

Schwandner O, Fürst A (2010) Assessing the safety, effectiveness, and quality of life after the STARR procedure for obstructed defecation: results of the German STARR registry. Langenbecks Arch Surg 395:505–513

Stelzner F (1984) Die Ursache des Pilonidalsinus und der Pyodermia fistulans sinifica. Langenbecks Arch Chir 362:105–118

Stelzner F, Staubesand J, Machleidt H (1962) Das corpus cavernosum recti – die Grundlage der internen Haemorrhoiden. Langenbecks Arch Chir 299:302–312

Tan KK, Kaur G, Byrne CM, Young CY, Wright C, Solomon MJ (2013) Long-term outcome of the anal fistula plug for anal fistula of cryptoglandular origin. Color Dis 15:1510–1514

Thin NN, Horrocks EJ, Hotouras A, Palit S, Thaha MA, Chan CL, Matzel KE, Knowles CH (2013) Systemic review of the clinical effectiveness of neuromodulation in the treatement of faecal incontinence. Br J Surg 100:1430–1447

Wannenmacher M, Wenz F, Debus J (2013) Strahlentherapie. Springer, Heidelberg

Willis S, Rau M, Schumpelick V (2000) Surgical treatment of high anorectal and rectovaginal fistulas with the use of transanal endorectal advancement flaps. Chirurg 71(7):836–840

Endocrine Organs

Franck Billmann, Courtney Elizabeth Gibson, and Robert Udelsman

Contents

The original version of the chapter has been revised. A correction to this chapter can be found at https://doi.org/10.1007/978-3-662-66735-4_17

F. Billmann, T. Keck (eds.), *Essentials of Visceral Surgery*,
https://doi.org/10.1007/978-3-662-66735-4_6

6.1 Anatomy and Physiology of the Thyroid Gland

F. Billmann

Key Points

Thyroid gland (Thyroid):
- Cervical endocrine gland (normal weight 15–20 g)
- Blood supply via 4 anastomosing arteries
- Closely related to: recurrent laryngeal nerve, parathyroid glands
- Regulatory circuit: TRH (thyrotropin-releasing hormone)—TSH (thyroid-stimulating hormone)—T3 (triiodothyronine), T4 (thyroxine)—TRH/TSH

6.1.1 Embryology and Anatomy

- Large cervical endocrine gland

Macroscopy

- Two lateral lobes connected by isthmus
- Pyramidal lobe: Cranial process from isthmus; inconstant (50% of cases)
- Total adult weight = 15–20 g

Microscopy

- Thyroid follicle = structural and functional unit
- follicular epithelium = source of thyroid hormones
- C cells: Release of calcitonin (= regulation of the blood calcium level; ► Sect. 6.1.2)

Localization

- Isthmus at the level of the 2nd–4th tracheal cartilage
- Lateral lobes adjacent to the cricoid and thyroid cartilage

Blood Supply

- 4 arteries + inconstant vessels
  - Superior thyroid artery: Paired, from external carotid artery
  - Inferior thyroid artery: Paired, from thyrocervical trunk (subclavian artery)
  - A. thyreoidea ima: Unpaired from aorta or truncus brachiocephalicus; inconsistent
- Venous drainage: Variable; drainage into internal jugular vein + brachiocephalic vein

Surgical-Relevant Anatomical Relationships
- Superior laryngeal nerve: from the inferior ganglion of the vagus nerve; divides at the level of the hyoid bone into the external branch (pharyngeal musculature) and internal branche (plica vocalis)
- Recurren laryngeal nerve: branch of the vagus nerve; course between trachea and esophagus, directly behind the thyroid gland; division into anterior branche (for Mm. vocalis) and posterior branche
- Parathyroid glands: dorsal to the thyroid gland; variable location (► Sect. 6.4)
- Lymph node groups (◘ Table 6.1 and ◘ Fig. 6.1)

Development

- During development, displacement of thyroid caudally with formation of thyroglossal duct.
- regression of the thyroglossal duct in the course (possible peristence = pyramidal lobe)

6.1.2 Physiology

Thyroid Hormones (Thyroxine, T4, and Triiodothyronine, T3)

- Production and release by follicular epithelial cells
- Active form = T3
- Function (on almost all body cells):
  - Metabolism increase
  - Important role in growth + development of the nervous system

Table 6.1 Classifications of locoregional thyroid lymph nodes (LN)

Compartment classification (Dralle et al. 1994)	US classification (Robbins et al. 2008)	UICC classification (Wittekind et al. 2003)	Japanese classification (Qubain et al. 2002)
Compartment 1 (1a cervicocentral right, 1b cervicocentral left)	Without side assignment: Level 1 (submental, submandibular), Level 6 (central), Level 7 (central caudal)	Without side assignment: LN groups 1 and 2 (submental, submandibular), and 8 (central)	Without side assignment: Regional LN groups 1–4
Compartment 2 (cervicolateral right) Compartment 3 (cervicolateral left)	Without side assignment: Level 2A, 2B (cranial jugular), Level 4 (caudal jugular), Level 5A, 5B (lateral jugular)	Without side assignment: LK groups 2, 3 (cranial jugular), 4 (middle jugular), 5 (caudal jugular), 6 (dorsal lateral), and 7 (lateral supraclavicular).	Without side assignment: Regional LN groups 5–7
Compartment 4 (4a upper infrabrachiocephalic mediastinum right, 4b left)	–	–	–

a

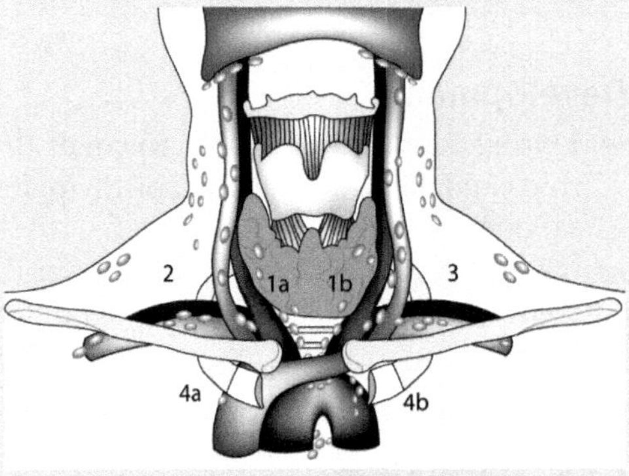

b

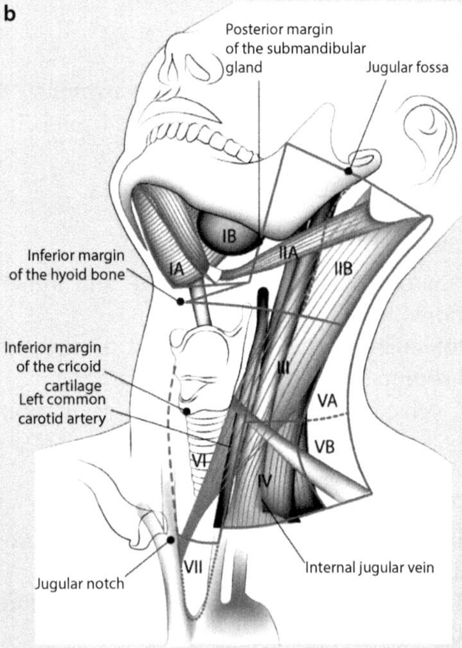

Fig. 6.1 **a**–**d** Classifications of locoregional thyroid lymph nodes. Comparison between **a** compartment classification according to Dralle, **b** US classification according to Robbins, **c** UICC/TNM classification and **d** Japanese classification

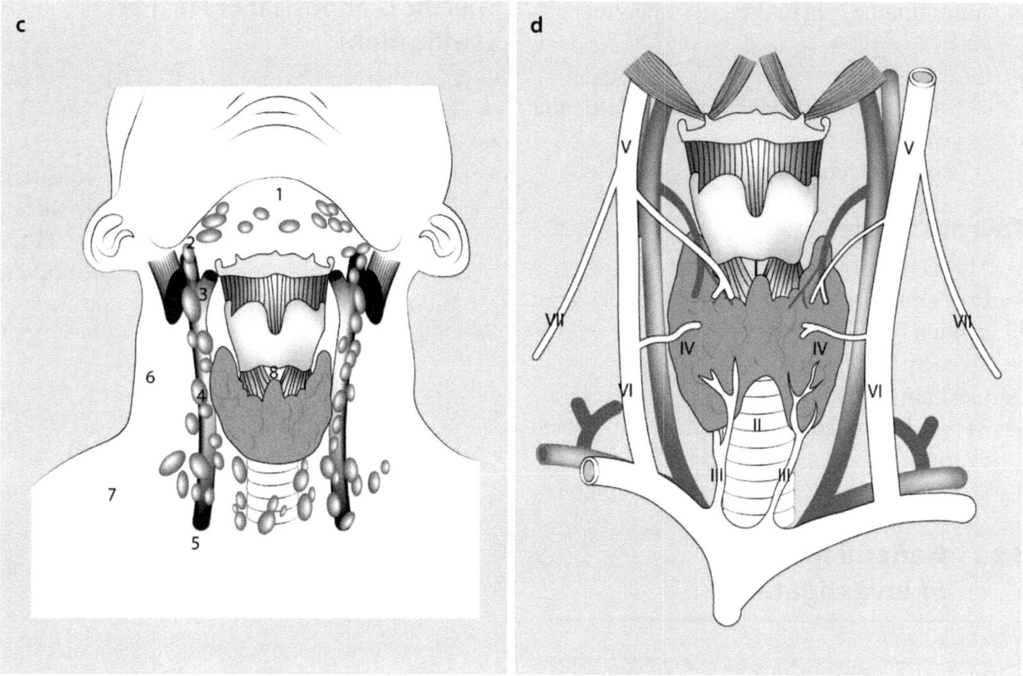

■ **Fig. 6.1** (continued)

Control Loop (Negative Feedback)

- Goal = accurate control of T3, T4
- Control of thyroid by hypothalamus + hypophysis (pituitary gland): mediators (TRF and TSH)

Calcitonin

- Produced and released by C cells
- Physiological antagonist of parathyroid hormone (PTH; ► Sect. 6.4 Parathyroid)
- Calcium regulation

6.2 Diseases of the Thyroid Gland

F. Billmann

6.2.1 Epidemiology

Goiter and Multinodular Goiter

- Prevalence: 33.1% of the working population
- Incidence of thyroid nodules:
  - 23.2% of patients with goiter (approx. 20 million people in Germany)
  - Age-dependent

Hyperthyroidism (Thyroid Autonomy)

- Prevalence: subclinical hyperthyroidism = 1.8%, manifest hyperthyroidism = 0.4%.
- Etiology:
  - Graves' disease: leading cause in regions without iodine deficiency
  - toxic nodular goiter/toxic adenoma: In regions with iodine deficiency
  - Iodine-induced hyperthyroidism (acute high iodine intake): Increasingly rare
  - Amiodarone (high iodine) induced hyperthyroidism: 30–40% of amiodarone treated patients

Autoimmune Diseases

- Prevalence: No precise data
- possibly associated with autoimmune diseases of other organs

- Autoimmune thyroiditis: women:men = 10:1
- Graves' disease:
  - 5–20 cases/100,000 inhabitants per year
  - Women:Men = 6–8:1

Thyroid Cancer

- Most common endocrine tumor
- Prevalence: men = 4/100,000 per year; women = 8.7/100,000 per year
- Women:Men = 2:1
- Germany: 5000 new cases/year
- Mortality declining (by 40% in recent years)

6

6.2.2 General Methods of Investigation

Key Points

- Standard examinations: clinical examination + laboratory thyroid function tests (TSH) + ultrasound (sonography)
- FNA (fine needle aspiration cytology): To exclude malignancy
- Scintgraphy, CT, MRT: Only for special questions

Clinical Examination

- Medical history: signs of hyper- or hypothyroidism (◘ Table 6.2)
- Inspection, palpation (position, size, consistency, swallowing displacement of the thyroid), auscultation (blood flow)
- Exclusion: globus sensation, voice change, stridor, dysphagia.
- Search for cervical lymph nodes

Laboratory Thyroid Function Tests

Basic Diagnosis (For Each Patient)

- TSH: Examination of thyroid function (see below: Overview of normal levels)
  - Euthyroid
  - Hyperthyroidism (subclinical/manifest)
  - Hypothyroidism (subclinical/manifest)

Specific Diagnosis (For Further Clarification)

- Free thyroid hormones (fT3, fT4)
- TRH test
- Thyroglobulin (Tg)
- Antibodies (in autoimmune thyroiditis): TRAb (TSH receptor autoantibodies), TgAb (thyroglobulin antibodies), TPO-MAb (thyroid peroxidase antibodies, microsomal antibodies)
- Calcitonin

Normal Levels of Thyroid Metabolism

- Serum TSH = 0.3–6 mU/L
- Serum fT3 = 3–9 pmol/L (2–6 ng/L)
- Serum fT4 = 9–29 pmol/L (7–23 ng/L)
- Serum calcitonin <2.8 pmol/L (<10 ng/dL)

Imaging Studies

Ultrasound

- Orienting study
- High resolution linear transducers (7.5–18 MHz)
- Display of nodules from 0.5–1 mm
- Special Techniques:
  - Color-coded duplex sonography: vascularization of the thyroid nodules
  - Elastography: degree of hardness of the thyroid/a nodule
  - Contrast-enhanced sonography (under evaluation)
  - "Acoustic Radiation Force Impulse-Imaging" (under evaluation)

Imaging Studies

- Ultrasound = key examination
- Cross-sectional imaging (CT/MRT) = environmental diagnosis + therapy planning
- CT, MRI, nuclear medicine procedures: Only for further clarification

Computer Tomography (CT)

- Assessment of the thyroid environment (trachea, esophagus, vessels)
- Good retrosternal/intrathoracic assessment

Table 6.2 Comparison of symptoms of hyperthyroidism and hypothyroidism

Symptoms	Hyperthyroidism	Hypothyroidism
General	Rapid fatigue	Fatigue
	Anorexia	
	Cycle Irregularity	
	Weight loss	Weight gain
	Weakness	Muscle weakness
	Heat intolerance	Hypothermia
	Increase appetite	Hypercholesterolemia
Cardiovascular	Tachycardia	Bradycardia
		Hypotension
Neurological	Nervousness/restlessness	
	Insomnia	
	Hyperreflexia	Hyporeflexia
	Tremor	
	Apathy	Adynamics
	Depression	Depression
	Confusion	
		Deep hoarse voice
Gastrointestinal	Diarrhea	
	Polydipsia	
	Constipation	Constipation
Pulmonology	Dyspnea	
Musculoskeletal	Muscular atrophy	
	Muscle cramps	
Dermatological	Sweating	Hair loss
		Facial Edema
		Pale yellowish skin coloration

- Detection of metastases (lymph nodes from 1 cm, lung +++)

Contrast Medium Containing Iodine

- In case of manifest autonomy/hyperthyroidism only approved in case of vital indication
- Radioiodine therapy through this administration for several months impossible

Magnetic Resonance Imaging (MRI)

- Mostly for surgery planning
- Good sensitivity with regard to compression/infiltration of adjacent structures
- Detection of abnormal lymph nodes
- Postoperative tumor follow-up: differentiation of scar vs. tumor recurrence

Nuclear Medicine Diagnosis

- Use of radioactively labelled substances (involved in the metabolism of Thyroid) (^{99m}Tc-pertechnetate scintigraphy)

Table 6.3 Possible causes of cold and hot nodules

Cold nodules	Hot nodules
Cancer	Compensated toxic thyroid adenoma
Cyst	Decompensated toxic thyroid adenoma
Hemorrhage	
Nonstoring adenoma	
Regressive change	
Focal inflammations	

6

- Exploration of the function of the thyroid/nodules (semiquantitative)
- Relatively poor image resolution
- Differentiation between cold and hot nodules (possible causes: Table 6.3)
- Specific investigations: for specific questions
  - ^{131}I-scintigraphy (whole body scintigraphy)
  - ^{18}F-fluorodeoxyglucose positron emission tomography (^{18} F-FDG-PET) (whole-body tomography, possibly CT-coupled)
  - ^{124}I-Positron Emission Tomography
  - "Medullary Thyroid Carcinoma" section: ^{111} indium-pentetreotide; ^{99} Tc-Tyr3-octreotide scintigraphy; ^{68} Ga-DOTATOC; ^{68}Ga-DOTATATE-PET; ^{18}F-DOPA-PET; ^{18}F-FDG-PET.

- Well-differentiated iodine-storing metastases = usually only low FDG enrichment
- De-differentiated metastases no longer storing iodine = intensive FDG enrichment

Fine Needle Aspiration Cytology (FNA)

- Objective = selection of lesions suspicious of malignancy to avoid unnecessary surgery
- Accuracy: Depending on the experience of the examiner/pathologist
- Inexpensive, easy to perform, low complications

Principle

- Contraindication = haemorrhagic diathesis
- Local anesthesia
- Puncture with disposable cannula (25–23 G)
- Ultrasonic control, monitoring
- Transfer of the punctate onto slides, air drying, staining

Interpretation of the Cytological Findings

- Quality control
- Interpretation: current consensus between Italian/UK Royal College of Pathologists/Bethesda classifications (Table 6.4)
- Diagnostic reliability (see malignancy rate Table 6.4)

Diagnostic Strategy

- Geographic variation in the prevalence of thyroid nodules = different strategies
  - USA: FNA = primary diagnostic procedure (with clinical examination and sonography)
  - Germany: FNA = additional method as part of a differentiated approach
- Clinical history-oriented procedure (▶ Sect. 6.2.6 Workup of a solitary thyroid nodule)

6.2.3 Basics of Surgical Therapy, Complications and Postoperative Care

Preoperative Measures

- Control/achievement of a euthyroid metabolic state
- Laboratory chemistry parameters: Blood count, electrolytes, coagulation, eventually blood type and Packed red blood cells (PRBCs) if large retrosternal goitre
- Calcitonin: For the early detection of medullary thyroid cancer
- Cervical ultrasound: complementary to the clinical examination
- FNA: For suspicious nodules >1.0 cm
- Preoperative laryngoscopy: examination of vocal cord function

Table 6.4 Interpretation of fine needle aspiration cytology (*FNA*; comparison (consensus) Italian/UK Royal College of Pathologists/Bethesda classifications)

Italian system	Bethesda System	UK Royal College of Pathologists System	Cytology category	Malignancy risk	Therapy recommendation
TIR 1	I	Thy 1	Non-diagnostic or insufficient test material[a]	1–4%	Repeat FNA under sonographic control[c]
TIR 1C	Ic	Thy 1c	Non-diagnostic with cystic fluid	dependent on clinical presentation	Repeat FNA under sonographic control[c]
TIR 2	II	Thy 2/Thy 2c	Benign	0–3%	Annual control: clinical examination+TSH + sonography Renewed FNA if size progression
TIR 3A	III	Thy 3a	Atypia of undetermined significance or follicular lesion of undetermined significance[b] (A/FLUS)	5–15%	Repeat FNA (3–6 months) Surgery for persistent A/FLUS, with frozen section examination
TIR 3B	IV	Thy 3f	Follicular or Hurtle cell neoplasia[b]	15–30%	Surgery due to high risk of malignancy Frozen section no further benefit
TIR 4	V	Thy 4	Suspicious for Malignancy[b]	60–75%	Surgery due to high risk of malignancy with frozen section
TIR 5	VI	Thy 5	Malignant	97–99%	Surgery with definitive thyroidectomy Preoperative sonography to exclude lymph node metastases (neck dissection)

[a] Non-diagnostic or inadequate if quality criteria not met: At least 6 groups, each group with at least 10 follicular cells, at least 2 aspirates for each nodule examined

[b] Categories III, IV and V are collectively referred to as "intermediate" and require repeat FNA (III) or surgical exploration (IV and V)

[c] After renewed non-diagnostic FNA, surgery should be performed (risk of malignancy = 8%)

- Imaging procedures for mechanical impairments (CT, MRI)
- chest X-ray
- Patient education
- Marking of the skin incision directly preoperatively

Basics of Surgical Therapy

Key Points

- Gold standard = open hemithyroidectomy/thyroidectomy (Table 6.5)
- Caution:
  - Protection of the parathyroid glands
  - Visualisation of the recurrent laryngeal nerve (= necessity of a dry operation field) to avoid injury
- Minimally invasive techniques: Cosmetic benefits only
- Lymphadenectomy: Compartmental/regional only
- Postoperative Complications (informed consent):
  - Bleeding
  - Recurrent laryngeal nerve lesion
  - Hypoparathyroidism
- Rarely thyrotoxic crisis, tracheomalacia
- Quality Criteria: Magnifying loupes/microsurgical technique.

Open Surgical Technique (= Procedure of Choice)

- Obligatory compromise: finding-oriented/preservation of function/minimization of complications (recurrent laryngeal nerve, parathyroid glands)

Table 6.5 Clinical factors in favour of/against initial total thyroidectomy

In favor of total thyroidectomy	1. Planned radioiodine therapy due to known (or suspicion of) differentiated thyroid cancer: a. Malignant FNA with lesion >4 cm b. Relevant extrathyroidal extension on US or intraop. c. Clinical, intraop. or ultrasound signs of LN metastases d. Known distant metastases e. Abnormal result of the molecular examination
	2. Medullary thyroid cancer
	3. Bilateral thyroid disease: a. Euthyroid/toxic goiter b. Graves' disease c. Contralateral dominant nodule d. Radiotherapy in anamnesis e. Familial predisposition syndrome f. Indication of contralateral parathyroidectomy
	4. Struma ovarii
Controversial/no consensus	1. Known or suspected unilateral differentiated thyroid cancer 1–4 cm with low-risk signs on ultrasound
	2. Index lesion under known thyroid hormone therapy
	3. Unilateral differentiated thyroid cancer with need for Tg/ultrasound surveillance
	4. Unilateral lesion in complex medical situation
	5. Unilateral lesion and patient preference for total thyroidectomy.
In favor of hemithyroidectomy with isthmus resection	1. Unilateral papillary thyroid microcarcinoma low-risk on ultrasound
	2. Unilateral lesion with inconspicuous molecular examination
	3. Unilateral goiter

- Standard technique = extracapsular lobectomy with isthmus resection
- Subtotal resection = inadequate (higher risk of injury to the recurrent laryngeal nerve and parathyroid glands).
- Ideal: Operation in centres with adequate expertise
- Rules:
  - Good exposure (= excellent visualization of the recurrent laryngeal nerve + parathyroid glands)
  - Systematic identification of the anatomical structures + careful dissection
  - Preoperative informed consent (operation, alternative procedures, possible complications)
  - Preoperative confirmation of the euthyroid metabolic state

Surgical Procedure

Open Hemithyroidectomy/Thyroidectomy

- General anaesthesia (only rarely locoregional anaesthesia possible)
- Cervical spine extension, roll or vacuum mattress under the shoulders
- Access: 4–5 cm Kocher collar incision, in skin fold approx. 1 finger width above the jugulum (preoperative marking)
- Transection of the platysma muscle, formation of a subplatysmal flap which is retracted cranially (holding suture)
- Incision of the linea alba, lateral retraction of the strap muscles (infrahyoid muscles)
- Preparation only on the side of the nodule(s)
- Neuromonitoring of the vagus nerve before resection
- Finding the right plane on the thyroid capsule (crucial)
- Dissection of the upper thyroid pole; visualization of the upper pole vessels: transection + ligation (close to the capsule); mobilization of the upper pole
- Mobilization to lateral + caudal; transection of the Kocher veins; mobilization of the lower pole
- Medial retraction of the thyroid and central preparation
- Exposure of the inferior thyroid artery and the recurrent laryngeal nerve; neuromonitoring prior to resection; exposure of the inferior thyroid artery (close to thyroid capsule)
- Identification of both parathyroid glands and assessment of blood flow; if insufficient blood flow: parathyroidectomy and autotransplantation into the sternocleidomastoid muscle
- Complete mobilization of the SD lobe while sparing the recurrent laryngeal nerve
- Subtle hemostasis; close to the nerve, PDS (polydioxanone)-6/0 sutures (no electrocoagulation)
- Final neuromonitoring of the recurrent laryngeal nerve and the vagus nerve after resection
- Thyroidectomy: Only justified if neuromonitoring is unremarkable on the primary side; analogous procedure on the opposite side
- Suture of the strap muscles; suture of the platysma muscle; continuous subcutaneous suture; skin closure (suture, glue)

Minimally Invasive Surgical Techniques

- Only in centres with adequate expertise
- Purely aesthetic benefits (evidence-based)
- New complications (vascular injury, nerve injury) = critical use of these techniques.
- 3 groups of procedures:
  - Purely endoscopic procedures (collar, prethoracic, axillary, perimammillary or supramandibular approach)
  - Open video-assisted procedures (MIVAT)
  - Open procedures with minimum incision length
- Indications, relative and absolute contraindications (◘ Table 6.6)

Table 6.6 Indications, relative and absolute contraindications for MI (minimally invasive) techniques

Indications	Absolute contraindications	Relative contraindications
Nodule, diameter < 3 cm	History of cervical surgery	History of neck irradiation
Thyroid volume < 20 mL	Large goiter	Hyperthyroidism
Benign nodule	Locally advanced cancer	Thyroiditis
Low-risk papillary carcinoma	Lymph node metastases	

6

Surgical Procedure

Minimally Invasive Video-Assisted Thyroidectomy (MIVAT) According to Miccoli

- General anesthesia
- No hyperextension of the cervical spine
- Access: 1–2 cm transverse skin incision, in jugular fossa (preoperative marking)
- transection of the platysma muscle and formation of a subplatysmal flap
- Incision of the linea alba (3 cm) and retraction of the strap muscles to the lateral side, medial retraction of the thyroid
- After exposure of the thyroid: Further preparation videoscopically-assisted (30°, 5-mm endoscope)
- Mobilization and resection of the thyroid: Following the rules of open surgery
- supply of the vessels: ligation impossible, therefore electrosurgery (bipolar vessel sealing devices, ultrasound dissection devices) or stapling devices
- Conversion to open surgery always possible
- Continuous subcutaneous suture; skin closure (suture, glue)

Surgical Procedure

Complete Endoscopic Thyroidectomy According to Gagner

- General anesthesia
- Moderate extension of the cervical spine
- Access: 5 mm transverse neck incision, above the jugulum (preoperative marking)
- Opening of the cervical fascia; preparation below the platysma
- Insertion of 5-mm trocar into the subplastysmal space; CO_2 insufflation (10 mmHg)
- Dissection along the anteromedial border of the sternocleidomastoid muscle (SCM), using a 0° endoscope via the 5 mm trocar; then use a 30° endoscope as soon as sufficient space is created.
- 3 additional working trocars: 3-mm trocar on the midline, 3-mm trocar on the ipsilateral SCM, 5-mm trocar on the anterior border of the SCM
- Opening of the linea alba; retraction of the sternohyoideus and sternothyroideus muscles medially
- Mobilization of the thyroid lobe
- Sealing/Transection of the Kocher veins (clip, ultrasound)
- Identification and dissection of the parathyroid glands and the laryngeal recurrent nerve
- Identification and Sealing/Transection of the inferior thyroid artery (clip, ultrasound)
- Isolation of the upper pole vessels and Sealing/Transection of the same (clip, ultrasound)
- Isolation of the lower pole vessels and Sealing/Transection of the same (clip, ultrasound)
- Transection of the Berry ligament and isthmus; extraction of the specimen
- Continuous subcutaneous suture; skin closure (suture, glue)

Cervical Lymphadenectomy (LAD) for Thyroid Cancer

SurGical Anatomy and Classification Systems

- ▶ Section 6.1, ◘ Fig. 6.1 and ◘ Table 6.1

Pathophysiology

- Lymphadenectomy for thyroid cancer (limited to the neck)
  - = curative intervention: resection of the LN (lymph node) metastases
  - = preventive intervention: prevention of LN metastases
- Lymphadenectomy: the most important curative treatment modality for locoregional LN metastases
- Indication + extent = depending on tumor biology
  - Tumour type (papillary, follicular, low-differentiated, undifferentiated, medullary)
  - Tumor extension (intrathyroidal vs. extrathyroidal; locoregional vs. distant metastases)
- Currently no consensus due to lack of studies: prophylactic vs. therapeutic LAD
- Adjuvant therapy modalities (= no replacement of surgery):
  - Radioiodine therapy (for differentiated thyroid cancers)
  - External radiation (for undifferentiated cancers or locally advanced differentiated cancers)

Sentinel Node Biopsy Technique

- Only in the context of studies
- Not routine use because of: High variability of lymphatic drainage/Frequent multiple primary tumours.

Selective LAD ("Berry Picking")

- Contraindicated
- In case of locoregional recurrence: after already performed compartment-oriented LAD

◘ **Table 6.7** Forms of cervical lymphadenectomies

Forms of neck dissection	Resection extension
Radical neck dissection	Removal of the lymph node groups 1–5 including the sternocleidomastoid muscle, internal jugular vein and vagus nerve
Modified radical neck dissection	Removal of lymph node groups 1–5 leaving at least one of the following structures: sternocleidomastoid muscle, internal jugular vein and vagus nerve
Selective neck dissection	Removal of groups of cervical lymph nodes, leaving at least one group intact. Classically, one distinguishes: Central neck dissection: removal of the lymph nodes of groups 1a and 1b according to Dralle (6 according to Robbins) Lateral neck dissection: removal of the lymph nodes of groups 2 and 3 according to Dralle (2–5 according to Robbins)
Extended neck dissection	The above resection procedures extended to include other groups of lymph nodes (deep mediastinal) or other structures (muscles or nerves)

Compartment-Oriented LAD

- Classification + definition of cervical lymph node dissections (◘ Table 6.7)
- Standard procedure for LN-positive thyroid cancer
- Surgical strategy: In case of preoperatively confirmed locally advanced thyroid cancer:
  - Centripedal tactics
  - Centrifugal tactics
  - Mediastinal LAD (sternotomy): Only in case of confirmed LN metastasis.

Surgical Procedure

Central Lymph Node Dissection

- General anesthesia
- Resection Boundaries:
  - Lateral = medial aspect of the carotid artery
  - medial = trachea
- Central LAD always with thyroidectomy (ideally "en bloc")
- Protection of the upper PG (parathyroid glands) extremely important (possibly autotransplantation)

Surgical Procedure

Lateral Lymph Node Dissection

- General anaesthesia; following thyroid resection or as an independent procedure
- sternocleidomastoid muscle, strap muscles pulled laterally dorsally
- transection of the omohyoid muscle
- Visualization of carotid artery, internal jugular vein, vagus nerve (vessel loop)
- Exposure of hypoglossal nerve (= cranial dissection landmark and border)
- Exposure of the accessorius nerve in its course (important for its protection) at the upper edge of the sternocleidomastoid muscle
- En bloc resection of the entire compartmental fibro-fatty tissue with LN
- Dorsal landmark and border = dorsal cervical fascia
- Dorsal to note and spare: C3 to C7 fibers of the brachial plexus…
- Dorsal to note and spare: cervical sympathetic trunc (mediodorsal; avoid Horner's syndrome).
- Visualization of the subclavian vein dorsal to the clavicle (= caudal dissection landmark and border)
- Caudomedial left: Protection of the thoracic duct…

Postoperative Complications

Bleeding Needing Revision

- Incidence = 0.3–5%
- Bleeding within a few hours to 24 h postoperatively
- Clinical signs: cervical swelling of the throat; dyspnoea; dysphagia
- Therapy: Immediate revision

Recurrent Laryngeal Nerve Lesion

- Temporary vs. permanent (passing after 6 months = permanent)
- Causes: transection, contusion, strain, electrocoagulation, pressure damage (edema, hematoma)
- High rate of spontaneous remission of the paresis
- Unilateral lesion: often late diagnosis/ unnoticed
  - Clinical signs: Absence of glottis closure on coughing; discrete hoarseness; deeper voice; usually only evident on postoperative laryngoscopy.
  - Therapy: Speech therapy
- Bilateral lesion: Usually early and markedly symptomatic
  - Clinical presentation: Stridor, dyspnea
  - Therapy: In mild clinical condition: conservative (calcium, glucocorticoids, if necessary NSAIDs, O_2 administration); in case of respiratory impairment (reintubation, if necessary translaryngeal laterofixation of the vocal cord, if necessary tracheotomy).

Parathyroid Hypofunction (= Hypoparathyroidism; ◘ Fig. 6.6)

- Temporary vs. permanent (passing after 6 months = permanent)
- Prophylaxis: Intraoperative exposure/ imaging of the parathyroid glands, autotransplantation in case of reduced blood flow
- Clinical presentation, diagnosis and therapy (► Sect. 6.5.1)

Thyrotoxic Crisis

- Rare; on the ground of hyperthyroidism.

■ **Table 6.8** Akamizu criteria for the diagnosis of thyrotoxic crisis

Main criterion 1	Main criterion 2	Secondary criterion 1	Secondary criterion 2
Elevated fT4 or fT3 levels	CNS manifestations (agitation, delirium, psychosis, seizure, impaired consciousness)	Body temperature ≥ 38 °C, heart rate ≥ 130, cardiac decompensation, gastrointestinal and hepatic manifestations	Thyroid disease in history, goiter, exophthalmos
Definite thyrotoxic crisis	Both main criteria + one of the Secondary criteria **or** main criterion 1 + at least three of the secondary criteria		
Suspicion of thyrotoxic crisis	Main criterion 1 and exactly two of the secondary criteria, **or** main criterion 2 + one of the secondary criteria 1 + all of the secondary criteria 2, **or** at least three of the secondary criteria 1 + all of the secondary criteria 2		

■ **Table 6.9** Staging of thyrotoxic crisis according to Hermann

Stage	Clinical criteria
1	Tachycardia, arrhythmias, hyperthermia, adynamia, diarrhea, dehydration, tremor, agitation, hyperkinesia, possibly increased thyroid hormone levels.
2	Stage 1 + disorientation, somnolence, stupor or psychosis
3	Stage 1 + coma
1–3a	Age < 50 years
1–3b	Age > 50 years

- Life-threatening due to decompensation of the organism
- Diagnosis: Purely clinical (Akamizu criteria ■ Table 6.8)
- Clinical presentation: (Classification according to severity: staging according to Hermann ■ Table 6.9)
- Prognosis: Overall lethality >15%; in stage 3 up to 30%
- Prophylaxis:
  - Consistent preoperative preparation in patients with hyperthyroidism (thyrostatic drugs, α/β-blockade if necessary) until euthyroidism is achieved.
  - Avoidance of Iodin exposure
  - Resection of all autonomies
- Therapy:
  - Interdisciplinary intensive medical treatment
  - Sedation + thyrostatic drugs + β-blockade + corticosteroids
  - Symptomatic measures: Reduction of temperature, fluid and electrolyte balance, high-calorie diet, possibly plasmapheresis
  - In case of uncontrollable crisis: emergency thyroidectomy

Tracheomalacia

- Rare
- Postoperative collapse of the trachea during inhalation
- Therapy:
  - Intraoperative: Atraumatic lateral submucosal stabilization sutures (pillar sutures) to sternocleidomastoid muscle
  - Postoperative: Postoperative mechanical ventilation
  - Endoluminal stenting

Postoperative Care

- Monitoring in the recovery room: HF (heart rate), SpO_2 (pulse oximetric oxygen saturation), neck circumference, hypocalcemia signs.
- Postoperative pain therapy (analogic pain scale)
- Workflow:
  - On the first postoperative day: calcemia and PTH
  - Calcium substitution if symptomatic hypoparathyroidism or very low level
  - Before discharge: Postoperative laryngoscopy

- 1 week postoperatively: clinical follow-up (with discussion of the definitive histopathology); possible initiation of substitution therapy; planning of possible radioiodine therapy
- 3–4 weeks postoperatively: TSH control and eventual adaptation of substitution
- Cervical ultrasound: after 6 months

6.2.4 Benign Thyroid Diseases

6

Hypothyroidism

Definition

- Insufficient central thyroid hormone production
- Limited peripheral activity of thyroid hormones

Symptoms

- During growth
  - Delayed growth to dwarfism
  - Mental retardation
  - Rare: Rectal prolapse, umbilical hernia…
- In adults (incidious and slowly progressive; ◘ Table 6.2)

Diagnosis

- Laboratory diagnosis: Elevated TSH, low fT3 and fT4

Therapy

- Purely substitution therapy (levothyroxine)

Hyperthyroidism

Key Points

- Increased thyroid hormone secretion: hypermetabolism
- Extrathyroidal vs. thyroidal (toxic nodules, Graves' disease, thyroiditis) causes
- Definitive therapy possible only under euthyroidism
- Therapy: Medical and/or radioiodine and/or surgical therapy

Definition

- Increased thyroid hormone secretion
- As a consequence = hypermetabolism

Etiology

- Diseases of the thyroid (toxic nodules, autoimmune thyreopathy)
- central nervous system disease (increased TSH secretion or thyroid hormone resistance)
- Exogenous thyroid hormone supply
- Molar pregnancy
- Thyroid cancer (▶ Sect. 6.2.5)

Symptomatology (◘ Table 6.2)

Toxic Nodules (= Autonomies)

Definition

- Thyroid cell clusters with autonomous (= TSH-independent) hormone secretion
- Forms: Unifocal vs. multifocal vs. multifocal disseminated

Epidemiology

- In regions with iodine deficiency: prevalence up to 65%
- In regions without iodine deficiency: prevalence <2–5%
- Prevalence increases with age

Symptoms

- Symptoms of hyperthyroidism (◘ Table 6.2) in up to 20% of patients (in Germany, 4.1%/year hyperthyroidism in patients with unifocal autonomy)

Diagnosis

- Laboratory tests:
  - TSH (low)
  - Exclusion of an immunothyreopathy (Graves' disease)
- Thyroid ultrasound: nodules; however, cannot prove/exclude an autonomic area
- Thyroid suppression scintigraphy with quantification of uptake: method of choice to prove/exclude functional autonomy (toxic nodules)

Normal TSH (in 70% of patients with relevant autonomy) does not exclude the diagnosis of hyperthyroidism.

Therapy

- Principle: Definitive therapy only in case of euthyroidism

Pretherapeutic/Preoperative Hyperthyroidism Treatment

- Thyrostatic agents: Thiamazole (initially 10–40 mg/day, then 2.5–10 mg/day), or carbimazole (initially 15–60 mg/day, then 5–15 mg/day), or thiouracil (initially 25–150 mg/day, then 10–50 mg/day)
- Inhibitors of iodine uptake: (e.g. perchlorate) Inhibition of iodine uptake prior to planned iodine contamination/contrast medium (CM) administration: Irenate drops (1 mL = 300 mg sodium perchlorate), 3 × 25 drops/day
- Adjunctive therapy: β-blockers (attenuation of sympathetic activity and reduction of peripheral conversion of T4; e.g. propranolol 3 × 20–40 mg/day for 3–6 days before surgery), possibly benzodiazepines (to alleviate symptoms)
- Lugol's iodine solution (Plummer and Boothby 1923): If thyrostatic not suitable because of side effects

- **Radioiodine Therapy**
  - Indications/contraindications (limit = goiter >80–90 mL; ◘ Table 6.10)
  - Low side effects + high success rate (85–95%)
  - Principle:
    - In-patient (2–5 days), with radiation protection measures (= isolation in special departments)
  - Per os intake from ^{131} I
- Risks/Side Effects:
  - Sialadenitis
  - Posttherapeutic hyperthyroidism (due to disintegration of the follicles)
  - Radiation-induced thyroiditis
  - Hypothyroidism: When excessive destruction of normal functional tissue
- **Surgical Therapy**
  - Medical pretreatment obligatory (see above; exception: uncontrollable thyrotoxic crisis)

◘ Table 6.10 Indications and contraindications for ^{131}I therapy

Indications	Contraindications
Small to medium sized autonomous goiter	Very large goiter with existing mechanical complications
Focal toxic nodules (autonomous volume treatable with one radioiodine session)	Very large volume of autonomous tissue
Toxic nodules in recurrent goiter	Low iodine uptake of the thyroid in scintigraphy
Toxic nodules in patients with increased surgical risk	Children and young people with toxic nodules
	Gravidity and lactation
	Large cold nodules with suspected malignancy

  - Indication for surgical therapy:
    - Large goiter (volume > 80 mL); small strumen with poor iodine uptake.
    - Goiter with persistent symptoms under medication
    - Goiter with additional cold nodules
    - For children, women of childbearing potential, pregnant women (when medication is no longer possible or desirable)
    - Autonomous adenomas (toxic nodules) with diameter > 3 cm
    - Refusal of radioiodine therapy
    - Iodine-induced thyrotoxicosis; thyrotoxic crisis that cannot be controlled despite drug therapy
    - Principle: High risk of recurrence: Therefore rather aggressive therapy
    - Complications of surgery (Section "Cervical Lymphadenectomy (LAD) for thyroid Cancer")
- Posttherapeutic/postoperative therapy: objectives: Prophylaxis of recurrence + treatment of postoperative hypothyroidism

Immunothyreopathy: Graves' Disease

Definition

- Merseburg Triassic
  - Goiter
  - Tachycardia (sinus tachycardia)
  - Exophthalmos
- Hyperthyroidism

Epidemiology

- Prevalence = 0.5–2%; second most common cause of thyroid hyperfunction (in Europe)
- Mostly between 20 and 50 years of age
- Most common reason for hyperthyroidism in children and adolescents
- Annual incidence = 40–60/100,000 population per year
- Women:Men = 5:1
- Association with other autoimmune diseases (5–10% of patients):
  - Vitiligo
  - Pernicious anaemia
  - myasthenia gravis
  - Diabetes mellitus type 1
  - Addison's disease
  - Rheumatoid arthritis

Pathophysiology

- Pathogenesis not fully understood
- Autoantibodies: anti-TSH receptor = increased hormone production = hyperplasia, hypertrophy
- Risk factors
  - Genetic predisposition (familial clustering)
  - Nicotine consumption
- Triggering factors: stress; iodine exposure to jodes; viral infection; influence of sex hormones

Symptoms

- **Caution:** Oligosymptomatic courses
- Clinical presentation: (◘ Table 6.2 Symptoms of hyperthyroidism), in addition:
  - Overheated moist skin
  - Systolic hypertension
  - Auscultatory murmur over the thyroid (increased blood flow)
  - Enlarged thyroid (80% of patients)
  - Endocrine ophthalmopathy (not always synchronous), pathognomonic
  - Pretibial myxedema, rare (4% of patients)
  - Hypertrophic osteoarthropathy, rare
  - Acropachy, rare

Diagnosis

- Laboratory Diagnosis:
  - Low TSH: Hyperthyroidism
  - Increased fT4 and/or fT3 (if TSH low and T4/T3 normal = subclinical hyperthyroidism)
  - Antibody determination: TSH receptor antibodies (= TRAb) elevated (grey range = 1–1.5 IU/L)
  - Blood count and liver values: Required if drug therapy is used
- Ultrasound:
  - Hypoechogenicity with/without goiter
  - Doppler: Diffusely increased perfusion
  - Exclusion of focal findings
- Complementary Diagnosis:
  - Scintigraphy: Not absolutely necessary
  - Ophthalmological examination of an ophthalmopathy: measurement of the protrusio
  - In case of symptoms: cardiological examination, osteodensitometry

Therapy

- Primary (initial manifestation): Thyrostatic long-term therapy
- After completion: regular follow-up to exclude recurrence
- In case of recurrence/unsuccessful therapy: definitive therapy (surgery vs. radioiodine therapy)
- **Thyrostatic long-term therapy**:
  - 30–60% remission after long-term thyrostatic therapy
  - Therapy duration at least 12 months (= better remission rate)
  - Contraindications:
    - Mechanical impairment due to thyroid volume
    - Suspicion of malignancy
    - Severe side effects
    - Multimorbid patient (if stable euthyroidism cannot be achieved by drug therapy)

  - Lack of compliance
  - Desire to have children (= relative contraindication)
  - Recurrence after long-term thyrostatic therapy
- Practical implementation (◘ Table 6.11)

- **Radioiodine Therapy**
  - Indications:
    - Graves' disease with small or moderate goiter
    - Increased risk of surgery, recurrent laryngeal nerve palsy, postoperative hypoparathyroidism
    - refusal of an operation
    - Special occupations (using the voice): Singer, teacher, speaker
  - Contraindications:
    - Pregnancy (should be avoided 4 months after therapy)
    - Breastfeeding women (wean at least 6–8 weeks before radioiodine)
    - Suspected malignancy
  - Practical implementation:
    - Ablative concept: Complete thyroid ablation (about 250 Gy)
    - Function-optimized concept: function-preserving therapy (about 150 Gy)

◘ Table 6.11 Thyrostatic long-term therapy of Graves' disease (practical implementation)

Substance	Initial therapy (mg/day)	Maintenance therapy (mg/day)
Monotherapy[a,b]		
Thiamazole	10–40	2.5–10
Carbimazole	20–60	5–15
Propylthiouracil	150–300	50–200
Combination therapy [a,b]		

[a] Combination therapy with thyroid hormones (levothyroxine 100 µg/day) possible: lower thyrostatic doses

[b] Pregnancy: Absolutely monotherapy, as only thyreostatics pass the blood-placental barrier. Multidisciplinary monitoring

- **Surgical therapy**:
  - Indications:
    - Compression symptoms (tracheomalacia, tracheastenosis, stridor)
    - Malignancy suspected
    - Need for immediate therapeutic effect (e.g. severe side effects to thyrostatic or radioiodine therapy)
    - Therapy refractory hyperthyroidism
    - Highly-active endocrine orbitopathy
    - Lack of patient compliance
    - Desire to have children
    - For children/adolescents (relative indication)
  - Preoperative preparation: (see above: Overview: Pretherapeutic/preoperative hyperthyroidism treatment); Glucocorticoids: In Graves' disease hyperthyroidism with suspicion of endocrine ophthalmopathy
  - Total/almost total thyroidectomy: therapy of choice
  - Intraoperative specific features:
    - Increased blood flow = bleeding tendency
    - Difficult identification of recurrent laryngeal nerve/parathyroid glands
  - Follow-up: Specific features:
    - Frequently postoperative hypocalcemia (disturbed bone metabolism)
    - Discontinue thyrostatic medication immediately postoperatively
    - Hormone replacement: levothyroxine (1.5 µg/kg BW/day)

Thyroiditis

Key Points

- Inflammatory diseases of the thyroid = histological evidence of inflammatory cells in the thyroid
- Diagnosis based on clinical presentation + laboratory diagnosis (+++) + ultrasound
- Therapy depending on entity (acute/subacute/Riedel's/autoimmune thyroiditis)

6

Acute Thyroiditis

Pathogenesis

- Rare
- Acute infection due to fungi/bacteria
- Especially in case of immunodepression (HIV, tuberculosis)
- Pathogen: Frequently Streptococcus pyogenes, Staphylococcus aureus

Symptoms

- Pain:
  - Mostly one-sided
  - Radiating pain (ears, lower jaw, retrosternal)
- Acute onset
- Fever
- Local redness, swelling, possible fluctuation
- Difficulty swallowing
- possibly hoarseness

Diagnosis

- Medical history: chronic diseases (HIV, tuberculosis)
- Palpation: pain/fluctuation
- Laboratory: leukocytosis, CRP elevation, temporary hyperthyroidism
- Ultrasound: Inhomogeneous image with hypoechogenic areas (= pus)
- CT: exclusion of a process involving more than one organ
- Contrast medium swallow: exclusion of a fistula with pyriform sinus/esophagus
- FNA: Confirmation of diagnosis + microbiological examination

Therapy

- No pus collection
  - i.v. antibiotics, pathogen-oriented, at least 14 days
  - Analgesia, cooling measures
- In case of pus collection
  - Additional surgical drainage

Subacute Thyroiditis (De Quervain)

- Granulomatous disease
- Inclusions of multinucleated giant cells

Pathogenesis

- Often a few weeks to several months after viral infection (especially respiratory tract)
- Predominantly women in the fourth and fifth decade
- Seasonal accumulation in early autumn
- Genetic predisposition (HLA B35)

Symptoms

- Acute onset with pain (radiating into the ears)
- subfebrile temperature
- Dysphagia
- Mild hoarseness
- Viral prodromes: muscle pain, general feeling of illness
- First mild hyperthyroidism then euthyroidism and possibly discrete hypothyroidism

Diagnosis

- Palpation: Firm consistency, pressure pain
- Laboratory: mild leukocytosis, CRP elevated, extremely accelerated blood sedimentation (>100 mm/h, almost pathognomonic), inflammation-related anemia
- Ultrasound: Typical: Map-like (hypo/hyperechogenic areas)
- Scintigraphy: Decreased Tc uptake (in the affected thyroid)
- FNA: Granulomatous change with multinucleated giant cells

Therapy

- Mild course: Aspirin 2–3 × 500 mg/day; alternatively, diclofenac 50–150 mg/day.
- Pronounced symptoms: glucocorticoid therapy (over 6–12 weeks)
- If hyperthyroidism: symptomatic (β-blocker, e.g. propranolol 3 × 40 mg).
- Surgical therapy: in case of therapy resistance (rarely necessary)

Autoimmune Thyroiditis

- Lymphocytic organ infiltration
- Women:Men =7–10:1

- Genetic predisposition (HLA DR3, DR4, DR5, B8), environmental influences, nutrition, infections, age, sex
- Autoimmune thyroiditis:
  - Hypertrophic autoimmune thyroiditis (Hashimoto's thyroiditis)
  - Atrophic autoimmune thyroiditis (primary myxedema)
  - Post-partum thyroiditis: In 3–11% of women after childbirth
  - Asymptomatic "silent thyroiditis": almost always an incidental finding
- Riedel's goiter: extracapsular and infiltrating thyroiditis

Symptoms

- Often incidental finding when organ enlargement is detected
- Feeling of pressure or slight pain
- Hypothyroidism symptoms (Hashimoto's and atrophic thryoiditis = most frequent cause of hypothyroidism in adults; ◘ Table 6.2)

Diagnosis

- Positive family history
- Presence of other autoimmune diseases
- Mild cervical pressure sensation
- Palpation: Firm consistency of the thyroid
- Laboratory tests:
  - Antibody elevation: anti-TPO (antithyroid peroxidase; frequent), anti-Tg (anti-thyroglobulin)
  - hyperthyroidism (at the beginning of the disease, short-term) then hypothyroidism
- Ultrasound: Diffuse hypoechogenicity
- Scintigraphy: Diffuse low uptake

Therapy

- If hypothyroidism: L-thyroxine substitution therapy
- If hyperthyroidism: symptomatic therapy
- If Riedel's thyroiditis: glucocorticoid therapy + surgery (to exclude cancer).

Special Forms of Thyroiditis

Traumatic Thyroiditis

- Thyroiditis induced by exogenous lesion (including radiation thyroiditis, radioiodin-induced thyroiditis)
- Therapy: analgesia + anti-inflammatory drugs, local cooling, rarely glucocorticoids

Drug-Induced Thyroiditis

- Drugs: e.g. cytokines such as interferons, Il-2, GM-CSF ("granulocyte macrophage colony-stimulating factor"), amiodarone
- In case of hyperthyroidism, surgical therapy may be necessary

Goiter and Nodular Goiter

Key Points

- Organ enlargement of the thyroid with/without nodule
- Etiopathogenesis: iodine deficiency + genetic predisposition
- Surgical therapy depending on: thyroid morphology, clinical presentation, nodule behavior, FNA

Definition

Goiter

- organ enlargement over 18 mL in women, 25 mL in men

Nodular Goiter

- Enlargement of the thyroid due to multifocal thyrocyte proliferation
  - Thyroid nodules: Clearly delineated clonal/polyclonal heterogeneous thyroid formation
  - Thyroid adenoma: histologically homogeneous monoclonal nodule with own structure + capsule

Pathogenesis

- Genetic predisposition + acquired alterations: Direct influence on the progenitor cells
- Iodine deficiency = hyperplasia-inducing

Diagnosis

Clinical Examination

- Inspection: Classification of goiter (grading, symmetry)
- Grading of goiter according to WHO
  - 0a: No goiter
  - 0b: Palpable, but not visible
  - 1: Palpable and visible with head reclination
  - 2: Visible goiter without reclination
  - 3: Large visible goiter
- Palpation: estimation of thyroid volume; relationship to landmarks (e.g., retrosternal goiter); number and consistency of nodules; swallowing displacement; presence of cervical lymph nodes.

Ultrasound

- Determination of the thyroid volume
- Localization, dimension and character (echogenicity, margins, vascularization, calcifications) of the nodules (◘ Table 6.12 Ultrasound signs of malignancy)

◘ **Table 6.12** Ultrasound signs of malignancy

Malignancy sign	Signs of benign node
Hypoechogenicity	Purely cystic mass
Increased intranodal vascularization	Spongiform mass
Irregular border	
Microcalcifications	
Absence of a halo	
Nodule larger than wide in transverse image	
Abnormal cervical lymph nodes	

Scintigraphy (► Sect. 6.2.2)

- Only if there's a nodule >1 cm on ultrasound…

Endemic euthyroid goiter: scintigraphy not required, neither for indication nor for planning surgery.

FNA

- For the differentiation of benign/malignant thyroid nodules
- Indications: ► Sect. 6.2.2

Laboratory (Standard Levels, ► Sect. 6.2.2, Laboratory Thyroid Function Tests)

- Basal TSH (sufficient if normal)
- In case of suppressed or elevated TSH: fT3 and fT4 for the detection of hyperthyroidism/hypothyroidism
- In case of disseminated functional autonomy (scintigraphy): TPO + TSH receptor antibodies to exclude Graves' disease
- If malignancy is suspected: calcitonin to exclude medullary thyroid cancer (**caution:** proton pump inhibitor (PPI) therapy and renal insufficiency)

Therapy

Medical Therapy and Prophylaxis

- Levothyroxine or iodide
  - Limited therapeutic influence on the progression of nodular goiter
  - Large nodules, large goiter = less sensitive to medical therapy
  - In iodine deficiency endemic areas: Early prophylaxis of nodular goiter indicated
- Radioiodine therapy: ultima ratio, only if surgical treatment is not possible

Surgical Therapy

- Procedure oriented to thyroid morphology and nodules
- Possible surgical procedures: Hemithyroidectomy, thyroidectomy…
- Indications:
  - Large thyroid volume (grade III, volume > 60 mL)
  - Suspicion of nodules (◘ Table 6.12)

  - Patient's request for pathology with smaller volume goiter
  - Waiver of the patient for long-term control examinations
- Section "Preoperative Measures"
- Procedural choice:
  - Hemithyroidectomy: When nodules localized on one side
  - Hartley-Dunhill procedure: hemithyroidectomy + contralateral subtotal resection
  - Thyroidectomy: standard procedure for euthyroid multinodular goiter

Highly Recommended For All Thyroid Operations

- Use of magnifying loupes
- Visual identification of recurrent laryngeal nerve (gold standard)
- Intraoperative neuromonitoring (recurrent laryngeal nerve + vagus nerve)
- Visual identification of the parathyroid glands

Recurrent Goiter

- Prophylaxis in case of incomplete resections = drug-based recurrence prophylaxis (administration of iodide/levothyroxine)
- Radical resection in primary surgery = thyroidectomy = most important factor for recurrence prophylaxis
- Surgery on recurrent goiter: only by very experienced surgeons; intraoperative neuromonitoring + readiness for frozen section obligatory

6.2.5 Malignant Thyroid Diseases

Key Points

- 1% of human malignancies
- 99% = epithelial tumours (carcinomas)
- Increase in incidence of thyroid cancers in the last 25 years (better diagnosis + absolute increase)
- Mortality declining (differentiated cancers = excellent prognosis)
- Evidence (RCT, meta-analyses): in the past 3 years in favour of limited resection or surveillance without surgery for "low-risk" differentiated thyroid cancers (not yet integrated in the current guideline)

German S3 guideline "Thyroid carcinoma": currently in development with planned completion by 30.04.2021.

Cancers of the Thyroid Gland

Definition (◘ Table 6.13)

- Differentiation: cancers with follicular epithelial cells vs. C-cell differentiation
- Distinction based on the different biological course:
  - Differentiated cancers (papillary = PTC, follicular = FTC)
  - Poorly differentiated cancers (medullary cancer = MTC, anaplastic carcinoma)
- Specific features of thyroid cancers:
  - Congenital (familial) or acquired in the course of life (sporadic)
  - From childhood to old age
  - Strong predominance in the female gender (especially PTC and FTC)
  - Geographical differences = genetic, environmental factors
  - Differentiated cancers = very good prognosis; anaplastic carcinomas = very poor prognosis
  - Incidence of thyroid microcarcinoma (carcinoma <1 cm) up to 35%.

Papillary Thyroid Cancer (PTC)

Epidemiology

- Most frequent malignant thyroid cancer (60–85%)
- Age peak = 40 years of age
- Women:Men = 3:1

Table 6.13 Classification of thyroid cancers

Carcinomas with follicular epithelial cell differentiation	Differentiation according to biological course	Cell differentiation	Subdifferentiation
	Differentiated carcinoma	Papillary carcinoma	Conventional type
			Variants
		Follicular carcinoma	Minimally invasive
			Broadly invasive
		Other	
	Anaplastic carcinoma[a]		
Carcinoma with C-cell differentiation	Medullary carcinoma[a]	Sporadic	
		Autosomal dominant inheritance (MEN 2, fam. MTC)	
	Mixed type (C-cell follicle differentiation)		
Rare primary thyroid carcinomas	Squamous cell carcinoma Mucinous carcinoma Mucoepidermoid carcinoma Mucoepidermoid carcinoma with eosinophilia Spindle epithelial tumor with thymus-like differentiation (SETTLE) Carcinoma with thymus-like differentiation (CASTLE)		

MEN 2 multiple endocrine neoplasia type 2, *MTC* medullary thyroid carcinoma
[a] Low-differentiated carcinoma = medullary + anaplastic carcinoma

6

Molecular Pathology BRAF Mutation: Approx. 50% of PTC

- RET/PTC rearrangements: 10–20% of the PTC
- NTRK1 rearrangements: 10% of the PTC

Prognosis

- Regional LN metastasis: Already with tumor sizes of a few mm (microcarcinoma)
- distant metastases significantly later (= mainly lung)
- Normal life expectancy even with metastases
- Prognostic factors:
  - Large PTC = poor prognosis
  - High age = poor prognosis
  - Radioiodine storage = good prognosis

Therapy Principles

- ► Section 6.2.3 "Principles of surgical therapy" and "Cervical lymphadenectomy for thyroid cancer":
- Total thyroidectomy + central lymphadenectomy
- Subsequent radioiodine therapy
- Lateral lymph node dissection:
  - if positive lateral LN
  - In case of special histology (poorly differentiated cancer)
- In case of recurrent PTC: primary therapy = surgery; in case of mediastinal LN metastases or distant metastases: Primary radioiodine therapy

Hemithyroidectomy = sufficient for papillary/follicular thyroid microcarcinoma (< 1 cm nodule) without extrathyroidal tumor manifestation.

Follicular Thyroid Cancer (FTC)

Epidemiology
- 10–30% of thyroid cancers
- High incidence in iodine deficient areas
- Women:Men = up to 5:1
- Age peak: 50 years of age

Molecular Pathology
- Adenoma-carcinoma sequence: FTC develops from an adenoma (genetic alterations)
- Vascular invasion/metastasis: From tumor size of 1–2 cm
- No specific genetic change (= no marker)

Prognosis
- Hematogenous metastasis mainly (lung, bone): 10% in encapsulated tumors, 50% of broadly invasive FTC
- Lymph node metastases together with organ metastases
- Minimally invasive FTC = excellent prognosis; broadly invasive FTC = 40–60% 10-year survival; oncocytic FTC = poorer prognosis.

Therapy Principles
- ► Section 6.2.3 "Principles of surgical therapy" and "Cervical lymphadenectomy for thyroid cancer"
- Total thyroidectomy + central lymphadenectomy
- Subsequent radioiodine therapy
- Lateral lymph node dissection:
  - if positive lateral LN
  - In case of special histology (poorly differentiated cancer)
- In case of FTC recurrence: primary therapy = surgery; in case of mediastinal LN metastases or distant metastases: Primary radioiodine therapy

Poorly Differentiated Thyroid Cancer

Epidemiology
- 4–7% of thyroid cancers (geographical differences)
- Women:Men = 2:0

Molecular Pathology
- Largest part = development de novo
- No specific genetic characteristic features

Prognosis
- 5-year survival rate = 50
- 10-year survival rate = 25–35%.

Therapy Principles
- ► Section 6.2.3 "Principles of surgical therapy" and "Cervical lymphadenectomy for thyroid cancer"
- Total thyroidectomy + central lymphadenectomy
- Lateral lymph node dissection
- Subsequent radioiodine therapy

Anaplastic Thyroid Cancer

Epidemiology
- <5% of thyroid malignancies; 90% of deaths from thyroid cancers
- Predominantly older people
- Mostly in nodular goiters
- Women:Men = 1.5:1

Molecular Pathology
- Often de novo

Prognosis
- Mortality >90%
- Mean survival <6 months (= one of the most aggressive human malignancies)
- Short history, rapid metastasis (hematogenous + lymphogenous)
- At diagnosis: already extensive extrathyroidal extension (trachea, esophagus, cervical vessels)

Therapy Principles
- Perioperative radiochemotherapy
- Operative therapy: If operable, ideally R0 resection
- Molecular genetic testing always indicated
- New targeted therapies/checkpoint inhibitor therapy: in evaluation within studies

Medullary Thyroid Cancer (MTC)

Epidemiology
- 1–3% of all thyroid cancers
- Sporadic MTC (75%): Mostly in patients >45 years
- Familial MTC (FMTC; 25%): In patients from childhood to old age

Molecular Pathology

- Tumor markers: calcitonin, chromogranin A, CEA
- Familial MTC: Autosomal dominant in the context of the MEN-2 syndrome (2a or 2b; ► Sect. 6.2.3)
- Familial MTC: detection/exclusion of the rearranged-during-transfection (RET)-protooncogene mutation obligatory

Prognosis

- MTC without metastasis: Excellent prognosis
- MTC with metastasis: generally poor prognosis

Therapy Principles

- Sporadic MTC: thyroidectomy + central LN dissection + ipsilateral lateral LN dissection ± contralateral lateral LN dissection (if calcitonin level > 200 pg/mL)
- Familial MTC: timing of therapy depends on mutation type: thyroidectomy + LN dissection; in MEN 2B: surgery immediately after diagnosis

Familial Non-Medullary Thyroid Cancer (► Sect. 6.3)

- 5% of the differentiated PTC, FTC
- In the context of defined autosomal dominant syndromes (e.g. Gardner syndrome, Cowden syndrome, Carney complex) or non-syndromic

Rare Thyroid Cancers

- Squamous cell carcinoma
- Mucinous carcinoma
- mucoepidermoid carcinoma
- Mucoepidermoid carcinoma with eosinophilia
- Spindle cell tumor with thymus-like differentiation (SETTLE)
- Carcinoma with thymus-like differentiation (CASTLE)

Primary Malignant Lymphoma of the Thyroid Gland

- Patients with Hashimoto's thyroiditis = 70 times higher risk
- Predominant part = extranodal mucosa-associated lymphoid tissue (MALT) marginal zone B-cell lymphoma
- Other lymphomas (non-Hodgkin or Hodgkin) very rare

Primary Sarcomas of the Thyroid Gland

- Rare
- Differential diagnosis with anaplastic thyroid cancer difficult
- Special type: angiosarcoma (poor prognosis)

Metastases in the Thyroid Gland

- Incidence of thyroid metastases in autopsies = 25%
- Origin tumors:
  - Lung Cancer
  - Breast Cancer
  - Renal cancer
  - Cancers of the GI tract
  - Malignant melanoma

6.2.6 Workup of a Solitary or Dominant Thyroid Nodule

Key Points

- High prevalence of thyroid nodes in Germany (25–50%)
- Necessity of a rational workup for differential diagnosis (workup diagram)
- Central = anamnesis + clinical examination + laboratory thyroid function tests + ultrasound
- Increasing importance: FNA

Epidemiology

- Prevalence (25–50%) depending on: Geography (endemic area), age, sex
- In Germany approx. 16 million people with nodules; 2/3 = cold nodules
- Diagnostic workup = **evidence-based rational approach** (◘ Fig. 6.2: ATA guideline 2015)

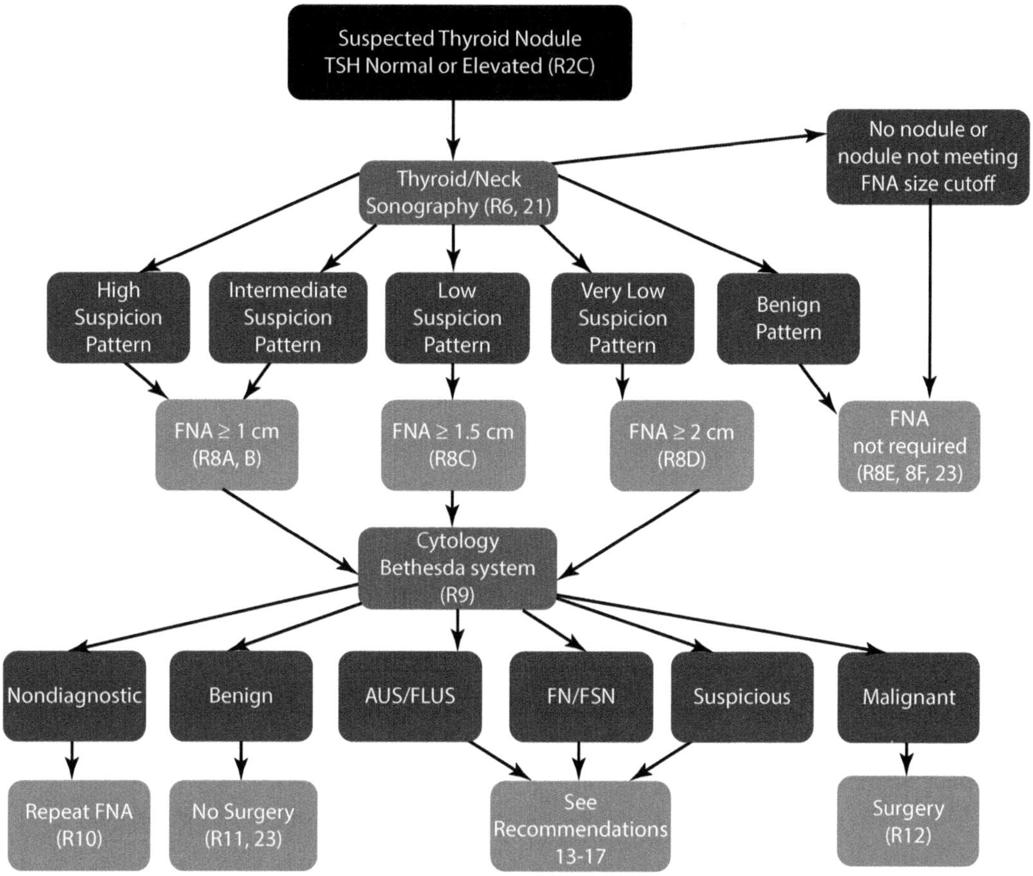

Fig. 6.2 ATA guidelines

- Prevalence-oriented differential diagnosis of the solitary/dominant thyroid nodule (with decreasing prevalence)
  - Colloid Nodules
  - Thyroid adenoma, hormonally inactive (mostly follicular adenoma)
  - Thyroid adenoma, hormonally active, toxic adenoma (autonomous adenoma)
  - Thyroid Cyst
  - Thyroiditis (Hashimoto)
  - Thyroid cancer (papillary, follicular)
  - Non-epithelial thyroid tumors and metastases
  - Abscess

Symptoms

- Mostly asymptomatic
- Mild symptoms/symptomatic: Only if large nodule
  - Subjective globus sensation
  - Swallowing disorders, to dysphagia
  - Stridor with tracheal compression

Diagnosis

- Rational approach

Medical History and Clinical Examination

- Age, sex, cervical radiation history, family history, familial thyroid disease patterns (► Sect. 6.3, e.g., MEN, poliposis coli, Gardner and Cowden syndromes).
- Time course of occurrence, growth
- Clinical examination:
  - Solitary nodule: Isolated nodular finding
  - Dominant nodule: Sudden change in a nodule in a nodular goiter.
  - Local symptoms

- Metabolic activity
- Exclusion of malignant signs

Clinical Signs of Malignancy in Thyroid Nodules

- Rough consistency
- Palpable cervical lymphadenopathy
- Non-displaceable Thyroid
- Hoarseness (expression of a recurrent laryngeal nerve impairment)
- Horner's syndrome = late sign

6

Laboratory Diagnosis (▶ Sect. 6.2.2 Laboratory Thyroid Functuon Tests)

Ultrasound

- Most sensitive examination method for solitary/dominant thyroid nodes
- Presentation of clinically inapparent nodules
- Best method for monitoring the progress of a nodule
- Guidance of the FNA
- Sonographic signs of malignancy (◘ Table 6.12)

Scintigraphy

- If low TSH
- In nodule endemic areas (even if TSH normal)
- To distinguish hot nodule (autonomous area) vs. cold nodule
- Diagnostic consequence: autonomous area (= no further diagnosis) vs. cold nodule (= indication for FNA); check possibility of radioiodine therapy

FNA (▶ Sect. 6.2.2 Fine Needle Aspiration Cytology) (◘ Fig. 6.3)

Therapy

- Oriented to:
  - Knowledge of the underlying disease/its prognosis (diagnosis)
  - Risk factors of the patient
  - Function of the thyroid
  - Expectations of the patient
  - Health condition of the patient

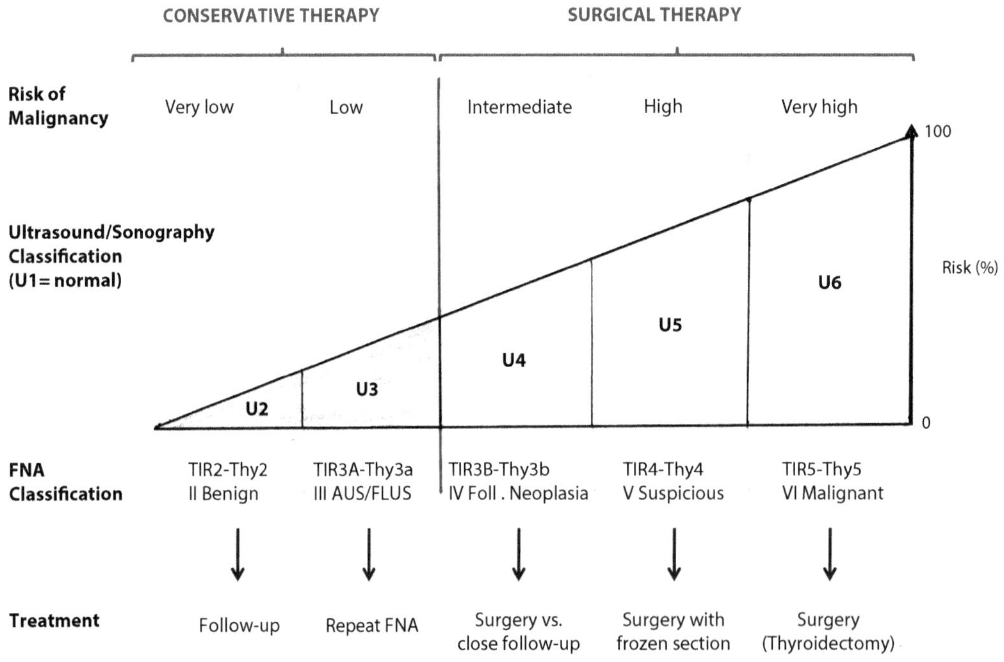

◘ **Fig. 6.3** Ultrasound and cytological FNA categories (classes) and recommended treatment

Indications for Surgical Therapy

- Higher-grade suspicion in FNA (Bethesda groups IV, V, and VI, TIR 3B/thy 3f to TIR 5/Thy 5 ◘ Table 6.4)
- Benign nodule with compression symptoms
- Newly appeared growing nodule with cervical radiation history
- Solitary autonomous adenoma >3 cm
- Suspicious nodule in the absence of follow-up

Indications for Conservative Therapy

- Operation criteria not fulfilled
- Patient not fit for anaesthesia/surgery

With conservative therapy:

- Always plan regular follow-up (interval = 6–18 months)
- In case of nodule growth: reschedule follow-uo sooner and possibly indicate surgery

Operative Therapy Principles

- Basically hemithyroidectomy + isthmus resection
- Enucleation: no longer justifiable; subtotal resection: actual controversial discussion
- In case of suspected malignancy: intraoperative frozen section
- In case of malignancy: thyroidectomy (exception = microcarcinoma)
- Prophylactic central lymphadenectomy: controversy

6.2.7 Guidelines

Gharib H, Papini E, Garber JR et al. (2016) American Association of Clinical Endocrinologists, American College of Endocrinology, and Associazione Medici Endocrinologi medical guidelines for clinical practice for the diagnosis and management of thyroid nodules—2016 update. Endocr Pract 22:S1–S60.

Haddad RI, Nasr C, Bischoff L et al. (2018) NCCN guidelines insights: thyroid carcinoma, version 2.2018. J Natl Compr Canc Netw 16:1429–1440.

Haugen BR, Alexander EK, Bible KC et al. (2016) 2015 American Thyroid Association Management Guidelines for adult patients with thyroid nodules and differentiated thyroid cancer. The American Thyroid Association Guidelines Task Force on Thyroid Nodules and Differentiated Thyroid Cancer. Thyroid 26:1–133.

Haugen BR, Sawka AM, Alexander EK et al. (2017) American Thyroid Association Guidelines on the management of thyroid nodules and differentiated thyroid cancer task force review and recommendation on the proposed renaming of encapsulated follicular variant papillary thyroid carcinoma without invasion to noninvasive follicular thyroid neoplasm with papillary-like nuclear features. Thyroid 27:481–483.

Musholt TJ, Bockisch A, Clerici T et al. (2018) Update of the S2k guideline Operative therapy of benign thyroid disease. Surgeon 89:699–709.

Patel KN, Yip L, Lubitz CC et al. (2020) The American Association of Endocrine Surgeons Guidelines for the definitive surgical management of thyroid disease in adults. Ann Surg 271:e21–e93.

Perros P, Boelaert K, Colley S, British Thyroid Association et al. (2014) Guidelines for the management of thyroid cancer. Clin Endocrinol 81:S1–S122.

S2k AWMF guideline (Register No. 088/007) Surgical therapy of benign thyroid disease. Version as of 03.10.2015. ▶ https://www.awmf.org/uploads/tx_s2leitlinien/088-007l_s2k_operative_Therapie_benigner_Thyroid_Diseases_2015-10-verlaegert.pdf

Wells SA, Asa SL, Dralle H et al. (2015) Revised American Thyroid Association Guidelines for the managements of medullary thyroid carcinoma. The American Thyroid Association Guidelines Task Force on medullary thyroid carcinoma. Thyroid 25:567–610.

6.3 Familial Malignant Syndromes of the Thyroid Gland

C. E. Gibson and R. Udelsman

6.3.1 Introduction (■ Table 6.14)

Genetics

- Thyroid cancer three times more frequent in women than men
- Earlier age at diagnosis in women (40–50 s) versus men (60 s–70 s)
- Certain inherited mutations associated with different types of thyroid cancer:
  - RET gene mutations: associated with medullary thyroid cancers/syndromes such as MEN 2A, MEN 2B and FMTC
  - APC gene mutations: associated with FAP and Gardner syndrome
  - PTEN gene mutations: associated with Cowden disease
  - PRKAR1A gene mutations: associated with Carney Complex, type I

6

6.3.2 Hereditary Medullary Thyroid Carcinoma

Medullary Thyroid Carcinoma (MTC)

Key Points

- Tumor of the parafollicular C cells
- accounts for ~5% of all thyroid cancers
- 25% = hereditary, 75% = sporadic
- responsible for disproportionate number of thyroid cancer deaths
- all patients with MTC should be screened for germline mutations:
  - linked to germ line activation of the Rearranged during Transfection (RET) proto-oncogene
  - several RET mutations identified; aggressiveness of MTC differs by mutation (i.e. genotype-phenotype correlation)

Clinical Presentation

- Neck mass; cervical lymphadenopathy
- Asymptomatic/incidental finding (e.g. during work-up for unrelated medical issues)
- Evidence of distant metastases: Liver, lung, bone and mediastinum

Diagnosis

- Neck ultrasound (US)
- Fine needle aspiration biopsy (FNA)
- Tumour markers: Elevated serum calcitonin + carcinoembryonic antigen (CEA) levels
- Cytology: plasmacytoid cell pattern, spindle cells, stromal amyloid deposits, positive calcitonin antibody

Treatment

- Surgery (total thyroidectomy; central and/or lateral neck lymph node dissection)
- External beam radiation (rarely used)
- Chemotherapy (rarely used)
- Tyrosine kinase inhibitor therapy

Multiple Endocrine Neoplasia 2A (MEN 2A)

Epidemiology

- Identified in <1000 kindreds to date
- High penetrance for the MTC
- accounts for 90% of MEN-2 cases

Genetics

- Germline mutation of the RET proto-oncogene
- Mutation in codon 609, 611, 618, 620, 630, 631 and 634 (most common; mutation at extracellular cysteine residues)
- Autosomal dominant (AD); localized on chromosome 10q11.2
- Neoplastic cell proliferation (C-cell hyperplasia) = precursor lesion
- Characteristic features:
- MTC (often multifocal and bilateral)
  - Pheochromocytoma
  - Parathyroid neoplasia (typically benign asymmetric multiglandul hyperplasia)
  - Hirschsprung's disease and cutaneous lichen amyloidosis (uncommon associations).

Table 6.14 Hereditary predisposition syndromes for thyroid cancer

	Familial adenomatous polyposis	PTEN hamartoma tumor (Cowden)	Carney complex type 1	RET-associated	DICER1
Gene	APC	PTEN	PRKAR1A	RET	DICER1
Pathognomonic criteria	>100 colorectal adenomatous polyps	Mucocutaneous lesions, cerebellar tumors (Lhermitte-Duclos)	Multiple pigmented skin lesions (e.g. nevi, blue nevi, lentiginous N)	Medullary thyroid carcinoma)	Pleuropulmonary blastoma)
Other main manifestations	–	Breast, endometrial, thyroid carcinoma, macrocephaly	Blue nevi, pigmented nodular adrenal gland, cardiac myxoma…	Primary hyperparathyroidism, pheochromocytom, mucous neuromas	Germline stromal tumors, cystic nephromas, multinodular goiter
Ancillary manifestations	Extracolic polyps, congenital hypertrophy of the retinal pigment epithelium, thyroid nodules, SD carcinoma, soft tissue tumors, desmoid tumors, osteomas	Fibrocystic mastopathy, gastrointestinal hamartomas, lipomas, fibromas, renal cell carcinomas, uterine fibromas	Thyroid nodules, melanotic schwanomas, adrenal or pituitary adenomas, HCC, pancreatic carcinoma	Hirschsprung's disease, cutaneous lichen, amyloidosis…	Wilms tumor, rhabdomyosarcoma, ciliary body medulloepithelioma, pituitary gland blastoma, nasal chondromesenchymal hamartoma
Prevalence of thyroid diseases	40%	75%	Up to 75%		Up to 30%
Benign	0.4–12%	35%	<5%	–	Up to 30%
Malignant subtypes	CMV-PTC 63% FV-PTC 25% PTC 12%	PTC 50% FV-PTC 28% FTC 14%	PTC FTC	100% MTC	FTC FV-PTC

CMV cribriform-morulare variant, *FV* follicular variant

Clinical Presentation

- Often asymptomatic
- If symptomatic, linked to hyperparathyroidism or pheochromocytoma.
- No correlation between extent of hypercalcemia and extent of symptoms

Diagnosis

- thorough family history
- Genetic testing = **gold standard** for diagnosis
  - can detect >30 variants of RET mutations
- FNA biopsy:
  - 85–99% specific for MTC
  - Cytologic features: Plasmacytoid cells, spindle cells, stromal amyloid deposits, eccentrically located nuclei, positive calcitonin staining.
- Tumor markers:
  - Calcitonin levels >100 highly suggestive of MTC
  - Elevated CEA levels may denote advanced disease

Treatment (■ Table 6.15)

- Mostly level 2 risk (codon 634):
  - Highest rate of pheochromocytoma and hyperparathyroidism
  - **Must rule out pheochromocytoma prior to neck surgery**
  - MTC development at earlier age than other codon mutations
  - Prophylactic total thyroidectomy (± central LN dissection) prior to age 5 recommended
- Modified radical (= functional) neck dissection --> if clinical or cytologic evidence of cervical metastases

Multiple Endocrine Neoplasia 2B (MEN 2B)

Epidemiology

- Less common cause of inherited MTC (<5% of cases)
- MTC presents at earlier age than in MEN 2A
- Worst prognosis

Genetics

- Germline mutation in the RET proto-oncogene
- mutation in codon 804, 806, 883 and 918 (most common: methionine → threonine)
- Autosomal dominant (AD); located on chromosome 10q11.2
- Neoplastic cell proliferation (C-cell hyperplasia); precursor lesion
- Characteristic features:
  - MTC (early onset; infancy—early childhood)
  - Pheochromocytoma (40% penetrance)
  - Mucosal neuromas, gangliomas, megacolon, Marfanoid-like body habitus.

Clinical Presentation

- Often asymptomatic
- If symptomatic, linked to tumor compressive symptoms, high calcitonin levels, or pheochromocytoma

Diagnosis

- Thorough family history

■ **Table 6.15** Management of patients with RET germline mutation detected on genetic screening. (From Revised American Thyroid Association Guidelines for the Management of Medullary Thyroid Carcinoma 2015)

MEN Type	RET mutation	Age at presentation (years)	Recommended procedure
MEN 2A	C609/F/G/R/S/Y	Variable	Thyroidectomy when serum calcitonin ↑, or based on patient/parent preference
MEN 2A	C611/F/G/S/Y/W	Variable	
MEN 2A	C618/F/R/S	Variable	
MEN 2A	C620F/R/S	Variable	
MEN 2A	C634F/G/R/S/W/Y	≤ age 5	Thyroidectomy by age 5 years
MEN 2B	A883F	≤ age 5	
MEN 2B	V804M + Y806C	20–30 years	Thyroidectomy when serum calcitonin ↑, or based on patient/parent preference
MEN 2B	V804M + S904C	20–30 years	
MEN 2B	V804M + E805K	20–30 years	
MEN 2B	V804M + Q781R	20–30 years	
MEN 2B	M918T	Infancy	Thyroidectomy ± Level VI LN dissection within first year of life

- Genetic testing = **gold standard** for diagnosis
- Can detect >30 variants of RET mutations
- FNA biopsy:
  - 85–99% specific for MTC
  - Cytologic features: Plasmacytoid cells, spindle cells, stromal amyloid deposits, eccentrically located nuclei, positive calcitonin staining.
- Tumor markers:
  - Calcitonin levels >100 highly suggestive of MTC
  - Elevated CEA levels may denote advanced disease

Therapy (◘ Table 6.15)

- Mostly level 3 risk (codon 918):
  - Highest rate of advanced disease (locally advanced or widely metastatic)
  - C-cell hyperplasia or MTC development during infancy
  - must rule out pheochromocytoma prior to neck surgery
  - Prophylactic total thyroidectomy (± central LN dissection) by age 1 recommended
- Total thyroidectomy + central neck dissection + modified radical (functional) neck dissection → if clinical or cytologic evidence of cervical metastases
- consider prophylactic functional neck dissection if clinically negative cervical LN but high calcitonin and/or CEA levels

Familial Medullary Thyroid Carcinoma (FMTC)

Epidemiology

- Clinical variant of MEN 2A
- Affected patients suffer **exclusively** from MTC

Genetics

- Germline mutation in RET proto-oncogene
- Similar codon mutations as those found in MEN 2A; also codons 768 and 790
- Autosomal dominant (AD); located on chromosome 10q11.2
- Neoplastic cell proliferation (C-cell hyperplasia); precursor lesion
- Least aggressive form of MTC

Clinical Presentation

- Often asymptomatic
- Incidentally found
- Presents in second or third decade of life

Diagnosis

- RET mutation
- Thorough family history
  - **Must** demonstrate the absence of pheochromocytoma or hyperparathyroidism in ≥2 generations within a family

Treatment

- Mostly level 1 risk (codon 918):
  - Total thyroidectomy ± central neck dissection
  - Add functional neck dissection → if clinical or cytologic evidence of cervical metastases

6.3.3 Familial Papillary Thyroid Carcinoma (FPTC)

Key Points

- First reported in monozygotic twins in 1955
- Now recognized as a distinct clinical entity
- Prevalence = 5–10% of well-differentiated thyroid cancer
- To date, no identifiable responsible genes, however heritability of FNMTC (familial non medullary thyroid cancer) considered to be one of the highest of all carcers

Clinical Presentation

- Neck mass; cervical lymphadenopathy
- May occur as a minor component of other familial cancer syndromes:
  - Familial adenomatous polyposis (FAP)
  - Gardner Syndrome
  - Cowden's disease
  - Carney complex type I

6

Diagnosis

- Neck ultrasound (U/S)
- Fine needle aspiration (FNA) biopsy
- **Genes: to date, none identified**
- Cytology: trabecular struma with oxyphilia (some cases)

Screening Recommendations

- all first degree relatives of affected families to be screened; consider screening of second degree relatives (nearly 50% of second degree relatives also affected)
- fine needle aspiration (FNA) biopsy
- Tumor markers: None
- Cytology: trabecular struma with oxyphilia (some cases)

Treatment

- Total thyroidectomy + prophylactic central neck lymph node dissection

FPTC felt to be more aggressive than sporadic cases:
- Earlier age of onset
- Higher incidence of:
  - Multifocality
  - Bilaterality
  - Nodal involvement
  - Intraglandular dissemination
  - Extrathyroidal invasion
  - Recurrence

6.3.4 Rare Genetic Syndromes Associated with Thyroid Cancer

Key Points

- 5% of well-differentiated thyroid cancers (WDTC) have familial disease, most of which are NMFTC
- Some rare syndromes associated with WDTC include familial adenomatous polyposis (FAP), Gardner syndrome, Cowden syndrome, and Carney complex I
- Inheritance is likely autosomal dominant with reduced penetrance
- Most common type of thyroid cancer associated with these syndromes is PTC

Familial Adenomatous Polyposis (FAP)

- ► Section 3.3.3

Epidemiology

- Occurs in approximately 1:10,000 to 1:30,000 live births
- Men:Women = 1:1
- Accounts for <1% of all colorectal cancer cases in the U.S.
- 0.5–2% of cases associated with thyroid cancer; cribriform variant classically associated with FAP

Genetics

- Germline mutation in the adenomatous polyposis coli (APC) tumor suppressor gene
- Autosomal dominant (AD); located on chromosome 5q21–q22
- Near complete penetrance of colonic manifestations; variable penetrance of extracolonic manifestations (◘ Table 6.16).

Clinical Presentation

- Often asymptomatic
- If symptomatic, linked to iron-deficiency anemia due to occult bleeding.

Diagnosis

- Suspect any patient with ≥10 colorectal polyps on colonoscopy

◘ Table 6.16 Colonic and extracolonic manifestations of familial adenomatous polyposis (FAP)

Colonic manifestation	Extracolonic manifestation
Adenomatous colorectal polyps (>100) by second to third decade of life Colorectal carcinoma: 100% of cases (if not treated)	Gastric polyps: Rarely progress to gastric cancer Duodenal polyps: Up to 12% risk of duodenal cancer Desmoid tumours Cysts Other benign tumors: lipomas, osteomas, fibromas, adrenal adenomas

- Genetic testing for germline mutation in the APC gene = required for **DEFINITIVE DIAGNOSIS**

Treatment

- total colectomy
- Excision of desmoid tumors:
  - Destruction of adjacent vital intra-abdominal organs
  - Leading cause of death in patients with FAP
- Thyroidectomy (if thyroid cancer present)

Gardner Syndrome

Definition and Epidemiology

- Considered a variant of FAP
- Combination of:
  - Inherited colonic adenomatosis
  - Along with extracolonic lesion (Table 6.17)

Genetics

- Germline mutation in adenomatous polyposis coli (APC) tumor suppressor gene
- Autosomal dominant (AD); located on chromosome 5q21–q22 (same as in FAP)

Clinical Presentation

- Based on which extra-intestinal manifestation(s) present

Diagnosis

- Suspicion in any patient with known FAP and additional extra-colonic lesion:

Table 6.17 Extracolonic and extraintestinal manifestations of Gardner syndrome

Benign extra-intestinal lesions	Extra-colonic malignancies
Osteomas, dental abnormalities Desmoid tumours Cutaneous lesions Adrenal adenomas Nasal angiofibromas Congenital hypertrophy of the retinal pigment epithelium	Duodenum/periampullary (5%) **Thyroid (2%)** Pancreastic (2%) Gastric (<1%) CNS (<1%) Hepatoblastoma (2%) Adrenal (rare)

- Genetic examination for germline mutation of the APC gene = required for **DEFINITIVE DIAGNOSIS**

Treatment

- Total colectomy (as in FAP)
- Additional therapy based on presence of other extra-intestinal lesions

Cowden Syndrome

Epidemiology

- First reported in 1963
- Estimated prevalence = 1/200,000–250,000

Genetics

- Germline mutation in phosphatase tensin homolog (PTEN) tumor suppressor gene
- Autosomal dominant (AD); located on chromosome 10q23
- Other mutations:
  - Hypermethylation of the promoter of the Killin (KLLN) gene, also located on chromosome 10q23
  - Mutations in succinate dehydrogenase (SDH) gene, subunits B and D
  - Germline PIK3CA and AKT1 mutations
- Characteristic features:
  - Enlarged cranium
  - Benign tumors on face, hands and feet
  - Breast, renal and thyroid malignancies

Clinical Manifestations

- Mucocutaneous
  - Distinctive and common manifestation of Cowden syndrome
  - Trichilemmomas, acral keratoses, facial papules
- Breast
  - Breast cancer = most common malignancy in Cowden syndrome
  - Early onset (third and fourth decades of life)
  - Lifetime risk = 25–50%
- Thyroid
  - Thyroid disease: incidence in >50% of patients
  - Risk of thyroid malignancy = 3–35%
  - incidence of non-medullary thyroid cancer (NMTC) = 70-fold increased

- Genitourinary
  - Endometrial Cancer
  - Renal Cell Cancer
- Gastrointestinal
  - Gastric, duodenal, colon polyps
  - Colorectal cancer
- Other manifestations
  - Macrocephaly
  - Mental retardation
  - Immune dysfunction
  - Vascular tumors

6

Diagnosis

- Thorough family history
- Genetic testing for PTEN, KLLN or other associated gene mutations

Management

- Genetic counselling
- Cancer surveillance:
  - Annual physical exam (PE): with particular attention to skin, breast and thyroid
  - Thyroid ultrasound: beginning at age 18
  - Colonoscopy: at age 35, then every 5 years
  - Consider renal ultrasound by age 40

Treatment

- Therapy based on organ system(s) involved

Carney Complex I

Epidemiology

- Approximately 600 cases reported to date
- Incidence: Men:Women = 1:1
- Mean age at diagnosis = 20 years

Genetics

- Germline mutation in PRKAR1A gene on chromosome 17q22–q24; codes for the type 1α regulatory subunit of protein kinase A
  - Other associated mutations: PDE11A gene mutation; involved in cAMP signaling
- Autosomal dominant (AD) inheritance; can also occur sporadically
- Characteristic features:
  - Multiple endocrine disorders: Cushing syndrome, adrenocortical hyperplasia, acromegaly, thyroid gland tumors (often WDTC= "well differentiated thyroid cancers")
  - Other features: Atrial myxomas, schwannomas, osteochondromyxomas, pigmented skin/mucosa lesions

Presentation

- Variable:
  - Cushing's
  - Acromegaly
  - Thyroid gland tumors
  - Other lesions (see characteristic features)
- Numerous pigmented lesions (lentigenes, blue nevi), noted during adolescence

Diagnosis

- Detailed patient history with identification of 2 or more of the following: (◘ Table 6.18)
- Genetic testing = **gold standard** for diagnosis:
  - PRKAR1A or PDE11A mutations
- Echocardiogram:
  - To detect cardiac myxoma = **life-threatening condition!**
- Biochemical analysis:
  - Hormones: cortisol, insulin-like growth factor, prolactin.

◘ Table 6.18 Diagnostic features of Carney complex I

Endocrine abnormalities	Non-endocrine abnormalities
Primary pigmented nodular adrenocortical disease (PPNAD) Thyroid tumors Acromegaly	Cardiac myxomas Lentiginosis Multiple Blue Nevi Testicular tumors Schwannoma Osteochondro-myxoma Skin myxoma

Treatment

- Treatement directed toward specific symptoms:
  - Cardiac myxoma requires open heart surgical removal
  - Pituitary adenoma → transphenoidal resection
  - thyoid cancer (typically well-differentiated) → Thyroidectomy ± lymph node dissection

6.3.5 Guidelines

Provenzale D, Gupta S, Ahnen DJ et al. (2018) NCCN Guidelines Insights: colorectal cancer screening, version 1.2018. J Natl Compr Canc Netw 16:939–949.

Kloos RT, Eng C, Evans DB et al. (2009) Medullary thyroid cancer: management guidelines of the American Thyroid Association. Thyroid 19:565–612.

Wells SA, Pacini F, Robinson BG et al. (2013) Multiple endocrine neoplasia type 2 and familial medullary thyroid carcinoma: an update. J Clin Endocrinol Metab 98:3149–3164.

Wells SA, Asa SL, Dralle H et al. (2015) Revised American Thyroid Association guidelines for the management of medullary thyroid carcinoma. Thyroid 25:567–610.

6.4 Anatomy and Physiology of the Parathyroid Gland

F. Billmann

6.4.1 Anatomy

- 4 Parathyroid glands (PG)

Localization

- Variable (embryological):
  - Lower PG: Posterior to the inferior pole of the thyroid gland, medial and anterior to the recurrent laryngeal nerve; wide variability.
  - Upper PG: posterior to the superior pole of the thyroid gland, lateral and superior to the recurrent laryngeal nerve (1 cm around the junction of the inferior thyroid artery and recurrent laryngeal nerve); relatively constant
  - approx. 90% of the PGs in "normal position

Blood Supply

- Inferior thyroid artery (A. thyroidea inferior)
- Variations = A. thyroidea superior/A. thyroidea ima

6.4.2 Physiology (◘ Fig. 6.4)

Parathormone (PTH)

- Production + distribution by PG
- Function: Regulation of calcium-phosphate balance together with vitamin D_3/calcitonin (thyroid gland)
- PTH receptors:
  - Type 1: Bones, kidneys, intestines
  - Type 2: brain, intestine

Calcium (Ca++)

- Functionally active calcium (Ca^{++}) = non-albumin-bound Ca^{++} = ionized Ca^{++}
- "CaSR" = Calcium Sensing Receptor (PG cells): Binding site for Ca^{++}
- Regulation of calcium = central to cell signaling pathways, cranial nerve function, muscle function, bone metabolism

Control Loop (Negative Feedback)

- Accurate control of calcium levels:
  - Hypocalcemia → lower Ca^{++} receptor binding → increase in PTH secretion.
  - Vitamin-D_3-receptor (PG cells): Vitamin D_3 deficiency → secretion of PTH
  - PTH → PTH receptor → bone resorption + absorption from small intestine + reabsorption in kidney → increase Ca^{++} level
  - Increase in Ca^{++} level → higher Ca^{++} receptor binding → reduction in PTH secretion

6

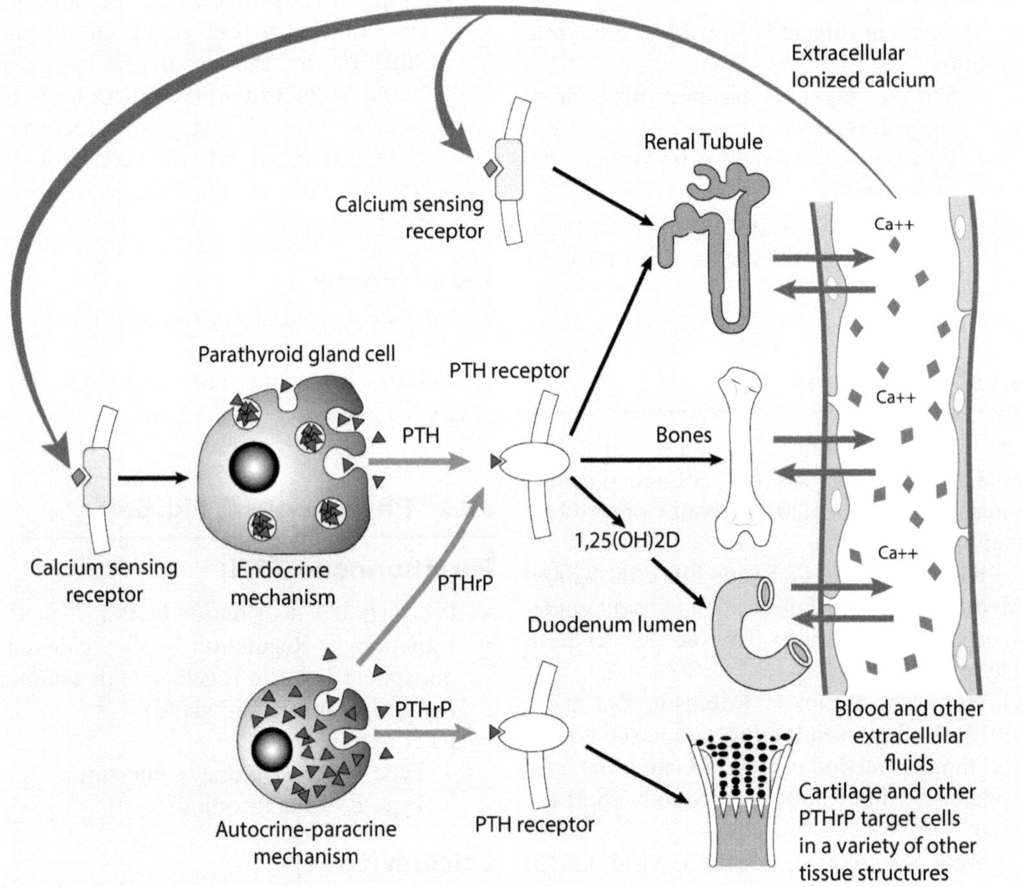

Fig. 6.4 Regulation of the calcium balance

Normal Levels of Calcium Metabolism

- Serum PTH: 1.5–6.0 pmol/L (12–72 ng/L)
- Serum calcitonin: <2.8 pmol/L (<10 ng/dL)
- Serum calcium (total): 2.15–2.75 mmol/L
- Serum calcium (ionized): 1.0–1.5 mmol/L
- Urine calcium: 4.02–4.99 mmol/L in 24-h urine
- Serum phosphate: 0.84–1.45 mmol/L

6.5 Diseases of the Parathyroid Gland

F. Billmann

6.5.1 Benign Parathyroid Diseases

Primary Hyperparathyroidism (pHPT)

Key Points

- Most common cause of hypercalcemia; prevalence = 1–5/1000 (increasing with age)
- Often asymptomatic

- Elevated/unexpected normal parathyroid hormone + elevated ionized serum calcium
- Imaging diagnosis for localization before planned parathyroidectomy
- Indication for parathyroidectomy:
  - Symptomatic pHPT patients
  - Asymptomatic pHPT patients with compliance with the guidelines (■ Table 6.20)
  - Monitoring impossible
- Monitoring without therapy = in asymptomatic patients (guidelines) = obligation of regular controls (progression of the disease)

Definition

- One or more hyperactive PG
- Continuous hypersecretion of PTH

Forms

Sporadic pHPT

- Solitary adenoma (65–85%)
- Multiglandular hyperplasia (10–30%)
- Double adenoma (5–10%)
- Carcinoma (approx. 0.1%)

Hereditary pHPT (▶ Sect. 6.3)

- Multiple endocrine neoplasia type 1 (MEN 1)
- Multiple endocrine neoplasia type 2A (MEN 2A)
- Neonatal severe hyperparathyroidism (NSHPT; mutation CaSR, chromosome 3q13.3–q21)
- Hyperparathyroidism jaw tumor syndrome (HPT-JT, mutation parafibromin, chromosome 1q25)

Epidemiology

- Prevalence: 1 per 1000 (USA), 3 per 1000 (Norway), 4.3 per 1000 (Sweden), 2–4 per 1000 (Germany)
- Incidence: 27–30 new cases/100,000 population years (increases with age)
- Third most common endocrinological disease (after thyroid disease, diabetes mellitus)
- Women:Men = 3:1
- Average age = 55 years

Caution

Radioiodine therapy = no pHPT incidence increase with currently used radioiodine doses.

Symptoms

- Associated with hypercalcemia (not with elevated PTH)
- Mostly few symptoms/asymptomatic (truly asymptomatic patients <5%)
- Affected systems ■ Table 6.19

■ **Table 6.19** Symptoms of pHPT

Bones and muscles	Muscle weakness Myalgia Bone pain Osteoporosis/penia Osteitis fibrosa cystica Brown tumor
Kidneys	Kidney stones/renal colic Nephrocalcinosis Dehydration/thirst Polyuria/oliguria/anuria Renal insufficiency
Neuropsychiatry	Concentration problems Poor memory Restlessness Depression Confusion Dementia/Paranoia Ataxia Hyporeflexia Coma
Gastrointestinal tract	Nausea/vomiting Abdominal pain Anorexia Ulcer disease Pancreatitis Constipation Weight loss
Cardiovascular system	Hypertension Vascular calcifications QT interval reduction Bradycardia Myocardial block Lethal arrhythmias
Other	Visual changes Linear keratopathy (corneal calcification) Conjunctivitis Pruritus

Caution

Hypercalcemic crisis:

- Metabolic emergency (calcium >3.5 mmol/L)
- Symptoms: Dehydration, metabolic encephalopathy (stupor to coma), gastrointestinal symptoms (distended abdomen, bloating, constipation, vomiting, ileus), renal (acute renal failure), cardiovascular symptoms (tachyarrhythmia)
- Intensive medical treatment (rarely haemodialysis necessary)

6

Diagnosis

- 2 stages (laboratory diagnosis + imaging diagnosis)

Laboratory Diagnosis (Fig. 6.5)

- Goal = Confirmation of the pHPT
  - In serum: Ionized Ca^{++} + PTH + Vitamin D
  - In urine: Ca^{++} + phosphate + creatinine
  - In 24-h urine: Ca^{++} + phosphate + creatinine (ratio creatinine clearance/Ca^{++} clearance)
  - 2 independent determinations (eventually after vitamin D deficiency treatment)
- Strategy:
  - PTH high/unusually normal = pHPT until proven otherwise.
  - Phosphate, electrolytes, creatinine, 24-h urine: calcium and phosphate: to exclude Differential diagnoses
  - s. Normal levels (► Sect. 6.4.2)

Diagnostic Imaging

- Goal = Localization: Essential for minimally invasive surgery (= no exploration of all 4 parathyroid glands)
- Standard = Ultrasound (US) + Scintigraphy
- Ultrasound (linear transducer 7.5–15 MHz)
  - Adenoma: Hypoechogenic, peripheral blood circulation (Doppler)
  - Possibility of US-guided fine needle aspiration (FNA)
- Scintigraphy: $^{99\,m}$Tc-Sestamibi-Scintigraphy
  - SPECT (Single Photon Emission Computed Tomography): Tomographic examination
  - Dual $^{99\,m}$Tc- and ^{123}I-scintigraphy: contrast enhancement by subtraction imaging (subtraction of thyroid uptake)
- 4D-CT/MRI (not first-line method)
- Fusion possible: SPECT + CT, SPECT + MRT, PET + CT
- Invasive investigations (not first-line methods): Selective vein sampling; Selective angiography; Fine needle aspiration (FNA)

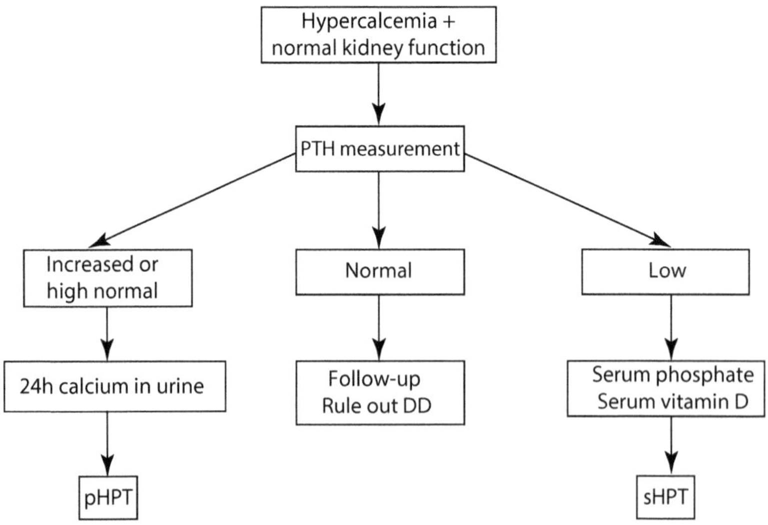

Fig. 6.5 Positive diagnosis of primary (pHPT) and secondary hyperparathyroidism (sHPT). *DD* differential diagnosis

Genetic Workup

- In young patient <40 years with pHPT + multiglandular disease + family history or syndromic signs

> **Ectopic Parathyroid Glands**
> - Ectopic location = 4–16% of cases
> - Necessity of a standardized neck exploration (localization OP technique)
> - If adenoma not identifiable by exploration: abort surgery + need for further imaging (MRI, CT, SPECT, selective vein sampling)

Differential Diagnosis (◘ Fig. 6.6)

Secondary (sHPT), Tertiary HPT (tHPT) (See Below)

Familial Hypocalciuric Hypercalcemia (FHH)

- Mutation of CaSR = loss of function of the receptor (kidney and parathyroid gland) leads to a reduction in calciuria
- Findings: hypercalcemia, PTH normal or high, 24-h calciuria decreased, Ca^{++}/Crea clearance <0.01

Milk-Alkali Syndrome

- Caused by an excess of easily absorbable alkalis (e.g. bicarbonates) + calcium (e.g. milk)

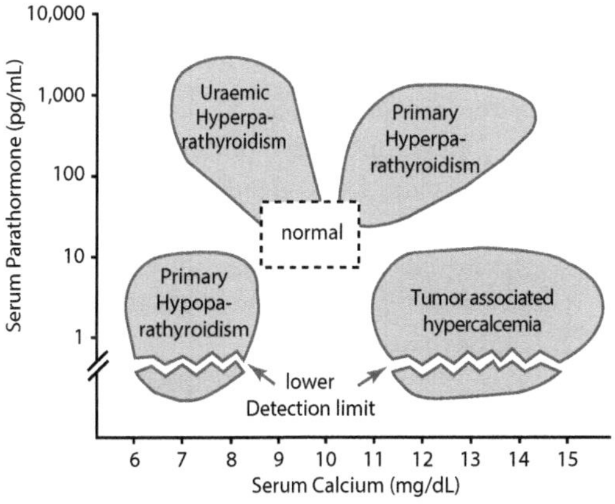

◘ **Fig. 6.6** Laboratory test results in hyper- and hypoparathyroidism

- Findings: hypercalcemia, metabolic alkalosis, decreased PTH, impaired renal function

Lithium Therapy

- Especially psychiatry: depression, mania, schizophrenia, cluster headaches
- Elevated PTH, increased bone turnover

Malignancy-Associated Hypercalcemia

- Calcium release by osteodestructive metastases of a malignant tumor or by tumor production and release of a parathyroid hormone-related peptide (paraneoplastic; PTHrP)
- Findings: Elevated tumor markers, elevated PTHrP and calcitriol

Granulomatous Disease

- e.g. sarcoidosis, berylliosis, tuberculosis, histoplasmosis
- Renal involvement = increased hydroxylation of vitamin D = hypercalcemia (increased absorption and reabsorption of calcium)
- Findings: hypercalcemia, PTH decreased, 24-h calciuria decreased

Endocrinopathies

- e.g. hyperthyroidism, adrenal insufficiency, pheochromocytoma, VIPoma
- Increased bone turnover
- Findings: Elevated calcium, low PTH

Drugs

- e.g. thiazides, vitamin D, calcium, vitamin A intoxication
- Elevated PTH, increased bone turnover.

Immobilization, Bed Rest

- Lack of stress on the musculoskeletal system = increased osteoclastic activity = hypercalcemia

Therapy

Indications for Medical Therapy

- OP criteria not met
- Patient not fit for anaesthesia/surgery
- Monitoring absolutely necessary: Ca^{++} + creatinine + PTH control every 6–12 months (once PTH target level is reached).
- Therapeutic options:

- Hormonal therapy (especially postmenopausal women): e.g. raloxifene 60 mg daily
- Bisphosphonates (e.g. alendronate): 70 mg once a week
- Calcimimetic (e.g. Cinacalcet): Starting at 30 mg/day (increase until PTH goal is reached).
- Dietary recommendations: Sufficient water intake (at least 2–3 L/day), calcium intake <1000 mg/day.

Indications for Surgical Therapy

- Symptomatic pHPT = always OP indication
- If monitoring is not desired/not possible
- For neurocognitive/neuropsychiatric symptoms
- Asymptomatic pHPT (75% of patients): Early surgery if OP criteria are met (■ Table 6.20), for prophylaxis of morbidity/mortality
- Multiglandular hyperplasia: persistence and recurrence rate high; sporadic or in the context of MEN; therapy = subtotal parathyroidectomy (± cryopreservation)

■ Table 6.20 Criteria for determining the indication for surgery in asymptomatic pHPT patients. (According to Wang and Udelsman 2007 and 2016 AAES guideline)

Measured level	Criteria for surgery	Monitoring without surgery
Serum calcium (above the upper normal level)	>1.0 mg/dL (0.25 mmol/L) above the upper normal level	Annual
24 h urine calcium	>400 mg/day (>10 mmol/day) or nephrocalcinosis on imaging	Annual
Creatinine clearance	Reduced <60 mL/min	Annual
Bone density	T-score < 2.5 (lumbar, femoral, or wrist), and/or fracture risk	Every 1–2 years (lumbar, femoral and wrist)
Age	<50 years	–

- Ectopic PG (up to 4–16% of patients): Treatment success depending on treatment algorithm (■ Fig. 6.7)

Guideline Criteria for Determining the Indication for Surgery (■ Table 6.20)

- Progressive disease (= only 25% of asymptomatic patients)
- Weighing morbidity/mortality of surgery vs. expected benefit
- If monitoring is not desired/not possible
- For neuropsychological/neuropsychiatric symptoms
- Caution: in Germany only S1 guideline

Operative Therapy Principles

- Bilateral neck exploration
  - Indication: No definite localization, or suspicion of 4-gland hyperplasia
  - Principle = exploration/visualization of all 4 parathyroid glands
  - Resection of enlarged, abnormal TG (based on morphology)
  - Intraoperative aids: Intraoperative PTH measurement, intraoperative frozen section, localization by gamma probe
- Minimally invasive parathyroidectomy:
  - Current method of choice
  - Only if positive localization (sonography, sestamibi scan)
  - Intraoperative aids: Intraoperative PTH measurement, intraoperative frozen section, localization by gamma probe

Surgical Therapy

- Need for careful hemostasis: "Only a dry situs guarantees the identification of the parathyroid glands"
- Advantage operative vs. medical: improvement of bone density and mass: back to baseline (lasts up to 10 years postoperatively)
- Early: prevention of cardiovascular morbi/mortality

- If 3 or more PGs are enlarged or PTH does not decrease adequately after removal of

Fig. 6.7 Treatment algorithm for intraoperative identification of missing parathyroid glands (failure to find a PG). (After Wang and Udelsman 2007)

Step 1
Opening and inspection of the thyroid capsule, palpation of the thyroid gland

Step 2
Dissection of the cervical thymus, paratracheal tissue, complete cervical thymectomy

Step 3
Mobilization of the pharynx and esophagus, Exploration of the para- and retropharyngeal and the paraesophageal area

Step 4
Opening of the carotid sheath, Exposure of the common carotid artery over its entire course in the neck

Step 5
Ligation of the ipsilateral inferior thyroid artery and ipsilateral hemithyroidectomy. All identified parathyroid glands must be precisely located and recorded in the OP report

Step 6
End surgery, monitor patient to show persistence of the Hypercalcemia, further localization diagnostics (4D-CT, MRT, invasive method) also outside the neck

the first PG = 3½-gland resection or total parathyroidectomy + autotransplantation of part of the most inconspicuous PG into sternocleidomastoid/brachioradialis muscle

- Postoperative aftercare
  - Postoperative calcium controls (1 time daily)
  - Search for clinical signs of hypocalcaemia (see “Hypoparathyroidism” below)
  - Eventual substitution of temporary hypocalcemia:
    - Calcium per os 1.5–3 g/day +1,25-dihydroxy vitamin D_3 0.5–2 μg/day
    - i.v. calcium administration in case of persisting symptoms
  - Before discharge: PTH determination + videolaryngoscopy

Surgical Procedure

Bilateral Neck Exploration

- General anaesthesia (rarely locoregional anaesthesia possible)
- Extension of the cervical spine, roll or vacuum mattress under the shoulders
- Access: 4–5 cm Kocher collar incision, in skin fold approx. 1 finger width above the jugular notch (preoperative marking)
- transection of the platysma muscle, formation of a subplatysmal flap (cranial retraction by suture)
- Opening of the linea alba and retraction of the strap muscles laterally
- Start surgery on the side of the localization (if negative localization, start on the right side)
- Visualization of the thyroid gland, ligation and transection of the middle thyroid veins, mobilization of the thyroid gland anteromedially
- Identification and sparing of the recurrent laryngeal nerve and inferior thyroid artery
- Lower PG = usually in the cervical thymus; upper PG = usually in a 1-cm radius around the point where the

recurrent laryngeal nerve inserts into the cricothyroid membrane.
- Removal of the conspicuous PG (+ intraoperative PTH determination + frozen section examination of the specimen)

Surgical Procedure

Minimally Invasive Open Parathyroidectomy
- Local/regional anaesthesia/general anaesthesia
- Moderate extension of the cervical spine
- Access: 2–4 cm Kocher collar incision, in skin fold approximately 1 finger width above jugular notch (preoperative marking)
- transection of the platysma muscle + formation of a subplatysmal flap (cranial retraction by suturing)
- Opening of the linea alba + retraction of the strap muscles to the lateral side
- Targeted preparation in the area of localization
- Mobilization of the thyroid gland (transection of the middle thyroid veins not necessary)
- Identification + protection of the recurrent laryngeal nerve and the inferior thyroid artery
- Visualization of the conspicuous PG, mobilization, ligation of the blood supply and excision of the adenoma
- Intraoperative PTH measurement

Surgical Procedure

Minimally Invasive Video-Assisted Parathyroidectomy (MIVAP)
- General anesthesia
- Thyroid positioning: Moderate extension of the cervical spine
- Access: 15 mm transverse neck incision, approx. 2 cm above the jugular notch (preoperative marking); lateral access possible in case of reoperation
- transection of the platysma muscle
- Opening of the linea alba over 3 cm + retraction of the strap muscles to the side
- Targeted dissection in the area of localization, mobilization of the thyroid gland + transection of the middle thyroid veins
- Insertion of a 5 mm 30° endoscope through the access and purely endoscopic continuation of the operation
- 2–3 surgeons required for surgery: Surgeon, first assistant (laparoscope guidance + suction), second assistant (holding the retractor).
- Identification + protection of the recurrent laryngeal nerve and the inferior thyroid artery (easier due to laparoscopic magnification effect)
- Visualization of the conspicuous PG, mobilization, ligation of the blood supply and exheresis of the adenoma
- Intraoperative PTH measurement

Complications (Section "Postoperative Complications")

Reoperation
- Indications
  - pHPT persistence: persisting hypercalcemia after neck exploration/recurrence of hypercalcemia within 6 months of initial surgery.
  - pHPT recurrence: recurrence of hypercalcemia later than 6 months after initial surgery
  - Causes of persistence/recurrence ◘ Table 6.21
- Preoperative strategy ◘ Table 6.22
- Surgical strategy ◘ Table 6.23

Table 6.21 Causes of pHPT persistence or recurrence

pHPT Persistence	Failure to identify or resect the PG adenoma Failure to identify or resect all adenomas or 4-gland hyperplasia Inadequate subtotal resection of a 4-gland hyperplasia Subtotal resection of a parathyroid adenoma Residual or metastatic parathyroid carcinoma Parathyromatosis Inadequate percutaneous ablation
pHPT Recurrence	Recurrent growth of hyperplastic PG tissue (especially familial pHPT) Recurrent growth of autotransplanted PG tissue Recurrence of PG carcinoma or metastatic PG carcinoma Parathyromatosis

Table 6.22 Preoperative strategy in case of reoperation

1. Reconfirmation of the diagnosis	Complete medical history and clinical examination again Repetition of laboratory diagnosis Exclusion of a differential diagnosis (see Differential diagnoses, Fig. 6.6)
2. Re-evaluation of the old localization diagnosis, operation report, pathology findings	(Essential information for planning the surgical strategy and the possible location of the adenoma)
3. Planning of additional localization examinations	(Only if 1. and 2. did not provide further information) Ultrasound + Sestamibi 4D CT/MRI Selective vein sampling Selective arteriography
4. Discussion of the operative risk with the patient	Injury to recurrent laryngeal nerve during reoperation 4–20% (preoperative laryngoscopy); if bilateral, need for tracheostomy Transient/permanent postoperative hypocalcemia (transient: 10–20%, permanent: 5–10% after reoperation)

Table 6.23 Surgical strategy for reoperation

1. Selection of an adequate time window and adequate access for the reoperation	Ideal time window: within the first week or 3 months after initial surgery Optimal strategy = targeted minimally invasive re-exploration (reducing the risk of laryngeal recurrent nerve injury and postoperative hypocalcaemia) Lateral access (“back door”): due to adhesions in the central neck Planning of the surgery on the basis of the localization diagnosis, the operation and pathology report
2. Exploration of ectopic and unusual PG localizations	Most unidentified PG (40%) are found in normal anatomical localization Fig. 6.7 in the other cases
3. Consider intraoperative localization methods	Intraoperative PTH measurement Intraoperative ultrasound examination Gamma probe examination (with radioactively labelled sestamibi)

Secondary Hyperparathyroidism (sHPT)

Key Points

- Renal etiology = 90% of patients with sHPT
- Mostly asymptomatic
- sHPT: elevated parathyroid hormone + low/normal ionized serum calcium; **caution:** differential diagnoses
- Primary therapy = conservative, medical
- Indications for surgical therapy:
  - Failure of conservative therapy
  - Hypercalcemia
  - Normocalcemia, if PTH > tenfold elevated, refractory hyperphosphatemia, advanced renal osteopathy, spontaneous fractures, calciphylaxis

6

Definition

- Compensatory hypersecretion of PTH in response to hypocalcemia

Etiology (◘ Table 6.24)

- Always outside the PG (= malfunction of one/several components of the calcium control loop)

Renal sHPT

- 90% of patients with sHPT
- Renal insufficiency → increased phosphate level → inhibition of renal calcitriol production → decreased serum Ca^{++} (hypocalcaemia) → stimulation of PTH production and release
- Renal insufficiency → hyperphosphatemia, acidosis, hyperuricemia → inhibition 1α-hydroxylase → hypocalcemia → compensatory hypersecretion of PTH + hyperplasia of PG

Extrarenal sHPT (= Differential Diagnosis) (◘ Table 6.23)

Symptoms

- Initially no symptoms
- Symptoms of pHPT (see above "Primary hyperparathyroidism")
- Extraosseous calcifications (perarticular with gout-like symptoms, vessels, kidneys, myocardium)
- Calciphylaxis: extreme form of extraosseous calcifications (vessels, subcutis) → vasculitis + paniculitis → necrosis

Diagnosis (◘ Fig. 6.5)

- Same as in pHPT (see above "Primary hyperparathyroidism")

Therapy

Conservative/Medical = Primary Therapy of sHPT

- Compensation of hyperphosphatemia: diet (reduction of intake) + phosphate binders + withdrawal by dialysis
- Calcium administration as required
- Vitamin D_3 substitution
- Calcimimetics (Cinacalcet): Receptor blockade of parathyroid cells (= prevention of PTH release).

Surgical Therapy

- Indication for surgery: Only 5% of patients with sHPT
- Indications:
  - Failure of conservative/medical therapy
  - Hypercalcemia = absolute indication for surgery
  - Normocalcemia and:
    - PTH > tenfold above the norm
    - Hyperphosphatemia resistant to therapy with extraosseous calcifications or
    - Advanced renal osteopathy or
    - Bone pain refractory to treatment or
    - Spontaneous fractures or
    - Calciphylaxis
- Standard operations
  - Subtotal parathyroidectomy: Smallest PG is left in situ with intact circulation (recurrence risk = 16%)
  - Parathyroidectomy + simultaneous orthotopic/heterotopic autotransplantation

Table 6.24 Differential diagnosis of sHPT

Gastrointestinal causes	Inadequate diet	Food intolerance Dietary restriction Phytic acid (legumes, cereals, oilseeds)
	Malabsorption	Celiac disease Pancreatic diseases (exocrine pancreatic insufficiency) Inflammatory bowel disease Cystic fibrosis (mucoviscidosis) Gastric bypass surgery Cortisone therapy Age
Vitamin D-associated causes	Lack of sunlight	Dark skin in northern latitudes Cultural habits, clothing
	Inadequate diet	Vegan or lactovegan diet
	liver or biliary disease	Malabsorption, 25-hydroxylase deficit. Liver cirrhosis Cholestasis
	Antiepileptic therapy	Modified vitamin D metabolism
Vitamin D-dependent osteomalacia		Hypophosphatemia
Nephrological causes	Chronic kidney disease	Hyperphosphataemia 1α-hydroxylase deficiency: Decreased 1,25-dihydrovitamin-D Reduction of PTH clearance: (C-terminal) PTH resistance
Cellular/tissue-associated causes	Bones	Growth
Genetic causes	Pseudohypoparathy-reoisism	Abnormal PTH receptor G protein/PTH resistance(s)
"Hungry Bone Syndrome"		
Bisphosphonate therapy		
Lactation, postlactation period		
Metastatic prostate carcinoma	Kidneys	Diuretics Increased natriuresis Idiopathic hypercalciuria
	Soft Tissue	Rhabdomyolysis: calcium deposition, hyperphosphatemia, acute renal failure. Acute pancreatitis Sepsis

Postoperative Follow-Up: Like pHPT (See Above "pHPT")

Surgical Procedure

Parathyroidectomy with Simultaneous Orthotopic/Heterotopic Autotransplantation

- General anaesthesia (rarely locoregional anaesthesia possible)
- Extension of the cervical spine, roll or vacuum mattress under the shoulders
- Bilateral neck exploration (see above)
- A portion of the least modified PG is divided into small, 1-mm pieces = implantation into the brachioradialis muscle of the non-shunt-bearing forearm; clip marking
- Thymectomy + central LK dissection (due to possibility of supernumerary PGs).

6

Tertiary Hyperparathyroidism (tHPT)

Definition

- PG function escaping the negative feedback within the framework of an sHPT
- Consequence of chronic sHPT (= PG hyperplasia):
  - Under-expression of CaSR
  - Reduction of vitamin D receptors

Etiology

- Chronic kidney disease (= most frequent cause)
- X-linked dominant hypophosphatemic rickets
- Autosomal dominant hypophosphatemic rickets

Therapy

- Always surgical therapy = parathyroidectomy + simultaneous orthotopic/heterotopic autotransplantation (see above "Surgical procedure")
- Postoperative follow-up like pHPT (see above "pHPT")

After kidney transplantation (= etiological treatment of sHPT)

- PG hyperplasia remains (= increased PTH secretion)
- Development of PTH-induced hypercalcemia in 1/3 of patients after kidney transplantation = risk for kidney transplant function!

Hypoparathyroidism

Epidemiology

- Incidence: Very controversial (especially for postoperative hypoparathyroidism)

Symptoms

- Symptoms of hypocalcemia:
  - Paresthesias
  - Muscle spasms (up to tetany) (Chvostek/Trousseau sign)
  - seizures (especially in acute hypoparathyroidism)
  - Chronic hypocalcemia: Mostly and long asymptomatic

Chvostek/Trousseau sign:

- Chvostek: contraction of facial muscles on tapping the facial nerve trunk (1 cm ventral to the ear lobe).
- Trousseau: carpopedal spasm (paw position) after inflation of a blood pressure cuff above systolic pressure for 3 min

Diagnosis

- Serum Ca^{++} + PTH levels

Etiology

- Intraoperative iatrogenic damage to the PG
  - Damage to PG blood flow
  - Unintentional parathyroidectomy
- Other: Developmental defect of parathyroid gland: autoimmune, genetic (e.g., mutation PTH gene).

Therapy

- Calcium + vitamin D (or vitamin D analogues)
- Thiazides: stimulation of renal calcium reabsorption
- In acute hypoparathyroidism (e.g. postoperative hypoparathyroidism): i.v. calcium and vitamin D administration
- PTH substitution in case of failure of other treatments

6.5.2 Parathyroid Cancer

Epidemiology

- Women:Men = 3:1
- Frequency peak: 40–60 years of age
- approx. 0.1–0.5% of HPT patients

Symptoms

- Symptoms of pHPT

Diagnosis

- Very high PTH levels
- Rarely preoperative diagnosis, mostly intraoperative (= infiltration of the tumor into the surrounding area)/postoperative diagnosis (= histology)

Therapy

- Always surgical therapy
  - Parathyroidectomy + ipsilateral hemithyroidectomy
  - En bloc resection of the infiltrated soft tissues
- Systematic ipsilateral lymphadenectomy
- Postoperative follow-up like pHPT (see above "pHPT")
- Palliative approach: chemotherapy ± radiotherapy

6.5.3 Guidelines

Bilezikian JP, Brandi ML, Eastell R et al. (2014) Guidelines for the management of asymptomatic primary hyperparathyroidism: summary statement from the Fourth International Workshop. J Clin Endocrinol Metab 99:3561–3569.

Wilhelm SM, Wang TS, Ruan DT et al. (2016) The American Association of Endocrine Surgeons Guidelines for definitive management of primary hyperparathyroidism. JAMA Surg 151:959–968.

German AWMF S1 guideline, registry no. 174–006. primary hyperparathyroidism. ►https://www.awmf.org/uploads/tx_szleitlinien/174-006l_S1_primaerer-Hyperparathyreoidismus_2016-05.pdf

6.6 Anatomy and Physiology of the Adrenal Gland

F. Billmann

6.6.1 Embryology

- Each adrenal gland = 2 different glands in one capsule
  - Adrenal cortex (cortex)
  - Adrenal medulla

Aberrant adrenal tissue is possible along the migratory route of the urogenital crest.

Extraadrenal chromaffin cells: Persistence of part of these cells = Zuckerkandl organ (usually left of aortic bifurcation) + possibly paraganglion.

6.6.2 Anatomy

Topographic Anatomy

- Pairs gland (endocrine cells)

Location

- Retroperitoneal position
- Superomedially from the upper pole of the respective kidney
- Right adrenal gland:
  - Often contact with right crus of the diaphragm
  - Close to inferior vena cava
- Left adrenal gland:
  - Between kidney and aorta
  - Contact/relationship with pancreas tail + splenic artery

Adrenal glands = usually not directly visible in the retroperitoneum. Therefore dissection + mobilization of the adjacent organs necessary.

Blood Supply

- Arterial blood flow:
  - Branches of the inferior phrenic artery + renal artery + aorta
  - Right adrenal gland: superior + inferior adrenal arteries
  - Left adrenal gland: middle + inferior adrenal arteries

- Venous drainage:
  - Right adrenal vein: drainage into inferior vena cava (short vein)
  - Left adrenal vein: drainage into the left renal vein (variant: directly into the inferior vena cava)
- Lymphatic drainage:
  - Lymphatic plexus of the adrenal gland
  - Drainage: Paraaortic + renal lymph node groups

Innervation

6

- Cortex: No direct innervation
- Medulla: Through preganglionic sympathetic nerves
- No parasympathetic component

Histological Anatomy

Adrenal Cortex

- 3 zones:
  - Zona glomerulosa (outer zone)
  - Zona fasciculata (intermediate zone)
  - Zona reticulata (inner zone)

Adrenal Medulla

- 10% of the weight of the adrenal gland
- Cells: Content = catecholamines (fix chromium salts = chromaffin cells).

Positional Relationships

- Right adrenal gland:
- Posterior: right diaphragmatic crus, diaphragm
  - Anterior: right lobe of the liver
  - Medial: Inferior vena cava (medial and anterior)
  - Cranial: diaphragm (cranial and posterior)
  - Caudal: Right renal upper pole
- Left adrenal gland:
  - Posterior: Left diaphragm, kidney
  - Anterior: peritoneum from the bursa omentalis (further: stomach, spleen)
  - Medial: left inferior phrenic artery, left gastric artery
  - Lateral: Left kidney
  - Cranial: diaphragm (cranial and posterior)
  - Caudal: pancreatic tail and splenic artery

6.6.3 Physiology

- Adrenal glands: Synthesis + secretion of 2 groups of hormones:
  - Steroid hormones (adrenal cortex)
  - Catecholamines (adrenal medulla)

Steroid Hormones

Glucocorticoids

Effects of Glucocorticoids

Regulation (Fig. 6.8)

- On almost all organ systems of the human body
- Alteration of the metabolism of proteins, lipids, carbohydrates: increase of blood sugar

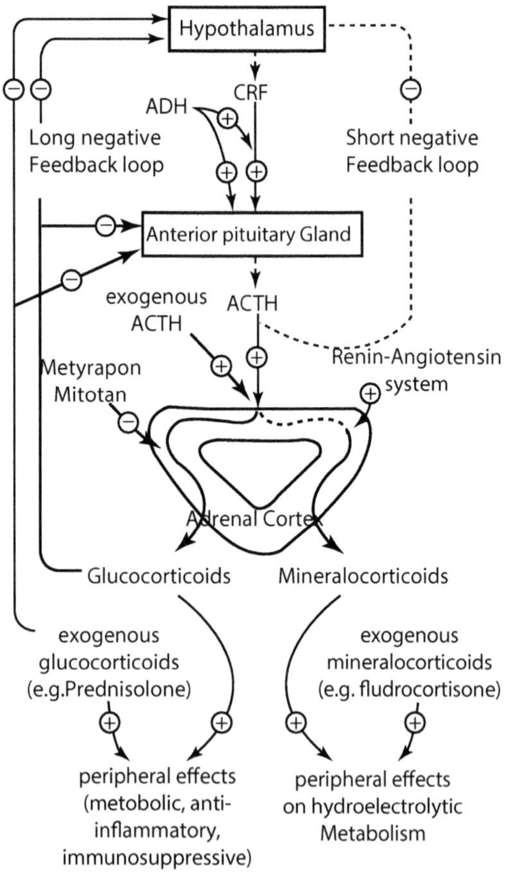

Fig. 6.8 Feedback regulation of glucocorticoid production and secretion in humans

- Preservation of intravascular volume, blood pressure
- Sensitization of β-adrenergic stimulation.
- Anti-inflammatory and immunosuppressive effect
- To summarize: Glucorticoids = response to stress
  - Short-term exposure = anabolism
  - Long-term exposure = catabolism

10–15% of cortisol in plasma unbound = active.

Mineralocorticoids

Effects of Mineralocorticoids

Regulation (Fig. 6.9)

- Regulation of water + electrolyte balance: expansion of intravascular volume

40% of aldosterone in plasma unbound = active.

Adrenal Sexual Steroids

Effects of Adrenal Sexual Steroids

- Regulation ACTH-dependent
- Other mechanisms (not yet fully understood)

Regulation

- In adults: Mild peripheral effects:
  - Development of secondary sexual characteristic features in men
  - female virilization
- During development:
  - development of the external male genitalia (vas deferens, epididymis, seminal vesicles, prostate)
- During puberty:
  - Development phallus, muscle mass, body hair

- Effects after peripheral transformation to testosterone
- Absence of androgens = development of female genitalia + vagina
- Adrenal gland = secondary source of secretion of sexual steroids (main source = gonads)

Catecholamines

Regulation

- Basal state: Low catecholamine secretion
- Autonomic sympathetic nervous system: stimulation = catecholamine secretion
- Activation of the autonomic sympathetic nervous system = response to stress
  - Physiological stress
  - Psychological stress

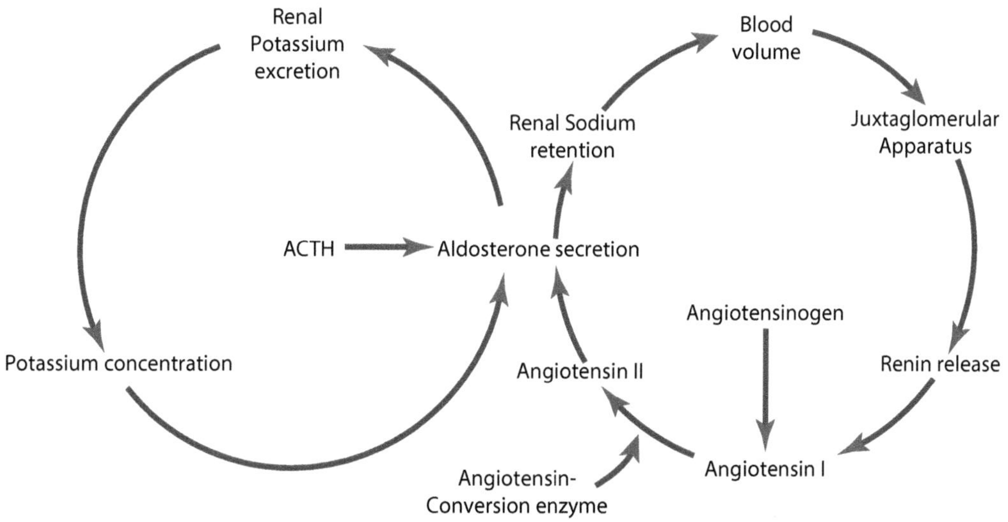

Fig. 6.9 Feedback regulation of mineralocorticoid production and secretion in humans

Effects of Catecholamines
- β-adrenergic effects:
  - Heart (β_1-receptors): Increase heart rate, increase contractility
  - Smooth muscle (uterus, bronchi, muscle vessels; β_2-receptors): Smooth muscle relaxation (= bronchodilation, increase muscle blood flow, etc.).
- α-adrenergic effects:
  - Vessels (skin, GI tract, etc.; α_1-receptors): Vasoconstriction
  - Presynaptic receptors (CNS; α_2-receptors): Reduction of sympathetic outflow

6

Action of the catecholamines
- Increase of blood supply and oxygen supply to brain, heart, muscle ("fight-and-flight response")
- Reduction of the supply to the other organs

6.7 Diseases of the Adrenal gland

F. Billmann

- In this chapter only adrenal diseases treated by surgery will be presented.

6.7.1 Primary Hyperaldosteronism (Conn Syndrome)

Definition

- Hypersecretion of aldosterone (► Sect. 6.6.3)
- Etiologies within or outside the adrenal gland

Etiopathogenesis

Etiologies
- Two main etiologies:
  - Unilateral aldosterone-producing adrenal adenoma (= Conn's adenoma) = 60%
  - Bilateral adrenal hyperplasia or idiopathic hyperaldosteronism = 40%
- Rare etiologies:
  - Unilateral primary adrenal hyperplasia
  - Adrenocortical carcinoma (aldosterone-producing)
  - Familial hyperaldosteronism
  - aldosterone-producing ovarian tumor

Pathogenesis (► Sect. 6.6.3)

Clinical Presentation

- Mostly mild/unspecific
- Most common symptoms:
  - Headache
  - Muscle weakness
  - Fatigue
  - Polydipsia, polyuria and nocturia
  - Arterial hypertension: Almost always, but mild (diastolic blood pressure usually <120 mmHg)

Diagnosis (See Algorithm ◘ Fig. 6.10)

Laboratory Adrenal Function Tests
- To confirm primary hyperaldosteronism

Caution
Discontinue all diuretics 2 weeks prior to blood sampling in cases of suspected hyperaldosteronism.

- aldosterone in plasma
- Plasma aldosterone/renin ratio

Aldosteronemia >20 ng/dL + plasma aldosterone/renin ratio > 30 (ng/dL:ng/mL/h); sensitive + specific in screening and diagnosis.
- Salt suppression test or 3-day sodium test: If aldosterone/renin not conclusive

Etiological Diagnosis
- To distinguish unilateral adenoma vs bilateral hyperplasia vs rare etiologies.
- Central to the decision-making process of therapeutic strategy:
  - Unilateral Conn's adenoma: surgery
  - Bilateral hyperplasia: non-surgical (medical) therapy

Diagnostic Imaging
- CT abdomen or MRI abdomen
- Visualization of a tumour/mass of the adrenal gland (suspicion of adenoma)

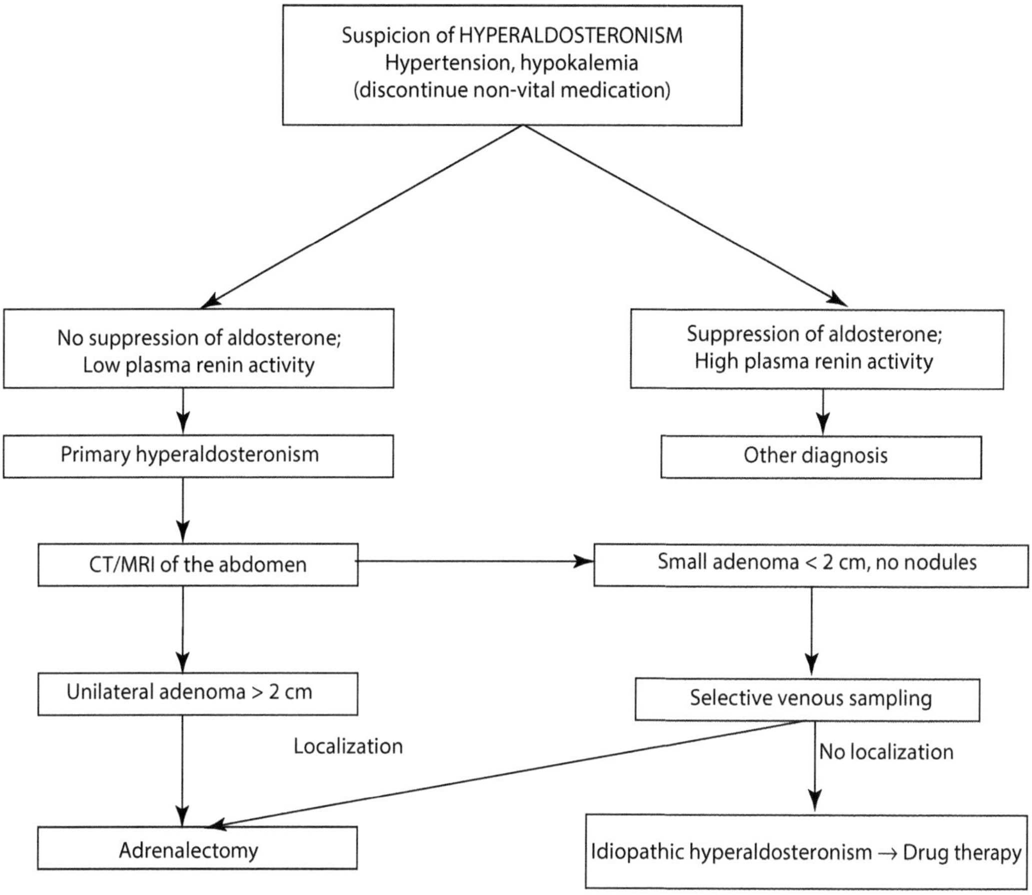

Fig. 6.10 Diagnostic algorithm in patients with suspected primary hyperaldosteronism

Caution
Adrenal tumour may also be nonfunctional (2–8%).

Selective Venous Sampling

- Invasive examination (only in centres with expertise)
- Localization (right/left) of aldosterone hypersecretion
- Indication:
  - None/Small adrenal tumor on imaging
  - Bilateral tumour of the adrenal gland
- Complications:
  - Adrenal Vein Thrombosis
  - Adrenal Infarction

Therapy

- Depending on etiology

Medical (Drug) Therapy

- In bilateral hyperplasia/idopatic hyperaldosteronism
  - Spironolactone (aldosterone antagonist) = therapy of arterial hypertension
  - Possible combination with other antihypertensive drugs

Surgical Therapy

- Indication = aldosterone-producing adenoma
- Preoperative Preparation:
  - Spironolactone: normalization hypertension
  - Potassium substitution: normalization of electrolyte/fluid balance
  - About 3–4 weeks
- Technique: (▶ Sect. 6.7.7) Minimal-invasive surgery

Aldosterone-producing adenomas = mostly small + benign: minimally invasive surgery = ideal modality.

- Low morbidity (fewer postoperative complications)
- Analogue success rate (vs. open)

Results

- Cure of hypokalemia: Almost all patients
- Cure of hypertension: 70% of patients (30% need further antihypertensives)

6.7.2 Cortisol-Producing Adrenal Adenoma

Definition

Cushing's Syndrome

- Hypercortisolism (overproduction of cortisol)
- Different etiologies (see below)

Exogenous steroid use = most common cause of Cushing's syndrome.

Cushing's Disease

- Hypercortisolism (overproduction of cortisol)
- Small pituitary adenoma: stimulation of the normal adrenal gland

ACTH Syndrome

- Ectopic ACTH secretion (outside the pituitary gland; 15% of Cushing's cases)
- Mostly malignant tumors (lung, pancreas, carcinoid tumor, thymoma)

Epidemiology and Etiology

- Exogenous steroid use (most common cause!)
- Endogenous causes:
  - Cushing's disease (pituitary adenoma, 70% of endogenous causes)
  - ACTH syndrome due to ectopic ACTH secretion (malignant tumors; 15% of endogenous causes)
  - Cortisol-producing adrenal disease (10–20% of endogenous causes).
    - Adrenal adenoma (50–60% of cases)
    - Bilateral adrenal hyperplasia (20–30% of cases)
    - Adrenocortical carcinoma (20–25% of cases)
  - Primary adrenal hyperplasia
  - Ectopic CRH (corticotropin releasing hormone) syndrome

Clinical Signs

- Weight gain = most common sign: Mostly on the trunk = centripetal obesity.
- muscular atrophy of the extremities
- Fat deposits on head ("moon face") + neck
- Dorsal kyphosis ("bull neck" = "buffalo hump")
- Abdominal striae (dark red, broad)
- Hypertonus
- Hyperglycemia

Subclinical Cushing's syndrome: Absent or poorly developed clinic, usually in patients with adrenocortical tumors.

Diagnosis

Laboratory Adrenal Function Tests

- To confirm Cushing's syndrome

Diurnal variation in cortisol secretion: cortisol high early morning, low evening: important for test interpretation.

Overnight Cortisol Suppression Test

- Most sensitive diagnostic test
- Principle: p.o. administration of 1 mg dexamethasone at 22 h or 23 h + cortisol determination in the blood the next morning at 8 h
- False negative = 3%; false positive = 30%.
- Interpretation:
  - Suppression (cortisol ≤5 μg/dL): Reliable exclusion of hypercortisolimsus
  - Absence of suppression: suspicion of hypercortisolism

Free Cortisol 24 h Urine Test

- In patients with suspected hypercortisolism in the suppression test
- Less sensitive, higher specificity
- Normal: Urinary cortisol <80 μg/day

48-h Low-Dose Dexamethasone Test

- For patients with ambiguous results
- Administration of 0.5 mg dexamethasone every 6 h for 2 days
- Determination of pre- and post-dexamethasone 24-h-cortisol in urine
- Interpretation:
  - No suppression: Autonomous cortisol secretion

Patients with adrenal incidentaloma: Always perform tests to exclude Cushing's syndrome.

Etiological Diagnosis

- To find the etiology

ACTH in Plasma

- ACTH secretion: diurnal variations parallel to cortisol (approx. 1–2 h earlier)
- Suppressed ACTH in patients with:
  - Adrenal Adenoma
  - Adrenocortical carcinoma
  - Cortisol-producing bilateral adrenal hyperplasia
- ACTH elevated/upper normal range: Cushing's disease
- ACTH markedly/very elevated: Ectopic ACTH secretion (tumor)

Therapy

- Depending on etiology

Surgical Therapy

Cushing's Disease

- Transsphenoidal pituitary adenoma resection (if resectable)
- Bilateral adrenalectomy:
  - In patients with no improvement after drug therapy + transsphenoidal pituitary adenoma resection.
  - In patients with end-organ insufficiency in relation to hypercortisolism.

Caution

In the case of bilateral adrenalectomy: perioperative steroid therapy (Table 6.25) + lifelong substitution.

Ectopic ACTH Secretion Syndrome

- Identification of the secreting tumor + treatment
- Bilateral adrenalectomy: Only if tumor irresectable or consequences of hypercortisolism not treatable with medication

Cushing's Syndrome in Adrenal Tumor (Adenoma or Carcinoma)

- Unilateral adrenalectomy (of the affected side)
- Adenoma: Almost all adenomas = resectable
- Adrenocortical carcinoma: resectable in only 25–35% of cases

Table 6.25 Recommendations for perioperative steroid therapy

Surgical stress	Example	Hydrocortisone Equivalency (mg).	Duration (days)
Small	Hernia surgery	25	1
Medium	Open cholecystectomy Revascularization of the lower extremity Segmental colon resection Total joint replacement Abdominal hysterectomy	50–75	1–2
Large	Pancreaticoduodenectomy Esophagogastrectomy Total proctocolectomy Cardiac surgery + cardiopulmonary bypass	100–150	2–3

Medical (Drug) Therapy

- Chemotherapy: Poor results
- In case of metastases/non-resectable tumor: drugs with direct effect on adrenal gland or on steroid synthesis (mitotane, aminoglutethimide, metyrapone, ketoconazole)

6.7.3 Pheochromocytoma

Definition

- Neuroectodermal tumor; from chromaffin cells of the adrenal medulla
- Treatable form of endocrine hypertension
- Secretion of catecholamines: symptoms
- High morbidity/mortality if not treated

6

Epidemiology

- Incidence = 0.005–0.1% of the general population
- Incidence = 0.1–0.2% of hypertensive adults
- Bilateral tumor = 10% of cases; possibility of multiple tumors
- Extraadrenal localization: 10% of cases (= paragangliomas)
- Non-functional pheochromocytomas = rare (mostly extraadrenal)
- Malignant pheochromocytoma: 10% of cases (metastases: bone, liver, lung, less frequently lymph nodes)
- 5-year survival rate:
- Benign phaeochromocytoma = 97%
- Malignant pheochromocytoma = 43%
- Familial pheochromocytoma: 10% of cases (currently more like 25%):
- MEN 2A or 2B (▶ Sect. 6.3): Often bilateral pheochromocytoma
- Neurofibromatosis type I or MEN 1 (▶ Sect. 6.3): Pheochromocytoma risk <1%
- Hereditary paraganglioma syndrome (mutations in SDHD, SDHB and SDHC genes)

In familial pheochromocytoma: Mandatory follow-up + regular screening.

Clinical Signs

- Variable clinical presentation: Over time and from one patient to another (up to dramatic situations)

Arterial Hypertension

- Constant hypertension + paroxysmal peaks (variable frequency and severity)
- Paroxysmal symptoms due to e.g. physical stress, food containing tyramine (chocolate, cheese, red wine)

Other Symptoms

- Excessive sweating
- Tachycardia
- Trembling
- Inner restlessness
- Thoracic pain
- Impaired glucose tolerance: with diabetes mellitus signs (polydypsia, polyuria)

Impaired glucose tolerance = consequence of catecholamine secretion.

Diagnosis

Laboratory Function Tests

- Confirmation of excessive catecholamine secretion
- In the blood:
  - Free metanephrines in plasma: more sensitive than punctual metanephrines in urine
- In the urine:
  - Free catecholamines + metabolites in 24-h urine: to confirm elevation in plasma
    - Free catecholamines: Dopamine, epinephrine, norepinephrine…
    - Metabolites: normetanephrines, metanephrines, vanillinmandelic acid
- Elevated levels in more than 90% of patients with pheochromocytoma

Phenylethanolamine-N-transferase = enzyme only in adrenal gland: conversion of norepinephrine to epinephrine; as consequence: extraadrenal pheochromocytoma = no epinephrine production.

Etiological Diagnosis = Localisation Diagnosis

- Goal = localization of the pheochromocytoma
- Only if laboratory diagnosis is confirmed (see above)

CT Scan

- Imaging of first choice for suspected pheochromocytoma
- Detects 95% of tumors >6–8 mm

MRI

- In selected cases
- T2 weighting: visualization of chromaffin cells (T2 adrenal/liver ratio > 3 in pheochromocytoma)

MIBG Scintigraphy

- Localization of extraadrenal pheochromocytomas + metastases + bilateral pheochromocytomas
- Method of choice in case of:
  - positive Laboratory function tests and negative CT + MRI examinations
  - Follow-up of patients with recurrent/metastatic disease

In (suspected) malignant pheochromocytoma: staging by standard imaging + MIBG scintigraphy.

Therapy

Preoperative Preparation

Background

- Preoperative preparation = central to prophylaxis of intraoperative cardiovascular crisis
- Intraoperative cardiovascular crisis: due to the release of catecholamines.

Principle

- α-adrenergic blockade
- β-adrenergic blockade for the prophylaxis of arrhythmias/tachycardia

Caution

β-adrenergic blockade: inhibition of α-blocker-induced vasodilation; β-blocker alone: increase in hypertension + left ventricular congestion.

- Restoration of a normal electrolyte-fluid balance

Dosages for Pheochromocytoma

- Phenoxybenzamine (non-selective α-blocker): 10 mg 3 times/day
- Prazosin (selective α_1 blocker): 0.5–1 mg titrated to 3–20 mg/day
- Metyrosine (tyrosine hydroxylase inhibitor): 250 mg 3 times/day titrated to a maximum of 1.5–4 g/day
- Propranolol (non-selective β-blocker): 10–40 mg 3 times/day.

Surgical Therapy

Strategy

- Laparoscopic/retroperitoneoscopic adrenalectomy:
  - In the case of unilateral small, benign appearing tumour with normal opposite side
  - Patients with MEN 2 or von Hippel-Lindau syndrome with small unilateral findings (<6 cm)
  - Bilateral minimally invasive adrenalectomy: For MEN 2 or von Hippel-Lindau syndrome with small bilateral findings

Adrenal cortex-sparing adrenalectomy (subtotal) = method of choice for bilateral benign disease (e.g. MEN 2 or von Hippel-Lindau syndrome): prophylaxis of adrenal insufficiency.

- Open adrenalectomy:
- For findings >6 cm (high risk of malignancy = approx. 25%)
- In case of primary suspicion of malignancy
- Malignant pheochromocytoma + limited metastasis: resection possible in well-selected patients

Principles of Surgical Therapy (▶ Sect. 6.7.7)

- Avoid intraoperative manipulation of the tumor
- Early ligation of the adrenal vein (interruption of the venous outflow of the tumor)

Postoperative Monitoring/Follow-Up

- 24-h monitoring: blood pressure (compensatory hypotension due to vasodilation), arrhythmias
- Annual: Plasmatic free metanephrines or urinary catecholamines

Chemotherapy

- Therapy regime
  - High dose streptozocin
  - Alternative: Cyclophosphamide + Vincristine + Darcarbazine
- Response rate = 50%

Radiotherapy

- For bone metastases

Palliative Therapy

- α-Methyltyrosine
- α-blockade + β-blockade

6.7.4 Adrenocortical Carcinoma

Definition

- Rare malignant endocrine tumor
- Surgical resection = only curative therapy

Epidemiology and Prognosis

Epidemiology

- Incidence = 0.5–2/1 million inhabitants per year in USA
- Bimodal age distribution:
  - Peak in young children <5 years
  - Peak in adults at 40–50 years

Prognosis

- Bad because of late diagnosis
- Most important prognostic factor = complete resection
  - With complete resection: 5-year survival = 40%, median = 43 months
  - In case of incomplete resection: Median survival = 12 months

Clinical Signs

Unclear Abdominal Complaints

- Secondary
- Due to progressive retroperitoneal mass.

Symptoms of Overproduction of Adrenocortical Hormones

- Majority of these tumors = functional
- Cushing's syndrome: due to cortisol secretion (50% of tumors)
- Virilization/Feminization/Hypertension: due to androgen/estrogen or aldosterone secretion (10–20% of tumors)

Diagnosis

Biochemical Screening

- Cortisol, aldosterone, androgens, estrogens
- Biochemistry = indicator for perioperative substitution therapy
- Exclusion of a pheochromocytoma: catecholamines + metabolites in plasma + urine

Imaging

- High-resolution CT/MRI:
  - MRI especially for the evaluation of a vena cava inferior infiltration
  - With thorax: For detection of pulmonary metastases
- PET-CT: For detection of metastases + recurrence

Therapy

- 50% of tumors = localized at the time of diagnosis

Surgical Therapy

Strategy

- Complete resection = only curative option for local adrenocortical carcinoma
- Open resection:
  - Adequate exposure
  - Reduction of malignant cell spillage
  - Better control of the vessels (inferior vena cava, aorta, renal vessels)
  - Radical en bloc resection (possibly multivisceral resection, if necessary)

- Laparoscopic resection technically possible, **but** high recurrence rate. **Caution:** tumor fracture + peritoneal contamination.
- Recurrence/Metastases: Complete resection of recurrence + metastases
- Prolonged survival
- Reduction of hormone-associated symptoms

Postoperative Follow-Up

- Regular control of hormone levels
- Abdominal CT examinations (thorax + abdomen)

Chemotherapy

- For unresectable cancer(s)/metastases
- No chemotherapy active in terms of improving survival
- Reduction of symptoms due to anti-hormonal effect
- Mitotan:
  - steroid inhibitor
  - Inducer of atrophy of adrenocortical cells
  - Side effects: Gastrointestinal + neuromuscular

Mitotan

- Need for close monitoring of hormone levels!
- Adjuvant mitotane therapy: currently being evaluated (in the context of studies)
- Neoadjuvant mitotane therapy: currently being evaluated (in the context of studies)
- Combinations of etoposide + doxorubicin + cisplatin + mitotane (EDP-M): Currently being evaluated (in the context of studies), possible advantages in recurrence-free survival/overall survival.
- Other active agents:
  - Suramin, Ketoconazole
  - Cisplatin, doxorubicin, vincristine

Radiotherapy

- Palliative therapy for bone metastases

6.7.5 Adrenal Incidentaloma

Definition

- Asymptomatic adrenal lesion as an incidental finding during imaging for another reason
- Increasing frequency with use of abdominal CT

Epidemiology

- Frequency = 4% of routine abdomen imaging
- Frequency = 9% in autopsy series
- Most lesions = benign; hormone active vs. hormone inactive.

Clinical Evidence

Functional Incidentalomas

- All incidentalomas >1 cm: need for Hormonal workup
- All hormone-active lesions: Resection
- In case of radiological suspicion of malignancy: resection
- In case of size progression during follow-up: resection

Non-functional Incidentalomas

- Malignancy risk dependent on:
  - Size of the mass: Best clinical indicator
    - <4 cm: risk of malignancy = 2%
    - 4.1–6 cm: risk of malignancy = 6%
    - >6 cm: risk of malignancy = 35%

- Nonfunctional incidentalomas <3 cm: surveillance; nonfunctional incidentalomas 3–5 cm: controversial.
- Radiological malignancy criteria/etiology (◘ Table 6.26)

Evaluation Algorithm

- In patients with adrenal incidentaloma (◘ Fig. 6.11)
- In patients with adrenal incidentaloma and extraadrenal carcinoma (◘ Fig. 6.12)

Therapy

- Therapy = surgical therapy vs. monitoring

Indications for Surgical Therapy

- Hormone-active incidentalomas
- Incidentalomas with radiological signs of malignancy (regardless of size)
- Incidentalomas >6 cm

Incidentalomas 3–6 cm: Individual decision for surgery based on age + general condition.

Table 6.26 Characteristic features of adrenal incidentalomas in imaging ("imaging phenotype")

	Adrenocortical adenoma	Adrenocortical carcinoma	Pheochromocytoma	Metastases
Size	Small, mostly ≤3 cm	Large, mostly >4 cm	Large, mostly >3 cm	Variable, often <3 cm
Form	Round or oval with smooth margin	Irregular with unclear margin	Round or oval with clear margin	oval, irregular with unclear margin
Texture	Homogeneous	Heterogeneous, with different densities	Heterogeneous, with cystic areas	Heterogeneous, with different densities
Laterality	Mostly solitary, one-sided	Mostly solitary, one-sided	Mostly solitary, one-sided	Often bilateral
Density (CT without CM)	≤10 HU	>10 HU (mostly >25)	>10 HU (mostly >25)	>10 HU (mostly >25)
Vessels in CM-CT	Not highly vascular	Mostly vascular	Mostly vascular	Mostly vascular
Washout	≥50% after 10 min	<50% after 10 min	<50% after 10 min	<50% after 10 min
MRI image	Isointens in T2 weighting	Hyperintensity in T2 weighting	Significantly hyperintensive in T2 weighting	Hyperintensity in T2 weighting
Necrosis, hemorrhage, calcification	Rarely	Frequently	Bleeding + cystic areas frequent	Regular bleeding + cystic areas
Size increase	Mostly stable in progression or very slow (<1 cm/year)	Mostly fast (>2 cm/year)	Mostly slow (0.5–1.0 cm/year)	Different, slow–fast

HU Hounsfield units, *CM* contrast medium

Strategy

- Laparoscopic adrenalectomy for:
  - Incidentalomas without malignancy criteria on imaging
  - Incidentalomas <4 cm
- Open adrenalectomy: All other incidentalomas with indication for surgery

Background = Risk of capsular rupture and cell spillage during laparoscopic adrenalectomy: Not adapted in the presence of malignancy.

6.7.6 Adrenal Metastases

Epidemiology

- Adrenal metastases = frequent
- In autopsies, adrenal metastases present in:
  - 42% of lung cancers
  - 16% of gastric cancers
  - 58% of breast cancers
  - 50% of malignant melanomas
  - High percentage of prostate and kidney cancers

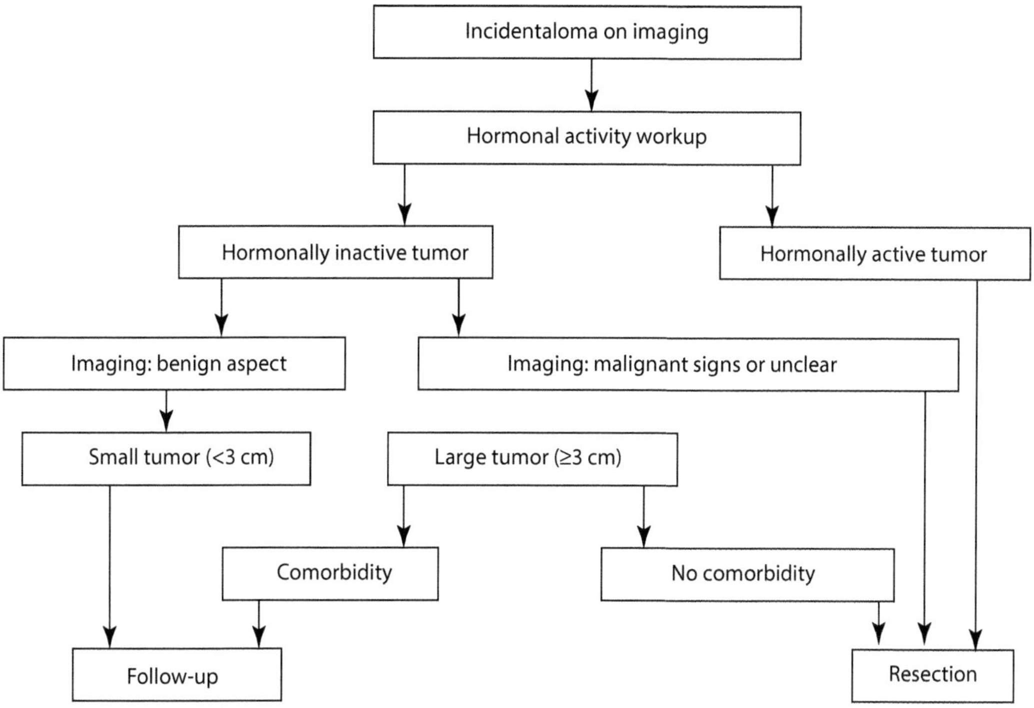

Fig. 6.11 Algorithm for the evaluation of a patient with an isolated adrenal incidentaloma

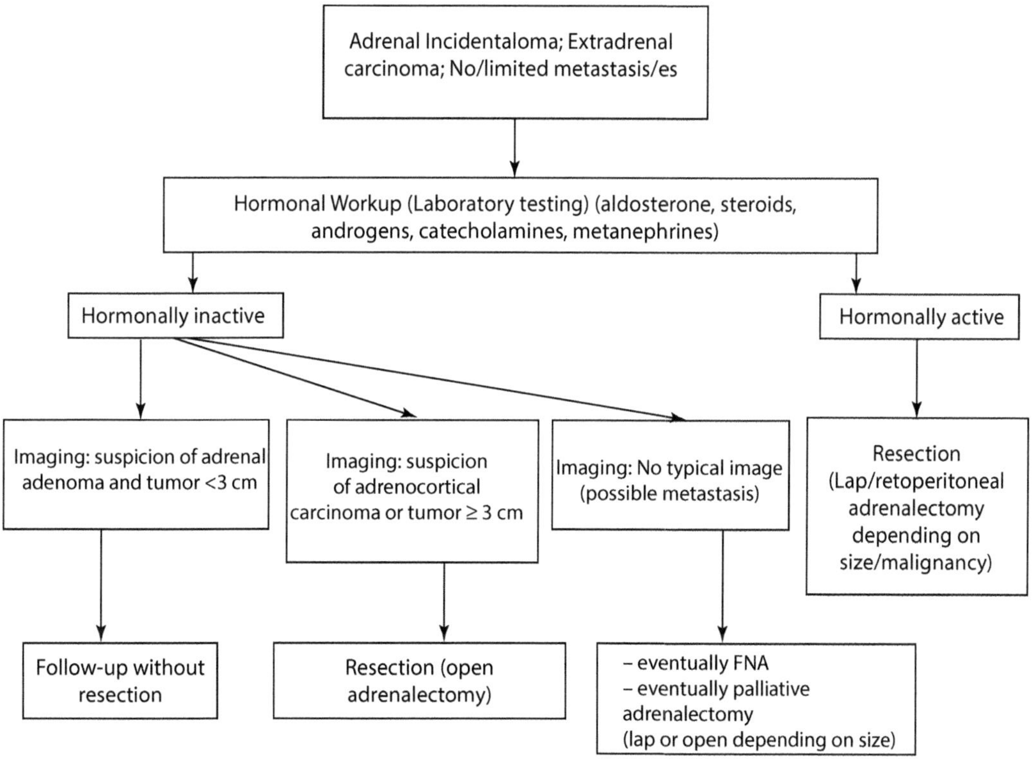

Fig. 6.12 Algorithm for the evaluation and therapy of a patient with an adrenal incidentaloma in the context of an extraadrenal carcinoma

Clinical Signs

- Mostly asymptomatic
- If symptomatic:
  - Unclear complaints
  - Adrenal insufficiency: Very rare

Adrenal insufficiency: At least 90% of the adrenal cortex affected (massive enlargement of the adrenal gland on CT).

Diagnosis

- Workup of patients with adrenal tumour in the context of extraadrenal malignant disease (◘ Fig. 6.12)

6

Therapy

Surgical Therapy

- Resection of adrenal metastasis: in selected patients
- Selection Criteria:
  - Prolonged disease-free interval
  - Adequate tumor biology: good response to systemic therapy, history of isolated metachronous metastasis, long disease-free interval
  - Primary tumour localisation: better results for metastases from lung, colon, kidney cancers and melanomas (worse for oesphagus, liver tumours or sarcomas)

6.7.7 Principles of Adrenal Surgery

General (◘ Fig. 6.13)

Decisive Factors for the Choice of a Procedure

- Size and localization of the tumor
- Malignant potential of the lesion
- Unilateral vs. bilateral lesion
- Presence of extraadrenal manifestations
- Surgical procedure in the anamnesis
- Habitus of the patient
- Surgeon's experience

General Rule

- Open access for large tumors and, if necessary, for tumors with malignant potential

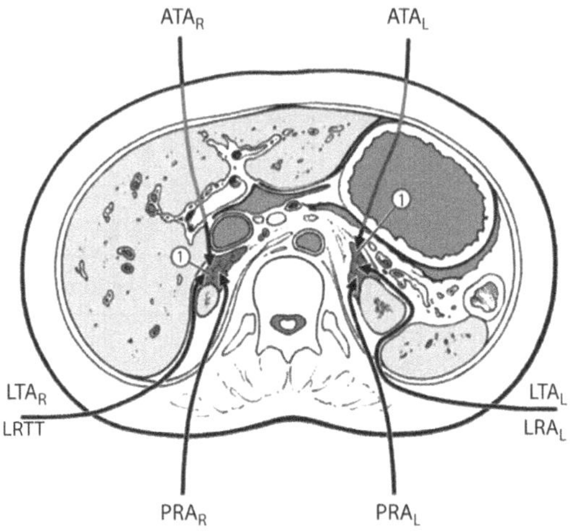

◘ **Fig. 6.13** Access routes in adrenal surgery. (After Walz 2012)

Open Adrenalectomy

Indications

- Known or suspected primary adrenocortical carcinoma
- Large tumors
- Tumor Recurrence
- Extension to adjacent organs

Technique

- 4 possible accesses:
  - Anterior: Preferred for adrenocortical carcinoma
  - Lateral: Ideal for obese patients
  - Posterior: Rarely used; for small tumors
  - Thoracoabdominal: Ideal for tumors requiring en bloc resection of adjacent organs + lymphadenectomy

Surgical Procedure

Open Anterior Left Adrenalectomy

- Mostly longitudinal laparotomy
- Mobilization of the left colonic flexure + descending colon
- Entering retroperitoneum through incision along the lower edge of the pancreas
- Medial visceral rotation of the spleen + pancreas tail (dissection on Gerota's fascia)

- Visualization of renal hilus and following renal vein to confluence with left adrenal vein
- Left adrenal gland = left to the aorta, above the left renal vein
- Early ligation of the adrenal vein
- Supply of thin-caliber collaterals of the aorta, inferior diaphragmatic vessels and renal vessels
- adrenalectomy
- No drainage

Surgical Procedure
Open Anterior Right Adrenalectomy
- Mostly longitudinal laparotomy
- Mobilization of the right ligamentum triangulare of the liver and anteromedial rotation of the liver = access to the right adrenal gland
- Kocher maneuver: mobilization of the duodenum if necessary; thereby better access to the right kidney + inferior vena cava
- Right adrenal vein: Mostly direct drainage into inferior vena cava; ligation of the adrenalvein
- Control of the arterial inflow of the adrenal gland
- adrenalectomy
- No drainage

Surgical Procedure
Open Posterior Adrenalectomy
- Patient in prone position; table bent 35°
- Oblique incision over the 12th rib; retraction of the sacrospinalis muscle medially
- Resection of the 12th rib; reflection on pleura cranially
- Left: Cranial resection border = diaphragm; Right: Cranial resection border = liver
- Adrenalectomy is performed like anterior technique

Surgical Procedure
Thoracoabdominal Approach
- Allows the best exposure: ideal for tumors requiring en bloc resection of adjacent organs + lymphadenectomy
- Incision over tenth rib on the right and 11th rib on the left, with rib resection
- If infiltration V. cava or hepatic veins: Need for additional sternotomy

Surgical Procedure
Lateral Access
- Patient in lateral decubitus: using gravity for organ retraction
- Extraperitoneal approach to the adrenal gland
- sparing of extensive adhesiolysis in patients with postop. Adhesions
- Vascular control usually more difficult

Laparoscopic Adrenalectomy

- Standard access for small benign adrenal tumors

Advantages (Compared to Open Access)

- Less pain and less postoperative restrictions
- Shorter hospital stay
- Faster recovery
- Better cosmetic result

Good Candidates for Laparoscopic Adrenalectomy

- Patients with Conn adenoma
- Small functional adrenal tumors (<4 cm)
- Unilateral sporadic benign tumors
- MEN 2 or von Hippel-Lindau syndrome, patients with unilateral pheochromocytoma
- Selected patients with adrenal metastasis

Laparoscopic Adrenalectomy
- Tissue-sparing subtotal adrenalectomy: Possible using laparoscopy
- In case of suspected malignancy: No laparoscopy
- In case of unclear incidentaloma: open approach recommended (potential malignancy)

Surgical Procedure
Laparoscopic Left Adrenalectomy
- Patient in right lateral decubitus
- Operating table adequately padded; abdomen and thorax washed down from areola to below the spina iliaca, and from right of umbilicus to spine
- Infracostal trocar 10–15 cm anterior to the anterior axillary line (open technique)
- 3 × 10 mm trocars under direct vision: anterior axillary line, posterior axillary line and one 5-cm posterior to posterior axillary line port, medial to left kidney
- Dissection (e.g., ligasure, ultracision): Mobilization left colonic flexure, using gravity; inferior and medial dissection
- Mobilization of the spleen by incision of the peritoneum lateral to the spleen
- Rotation of the spleen medially with pancreatic tail
- Dissection of the left adrenal gland from retroperitoneal fat
- Transection of the adrenal vein after mobilization of the gland and shortly before complete resection (difference to the open technique): Vascular stapler, energy sealing device (e.g.Ligasur) or clip (currently some authors advise against clips: slippage of clips)
- Extraction of the adrenal gland in sterile plastic bag via umbilical caltrocar

Surgical Procedure
Laparoscopic Right Adrenalectomy
- Patient in left lateral decubitus
- Trocar positions analogous to left
- Medial port for liver retraction
- Dissection of the adrenal gland caudally along the renal vein and medially along the inferior vena cava
- Right adrenal vein usually short and thick-lumened
- Transection of the adrenal vein obligatory, by means of vessel stapler, energy sealing (Ligasur), or vessel clips (currently some authors advise against clips: slipping of the clips)
- Remaining dissection analogous to left

Retroperitoneoscopic Adrenalectomy

Indications
- Small benign adrenal tumors
- Isolated adrenal metastases

Caution
Positioning in knee-elbow position.

Advantages
- Minimally invasive method
- Reduction of hemodynamic or respiratory instability (vs. capnoperitoneum)
- No need for adhesiolysis or transperitoneal access
- Possibility of hemostasis by increasing the pressure (insufflator pressure up to 20–25 mmHg)
- Possibility of bilateral adrenalectomy without repositioning the patient

Contraindications
- Suspicion of adrenocortical carcinoma/ malignant pheochromocytoma
- Adjacent Organ Infiltration
- Lesion >6 cm
- Morbid obesity
- Limited distance between costal arch and iliac crest

Surgical Procedure

Retroperitoneoscopic Adrenalectomy

- Patient in knee-elbow position
- Palpation of the 12th rib, 1.5-cm incision just below the tip of the 12th rib.
- Opening of the retroperitoneum with scissors and widening of the access with the finger
- Palpation with index finger and insertion of the 10 mm and 5 mm trocar (possibly also possible under visual control): Medial trocar 5 cm medial to the 12-mm trocar, lateral to the paraspinal muscles; the lateral trocar 5 cm lateral to the 12-mm trocar under the tip of 11th rib.
- Insertion of a 12 mm trocar with balloon and CO_2 insufflation with pressure 20–24 mmHg
- 30° 10 mm videoscope into the 12 mm trocar and start of blunt dissection: retroperitoneal space
- Opening of the Gerota fascia + visualization of the renal upper pole. Visualization of landmarks: paraspinal muscles, diaphragm, liver, peritoneum parietale, inferior vena cava
- videoscope into paravertebral trocar
- Dissection along the renal upper pole
- Identification of inferior vena cava on right side
- Exposure of adrenal vein and supply by means of sealing (e.g. Ligasur)
- Complete mobilization of the adrenal gland and salvage using a plastic salvage bag via 12-mm access
- haemostasis after reduction of pressure
- Removal of the trocar and closure of the accesses

6.7.8 Guidelines

AWMF S2k guideline, registry no. 088–008—Surgical therapy of adrenal tumors. ► https://www.awmf.org/uploads/tx_szleitlinien/088-008_S2k_operative-Therapie_Nebennierentumoren_2019-07.pdf

Fassnacht M, Arlt W, Bancos I et al.(2016) Management of adrenal incidentalomas: European Society of Endocrinology clinical practice guideline in collaboration with the European Network for the Study of Adrenal Tumors. Europ J Endocrinol 175:G1–G34.

Funder JW, Carey RM, Mantero F (2016) The management of primary aldosteronism: case detection, diagnosis, and treatment: an Endocrine Society clinical practice guideline. J Clin Endocrinol Metab 101:1889–1916.

Gaujoux S, Mihai R, Joint working group of ESES and ENSAT (2017) European Society of Endocrine Surgeons (ESES) and European Network for the Study of Adrenal Tumors (ENSAT) recommendations for the surgical management of adrenocortical carcinoma. Br J Surg 104:358–376.

Lenders JWM, Duh QY, Eisenhofer G et al. (2014) Pheochromocytoma and paraganglioma: an Endocrine Society clinical practice guideline. J Clin Endocrinol Metab 99:1915–1942.

Nieman LK, Biller BM, Findling JW et al. (2015) Treatment of Cushing's syndrome: an Endocrine Society clinical practice guideline. J Clin Endocrinol Metab 100:2807–2831.

Zeiger MA, Thompson GB, Duh QY et al. (2009) The American Association of Clinical Endocrinologists and American Association of Endocrine Surgeons medical guidelines for the management of adrenal incidentalomas. Endocr Pract 15:S1–S20.

References

Dralle H, Damm I, Scheumann GF, Kotzerke J, Kupsch E, Geerlings H, Pichlmayr R (1994) Compartment-oriented microdissection of regional lymph nodes in medullary thyroid carcinoma. Surg Today 24: 112–121

Plummer HS, Boothby WM (1923) The cost of work in exophtalmic goiter. Am J Phys 63:406

Qubain SW, Nakano S, Baba M, Takao S, Aikou T (2002) Distribution of lymph node micrometastasis in pN0 well-differentiated thyroid carcinoma. Surgery 131:249–256

Robbins KT, Shaha AR, Medina JE, Califano JA, Wolf GT, Ferlito A, Som PM, Day TA (2008) Consensus statement on the classification and terminologie of neck dissection. Arch Otolaryngol Head Neck Surg 134:536–538

Walz MK (2012) Minimal-invasive Nebennierenchirurgie. Transperitonealer oder retroperitonealer Zugang? Chirurg 83:536–545

Wang TS, Udelsman R (2007) Remedial surgery for primary hyperparathyroidism. Adv Surg 41:1–15

Wittekind C, Greene FL, Henson DE et al (2003) TNM supplement, 3. Aufl. Wiley-Liss, New York, pp 25–33

Further Reading

Abraham DT, Low T, Messina M et al (2011) Medullary thyroid carcinoma: long-term outcomes of surgical treatment. Ann Surg Oncol 18:219–225

Brindel P, Doyon F, Bourgain C et al (2010) Family history of thyroid cancer and the risk of differentiated thyroid cancer in French Polynesia. Thyroid 20: 393–400

Chen H, Wang TS, Yen TW, Doffek K, Krzywda E, Schaefer S, Sippel RS, Wilson SD (2010) Operative failure after parathyreoidectomy for hyperparathyroidism: the influence of surgical volume. Ann Surg 252:691–695

Crippa S, Saletti P, Barizzi J et al (2012) The clinical management in familial adenomatous polyposis deserves continuous monitoring for thyroid carcinoma. BMJ Case Reports 2:1–3

Elisei R, Schlumberger MJ, Muller SP et al (2013) Cabozantinib in progressive medullary thyroid cancer. J Clin Oncol 31:3639–3646

Feig BW, Ching CD (2012) The MD Anderson surgical oncology handbook, 5. Aufl. Lippincott Williams & Wilkins, Philadelphia/Baltimore

Frazer WD (2009) Hyperparathyroidism. Lancet 374:145–158

Kunstman JW, Kirsch JD, Mahajan A, Udelsman R (2013) Parathyroid localisation and implications for clinical management. J Clin Endocrinol Metab 98:902–912

Lappas D, Noussios G, Anagnostis P, Adamidou F, Chatzigeorgiou A, Skandalakis P (2012) Location, number and morphology of parathyroid glands: results from a large anatomical series. Anat Sci Int 87:160–164

Liaw D, Marsh DJ, Li J et al (1997) Germline mutations of the PTEN gene in Cowden disease, an inherited breast and thyroid cancer syndrome. Nat Genet 16:64–67

Lie S, Wang D, Ge J et al (2015) Single-center study of familial papillary thyroid cancer in China: surgical considerations. W J Surg Onc 13:115–121

Leonhardt H, Tillmann B, Töndury G, Zilles K (2003) In: Rauber A, Kopsch F (Hrsg) Lehrbuch und Atlas der Anatomie des Menschen. Band 2: Innere Organe, 3. Aufl. Thieme, Stuttgart

Lorenz K, Dralle H (2003) Chirurgie des Hyperparathyreoidismus. Chirurg 74:593–615

Lorenz K, Dralle H (2010) Intraoperative Parathormonbestimmung beim primären Hyperparathyreoidismus. Chirurg 81:636–642

Marcocci C, Cetani F (2011) Primary hyperparathyroidism. New Engl J Med 365:2389–2397

Marx SJ (2000) Hyperparathyroid and hypoparathyroid disorders. New England J Med 343(25):1863–1875

Miccoli P, Berti P, Conte M, Bendinelli C, Marcocci C (1999) Minimally invasive surgery for small thyroid nodules: preliminary report. J Endocrinol Investig 22:849–851

Moreno MA, Callender GG, Woodburn K, Edeiken-Monroe BS, Grubbs EG, Evans DB, Lee JE, Perrier ND (2011) Common locations of parathyroid adenoms. Ann Surg Oncol 18:1047–1051

Navas-Carrillo D, Rios A, Rodriguez JM et al (2014) Familial nonmedullary thyroid cancer: screening, clinical, molecular and genetic findings. Biochim Biophys Acta 1846:468–476

Oertli D, Udelsman R (2007) Surgery of the thyroid and parathyroid glands. Springer, Berlin/Heidelberg/New York

Ohgami M, Ishii S, Arisawa Y, Ohmori T, Noga K, Furukawa T, Kitajima M (2000) Scarless endoscopic thyroidectomy: breast approach for better cosmesis. Surg Laparosc Endosc Percutan Tech 10: 1–4

Pacini F, Castagna MG, Cipri C, Schlumberger M (2010) Medullary thyroid carcinoma. Clin Oncol 22:475–485

Pan L, Peng L, Jean-Gilles J et al (2010) Novel PRKAR1A gene mutations in Carney complex. Int J Clin Exp Pathol 3:545–554

Paschke R (2009) Abklärung des euthyreoten Schilddrüsenknotens: Wann punktieren? Stellenwert der Sonographie. Dtsch Med Wochenschr 134: 2498–2503

Rawat N, Khetan D, Williams W, Baxter JN (2005) Parathyroid carcinoma. Brit J Surg 92:1345–1353

Sackett WR, Barraclough BH, Sidhu S, Reeve TS, Delbridge LW (2002) Minimal access thyroid surgery: is it feasible, I it appropriate? ANZ J Surg 72:777–778

Schardey HM, Schopf S, Kammal M, Barone M, Rudert W, Hernandez-Richter T, Pörtl S (2008) Invisible scar endoscopic thyreoidectomy by the dorsal approach: experimental: experimental development of a new technique with human cadavers and preliminary clinical results. Surg Endosc 22: 813–820

Schmid KW (2010) Molekularpathologie von Schilddrüsentumoren. Pathologe 31:229–233

Sebag F, Palazzo FF, Harding J, Sierra M, Ippolito G, Henry JF (2006) Endoscopic lateral approach thyroid lobectomy: safe evolution from endoscopic parathyroidectomy. World J Surg 30: 802–805

Shimazu K, Shiba E, Tamaki Y, Takiguchi S, Taniguchi E, Ohashi S, Noguchi S (2003) Endoscopic thyroid surgery through the axillo-bilateral-breast approach. Surg Laparosc Endosc Percutan Tech 13:196–201

Standring S (2009) Gray's anatomy. The anatomical basis of clinical practice, 40. Aufl. Churchill Livingstone, Elsevier, London

Thomusch O, Dralle H (2000) Endokrine Chirurgie und evidenzbasierte Medizin. Chirurg 71:635–645

Sansal I, Sellers WR (2004) The biology and clinical relevance of the PTEN tumor suppressor pathway. J Clin Oncol 14:2954–2963
Steinhagen E, Guillem J, Chang G et al (2012) The prevalence of thyroid cancer and benign thyroid disease in patients with familial adenomatous polyposis may be higher than previously recognized. Clin Colorectal Cancer 11:304–308
Sung TY, Lee YM, Yoon JH et al (2015) Surgical management of familial papillary thyroid microcarcinoma: a single institution study of 94 cases. World J Surg 39:1930–1935
Vargas-Barron J, Vargas-Alarcon G, Roldan FJ et al (2008) Cardiac myxomas and the Carney complex. Rev Esp Cardiol 61:1205–1209
von Lanz T, Wachsmuth W (1955) Die Schilddrüse. In: von Lanz T, Wachsmuth W (eds) Praktische Anatomie, Band 1, Teil 2 Hals. Springer, Berlin/Göttingen/Heidelberg
von Lanz T, Wachsmuth W (2004) Praktische Anatomie. Hals, Springer, Berlin/Heidelberg
Walz MK (1998) Minimal-invasive Nebennierenchirurgie. Chirurg 69:613–620
Weber A, Randolph G, Aksoy F (2000) The thyroid and parathyroid glands. CT and MR imaging and correlation ith pathology and clinical findings. Radiol Clin N Am 38:1105–1129
Wheeler MH (1998) Total thyroidectomy for benign thyroid disease. Lancet 351:1526–1527
Witzel K, von Rahden BH, Kaminski C, Stein HJ (2008) Transoral access for endoscopic thyroid resection. Surg Endosc 22:1871–1875
Young WF (2007) The incidentally discovered adrenal mass. New Engl J Med 356:601–610
Zilles K, Tillmann B (2010) Anatomie. Springer, Berlin/Heidelberg

Bariatric and Metabolic Surgery

Michel Gagner and Franck Billmann

Contents

F. Billmann, T. Keck (eds.), *Essentials of Visceral Surgery*,
https://doi.org/10.1007/978-3-662-66735-4_7

7.1 Epidemiology

7.1.1 Incidence

- Obesity = epidemic worldwide
- Obesity definition:
  - Overweight (preadiposity): BMI (Body Mass Index) = 25–29.9
  - Obesity grade 1: BMI = 30–34.9
  - Obesity grade 2: BMI = 35–39.9 ("severe obesity")
  - Obesity grade 3: BMI ≥ 40 ("morbid obesity")
  - "Superobesity": BMI ≥ 50
- Obesity in USA:
  - Prevalence increase 15.3% of population (1995), 23.9% (2005), 27.2% (2010), 39.8% (2016)
  - 4.8% with BMI > 35, 3.7% with BMI > 40
  - Prevalence development (■ Figs. 7.1 and 7.2)
- Obesity worldwide (WHO data 2016):
  - Delayed increase
  - approx. 13% of the population obese; 39% overweight

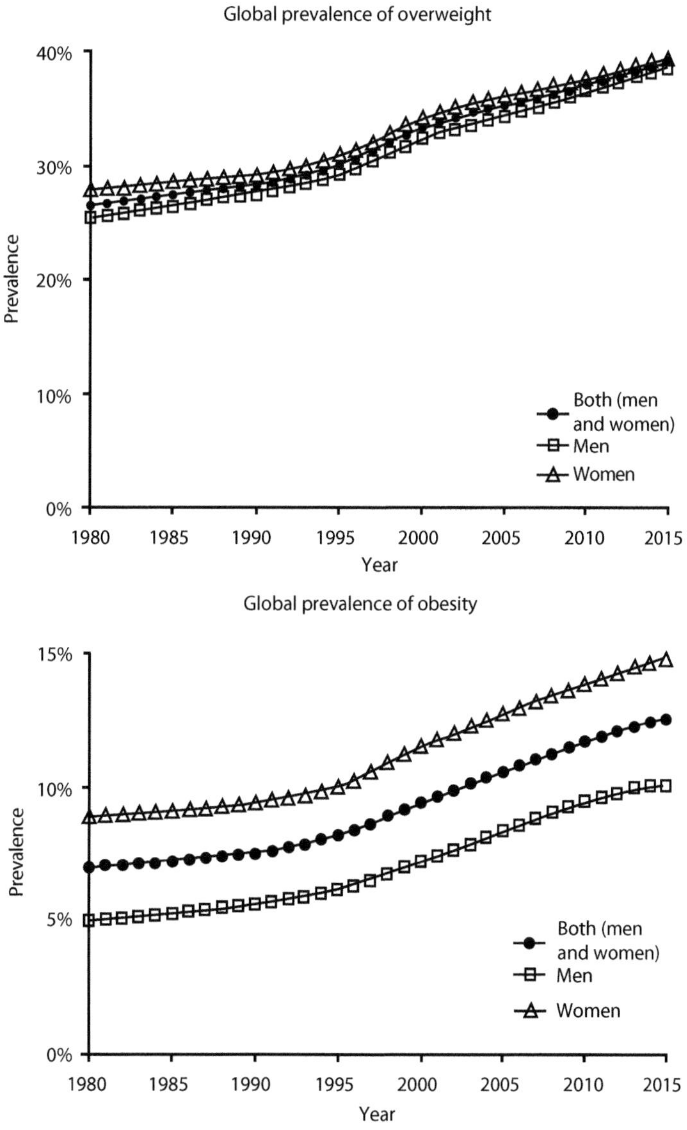

■ **Fig. 7.1** Age-standardized overall prevalence of overweight (upper curve) and obesity (lower curve) in men and women (age > 20 years) (during 1980–2015). (From Chooi et al. 2019; courtesy of Chooi et al.)

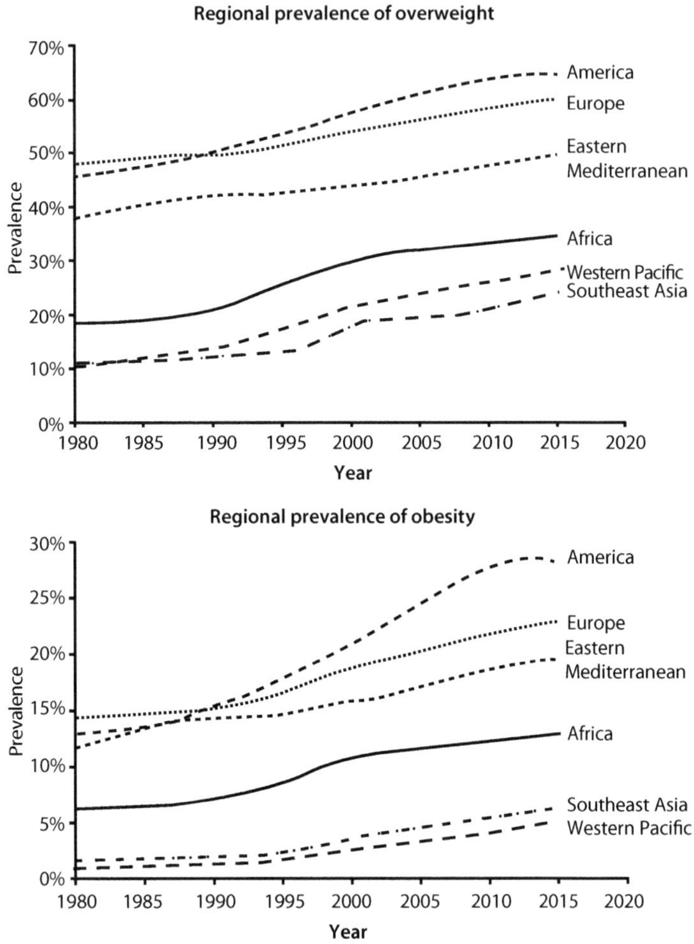

Fig. 7.2 Age-standardized regional prevalence of overweight (upper curve) and obesity (lower curve) in men and women (age > 20 years) (over the period 1980–2015). (From Chooi et al. 2019; courtesy of Chooi et al.)

7

7.1.2 Health Economic Consequences

- Obesity-associated morbidity (especially abdominal obesity): Increased risk of
  - Arterial hypertension
  - Type-2 diabetes mellitus
  - Hyperlipidemia
  - Sleep Apnea Syndrome
  - Coronary heart disease, steatosis hepatis and myocardial infarction
- Costs associated with obesity:
  - Compared to normal weight: 30% higher costs in obese patients, 81% higher costs in morbidly obese patients
  - 147 billion $ annually in the USA (2008)
  - 420,000 deaths in 2016 in U.S.

7.2 Pathophysiology and Principle of Action of Bariatric Surgery

Key Points

- Pathophysiology of obesity = complex + not completely understood
- Operating principle of bariatric surgery:
  - Gastric Restriction
  - Intestinal malabsorption
  - Learned behavioral changes
  - Neural and endocrine signal change (postoperative)

7.2.1 Pathophysiology

- Complex and not completely understood
- Contributing factors:
  - Genetic factors (approx. 67% of BMI variability)
  - Behavioural factors (decrease in physical activity, increase in intake of high calorie food)
  - Psychological factors
  - Other, e.g. economic, socio-educational factors

7.2.2 Working Principle of Bariatric Surgery

- Bariatric surgery = altering the anatomy of the GI tract: reducing caloric intake
- Simplified: 3 operating methods/principles:
  - Restrictive methods
  - Hormonal (hypoabsorptive) methods
  - Combined methods (restrictive + hormonal)
- In reality: active principle of bariatric surgery = complex and interaction of:
  - Gastric Restriction
  - Intestinal hypoabsorption
  - Learned behavioural changes (e.g. after excessive food intake following gastric restriction: nausea and vomiting lead to adaptation of eating habits)
  - Neural and endocrine signal change (postoperative)
    - For example, gastric bypass: suppression of grhelin secretion leads to a reduction in appetite
  - Other hormones with implications after bariatric surgery: cholecystokinin, peptide YY, GLP (*glucagon-like peptide*)-1

Restrictive Methods

- Principle of action of the gastric pouch: By reaching the feeling of satiety early + delayed gastric emptying to limit food intake (volume limitation)
- Basic principle of the operation: Formation of a small gastric reservoir with reduced outflow
- surgical procedures (◘ Fig. 7.3):
  - Gastroplasty (e.g. sleeve gastrectomy)
  - Gastric Balloon Insertion
  - Laparoscopic gastric plication (new method under study)
  - Endoscopic Sleeve Gastroplasty
- Historical method: adjustable gastric banding ("vertical banded gastroplasty")

Hypoabsorptive Methods

- Active principle: Limitation of nutrient uptake
- Basic principle of the operation: forming a bypass of different portions of the small intestine
- surgical procedures (◘ Fig. 7.3): Currently no purely hypoabsorptive method
- Historical methods: Purely hypoabsorptive methods
- For example, jejunoileal bypass.

Combined Methods

- Principle of action: Limitation of food intake (volume limitation) + Limitation of nutrient intake
- Basic principle of the operation: formation of a small gastric reservoir with reduced outflow + formation of a bypass of different portions of the small intestine
- Surgical procedures (◘ Fig. 7.3):
  - Proximal Roux-Y-Gastric Bypass
  - "Banded Gastric Bypass"
  - Biliopancreatic diversion with/without duodenal switch
  - Mini gastric bypass (new method under study)
  - "single anastomosis duodeno-ileal bypass with sleeve gastrectomy" (SADI-S); (new method under study)

7

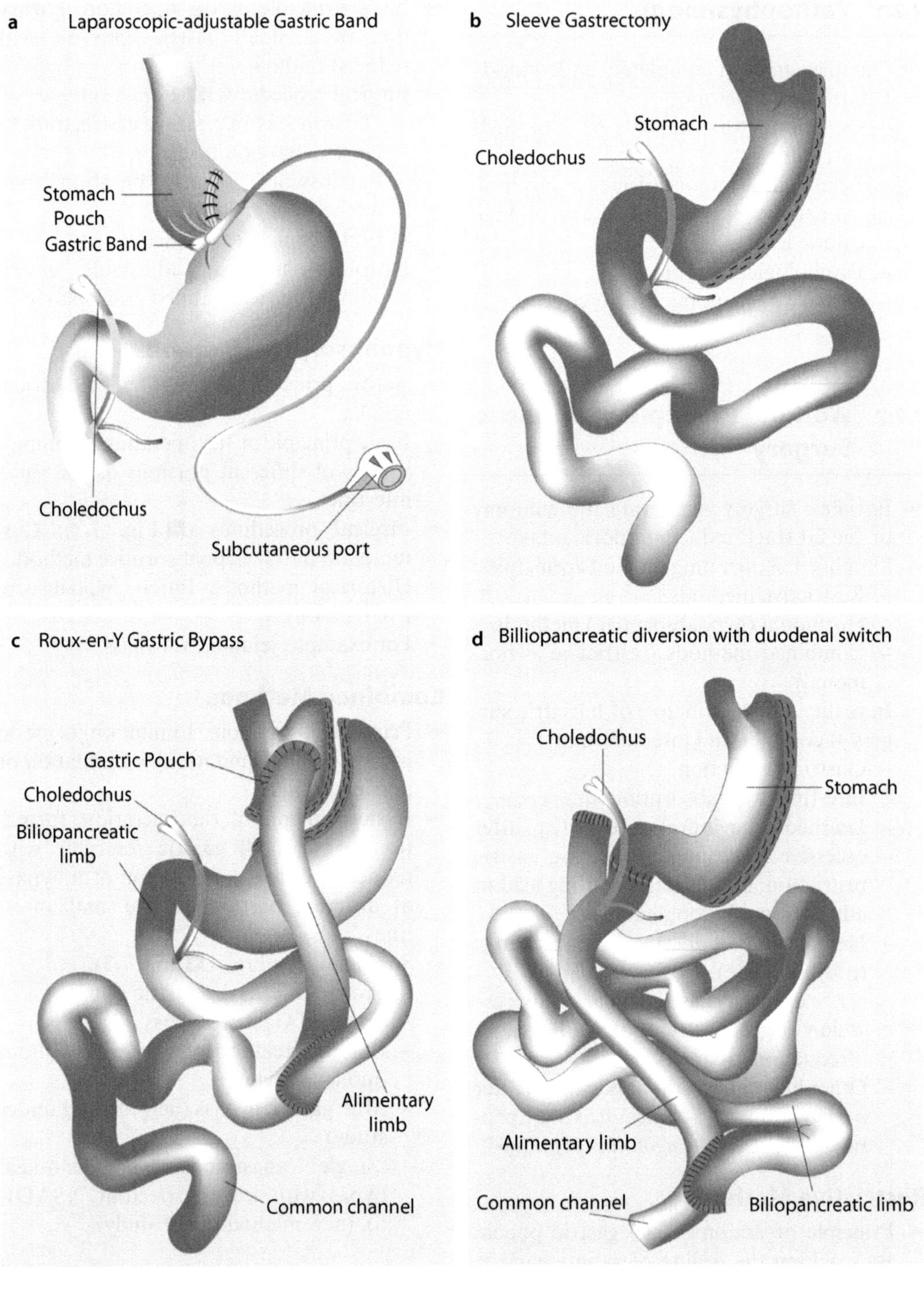

Fig. 7.3 a–d Currently most frequent specific bariatric interventions

7.3 Clinical Evidence

7.3.1 Bariatric Surgery: Laparoscopic Versus Open

- Reduced postoperative pain
- Reduction of morbidity:
  - In particular, fewer pulmonary complications
  - Fewer incisional hernias
  - Fewer wound complications (infections, wound healing disorders)
- Reduction of hospital stay
- Faster recovery time

7.3.2 Bariatric Surgery: Prospective Controlled Studies

- No large randomized trial comparing bariatric surgery vs. medical therapy
- Only 2 small randomized trials +3 cohort studies (all at high risk for bias) + meta-analyses:
  - Bariatric surgery: weight loss on average = 20–50 kg
  - Non-surgical therapy: Minimal weight loss
- A large prospective controlled case-control study (Swedish SOS study; Sjöström 2013):
  - Significantly better weight loss in surgery vs. non-surgery group after 2 years, and after 10 years
  - Combined procedures better than purely restrictive procedures
  - Median BMI decrease at 2 years after bariatric surgery: 50.0 (combined) to 32.6 (restrictive)
  - Significantly lower morbidity after surgery (HR = 0.56; P = 0.01)
  - Significantly fewer cardiovascular events after surgery (HR = 0.83; P = 0.05)

7.3.3 Metabolic Consequences of Bariatric Surgery

- Randomized controlled trial and meta-analysis results
- Diabetes mellitus:
  - Diabetes remission: 0% after no surgery vs. 22.4% after surgical therapy (after 5 years)
  - Diabetes-associated medication use: no treatment after 5 years: 0% after no surgical vs. 45% after surgical therapy
  - Effects independent of BMI at baseline
- Hyperlipidemia: treatment of 83% of patients
  - NAFLD/NASH: improvement steatosis index/fibrosis index (tubular stomach better than gastric bypass) (Billmann et al. 2021)
- Arterial hypertension: treatment of 66% of patients
- Sleep apnea: treatment of 88% of patients
- Improvement of end organ damage (especially those linked to Type-2 diabetes; e.g. diabetic kidney disease)

7.3.4 Mortality: Bariatric Surgery Versus Drug Therapies

- Matched case control studies only
- Last-published large study (Aminian et al. 2019): significantly lower all-cause mortality in the surgery Group (10.0%) vs. no surgery Group (17.8%)
- SOS study: Significant reduction in all-cause mortality of 31.6% in surgery group vs. non-surgery group

7.4 Specific Current Bariatric Interventions

7.4.1 Roux-Y Gastric Bypass "Gastric Bypass"

- Combined method
- Procedure basis: division of the stomach – small gastric pouch (20–30 mL); Roux-Y gastrojejunostomy + jejunojejunostomy with formation of a:
  - Biliopancreatic limb: Jejunal limb from Treitz ligament to jejunojejunostomy (confluence of biliary, pancreatic secre-

tions and alimentary flow); length = 30–100 cm
- Alimentary limb: Roux limb from gastrojejunostomy to jejunojejunostomy; the limb passes food; length = 75–150 cm
- Common channel: rest of the small intestine after jejunojejunostomy to ileocecal valve

Surgical Procedure
Roux Y Gastric Bypass
- Incision of the omentum minus 6 cm distal to the gastroesophageal junction
- Dissection dorsolaterally along the posterior wall of the stomach and finding the omental bursa
- Transsection of the stomach using the Endo-GIA device and formation of the stomach pouch (volume target of the pouch = 20 mL)
- Performing a CEEA ("circular end-to-end anastomosis") pressure plate 25 mm by means of a gastric tube through the gastric pouch; alternative = gastrojejunostomy by means of an Endo-GIA device, or completely hand-sewn
- Division of the omentum majus
- Measurement of the small intestine from Treitz ligament
- Antecolic end-to-side gastrojejunostomy by means of CEEA (device transabdominal through lumen of distal jejunum)
- Test for leakage
- Measurement of the Roux thigh and side-to-side jejunojejunostomy
- Standard lengths: Roux length = 75–100 cm; distance between Treitz ligament and jejunojejunostomy = 30–100 cm.
- Extended lengths: Roux and Treitz jejunostomy lengths 150 cm and 100 cm respectively
- Closure of mesenteric defects
- Leak-testing (not mandatory) and closure of the accesses

7

7.4.2 Banded Gastric Bypass

- Restrictive method
- Procedure basis: In addition to gastric bypass, a gastric band to prevent regain of weight.
- Complications: Complications of vertical banded gastroplasty (s. ► Sect. 7.6.1)

7.4.3 Laparoscopic Adjustable Gastric Banding (LAGB)

- Restrictive method
- Procedure basis: Placement of an adjustable band (connected to a subcutaneous port) approximately 1–2 cm aborally of the gastroesophageal junction and formation of a 30 mL gastric pouch

Surgical Procedure
Laparoscopic Adjustable Gastric Banding
- Placement of the tape 1 cm below the esophagogastric junction
- Formation of a tunnel for placing the ligament through the pars flaccida in the area of the small gastric curvature above the bursa omentalis
- Using an intragastric calibration probe
- Tape is left blank at the beginning
- Anterior extensive fixation of the ligament, especially at the large curvature (fundus)
- Gastrogastric sutures for fixation of the ligament below the virtual pouch, directly below the esophagogastric junction
- Port chamber placed on the rectus abdominis or epigastric muscle
- Adaptation of the band volume possible in the consultation (depending on weight loss and symptoms)

7.4.4 Biliopancreatic Diversion (BPD)

- Combined method

- Basic principle of the operation: Distal subtotal gastrectomy (50–80%) with reconstruction like gastric bypass; difference: enteroenterostomy clearly more distal with formation of a common channel of approx. 50–100 cm length

Surgical Procedure

Biliopancreatic Diversion (BPD)

- Devascularization of the large gastric curvature (mostly preservation of the gastricae-breves vessels) + first part of the duodenum
- Transection of the duodenum with stapler, after isolation and transection of the right gastric veins
- transection of the omentum minus along the small curvature up to approx. 2 cm below the left gastric veins
- Horizontal gastrectomy (residual stomach = approx. 300 mL; approx. 5 cm from cardia along the small curvature), by means of endo-GIA stapler
- Cholecystectomy
- Measure the common limb, mark 50 cm from the ileocecal valve.
- Cutting of the small intestine approx. 250 cm orally of the ileocecal valve (formation of the alimentary limb)
- Anastomosis between biliopancreatic and alimentary limb by means of side-to-side anastomosis at the level of the 50 cm marker
- Formation of a window in the mesocolon transversum and passage of the gastric stump to the submesocolic region
- Enterotomy of the distal intestinal stump and posterior gastric wall and gastroenterostomy using endo-GIA stapler
- Closure of the common defect by means of hand suture (closure of the mesenteric defects with non-absorbable suture)
- Exclusion of leakage/bleeding
- Irrigation, possibly drainage (not absolutely necessary), closure of the accesses

7.4.5 Biliopancreatic Diversion with Duodenal Switch (BPD/ DS)

- Combined method
- Basic principle of surgery: like BPD with sleeve gastrectomy and preservation of the pylorus, ileoduodenostomy behind the pylorus; alimentary limb approx. 150 cm and biliopancreatic limb (different lengths)

Surgical Procedure

Biliopancreatic Diversion with Duodenal Switch

- Devascularization of the large gastric curvature + first part of the duodenum
- Transection of the duodenum with stapler
- Vertical gastrectomy (70% of the stomach), starting 6 cm proximal to the pylorus parallel to the small curvature, using a 60 Fr.(French)-nasogastric tube (placeholder)
- Exclusion of leakage of the stapler line (after duodenoileal anastomosis)
- Measure the common limb, mark 100 cm from the ileocecal valve
- Cutting of the small intestine approx. 250 cm orally of the ileocecal valve (formation of the alimentary limb)
- Antecolic anastomosis between biliopancreatic and alimentary limb by means of side-to-side anastomosis at the level of the 100 cm marker
- Duodenoileal anastomosis end-to-side
- Closure of the common defect by means of hand suture (closure of the mesenteric defects with non-absorbable suture)
- Irrigation, possibly drainage (not absolutely necessary), closure of the accesses

7.4.6 Gastric Sleeve Resection

- Restrictive and hormonal method (especially in patients with high perioperative risk)

- Basic principle of the operation: By means of splinting (32 to 40 Fr probe) of the small curvature resection of the large gastric curvature:
  - As definitive bariatric surgery
  - In preparation for the BPD/DS
- Currently the most performed bariatric surgery worldwide

Surgical Procedure

Gastric Sleeve Resection "Sleeve Gastrectomy"

- Retraction of the liver (especially left lobe) and visualization of the pylorus and the large curvature of the stomach
- Dissection of the greater omentum to open the lesser sac
- Dissection of the large curvature (starting 2–3 cm proximal to the pylorus) and division of the short gastric vessels up to the gastroesophageal junction
- Splinting of the small curvature of the stomach by means of a thick gastric tube (approx. 36 Fr.) and vertical sleeve gastrectomy (by means of an endo-GIA stapler) starting 4 cm orally of the pylorus up to the gastroesophageal junction.
- Extraction of the resected part of the stomach
- Exclusion of leakage or bleeding along the stapler line
- Leak testing and closure of the accesses

Results Weight Loss

- 80% of gastric bypass patients achieve a weight loss of 60–80% of the excessive weight in the first year; in the longer term stabilization at 50–60% of the excessive weight
- Average weight loss: 30.19 kg for adjustable gastric band; up to 51.93 kg for BPD; after 10 years, stabilization of weight loss at 20–30 kg.
- 10–40% of patients do not achieve long-term weight loss

7

7.5 Complications

7.5.1 Mortality

- Between 0.1 and 2.0% in large studies
- No significant difference compared to non-op. General population (long-term study)
- In Meta-analyses:
  - After gastric bypass: 0.5%
  - After gastric banding: 0.1
  - After hypoabsorptive surgery: 1.1%

Causes of Mortality

- Pulmonary Embolism
- Anastomotic leakage and sepsis
- Myocardial Infarction
- Malignant/non-malignant neoplasms
- Ileus/gangrene due to hernias

Risk Factors

- Experience of the surgeon/department
- Advanced patient age
- Male gender
- Super obesity (BMI > 50)
- Comorbidities

7.5.2 Gastrointestinal Complications

- Relatively often

Nausea and Vomiting

- In more than 50% of patients with restrictive method
- Mostly because of dietary errors (too much, too fast)
- Anastomotic stenosis = other cause

Dumping Syndrome

- Neurohormonal syndrome
- Triggered by the ingestion of sugar
- Clinical presentation:
  - Flush phenomenon of the face and upper half of the torso
  - Drowsiness/dizziness

  - Tachycardia
  - Fatigue
  - Diarrhea
- Incidence = 70% of patients after Roux-Y gastric bypass

Deficiency Symptoms

- After hypoabsorptive methods (e.g. gastric bypass): Iron, calcium, folic acid, vitamin B_{12}, possibly other nutrients
- After BPD: proteins, fat-soluble vitamins (A, D, E and K)
- Therefore, the need for regular laboratory control + substitution

Other Gastrointestinal Complications

- Dehydration
- Intestinal obstruction, ileus
- Anastomosis leaks and fistulas
- Strictures/stenoses
- Incisional hernias or internal hernias
- Cholecystolithiasis and choledocholithiasis

7.5.3 Other Complications

- Venous thromboembolism
- Wound infections
- Bleeding
- Splenectomy after injury (rare)
- Incisional hernias or internal hernias
- Early postoperative ileus
- Gallstones

Complications in the SOS Study (Sjöström 2013)

- Postoperative complications = 13% of patients, of which
  - Bleeding = 0.5
  - Embolism/thrombosis = 0.8%
  - Wound complications = 1.8
  - Pulmonary complications = 6.1

7.6 Historical Interventions and Interventions in the Context of Studies

7.6.1 Historical Interventions

Jaw Wiring

- Historical intervention, no current application

Adjustable Gastric Banding (Vertical Banded Gastroplasty)

- Restrictive method
- Basic principle of the operation: Vertical partitioning of the stomach with attachment of a gastric band ("mesh") to control the diameter of the gastric outlet.
- Complications:
  - No long-term weight control
  - Intolerance of gastric constriction: vomiting, gastroesophageal reflux
  - Inflammatory reaction to the Band/Tube/Mesh: gastric stenosis
  - Free perforation due to erosion of the band

Jejunoileal Bypass (Intestinal Bypass)

- Hypoabsorptive method
- Procedure basis: Purely intestinal bypass; transection of the proximal jejunum, which is anastomosed distally to the ileum = bypass of up to 90% of the small intestine
- Complications:
  - perioperative complications, hypoproteinemia
  - Electrolyte dysregulation (loss via stool)
  - hepatic insufficiency, nephrolithiasis, autoimmune complications
  - bacterial overgrowth (SIBO)
  - Due to high complication rate = abandoned technique

Stomach Partitioning

- Restrictive method
- Basic principle of the operation: exclusion of a part of the stomach by double-row stapling to reduce the passage (no transection)
- Failure of this technique due to reopening of the stapler row or dilatation of the oral part of the stomach

7.6.2 Interventions in the Context of Studies

Laparoscopic Gastric Plication "Gastric Plication"

- Restrictive method
- Basic principle of the operation: reduction of the size of the stomach by inversion of the large curvature of the stomach internally
- Pros:
- Preservation of full stomach structure and function
- Comparable restriction as with sleeve gastric resection (see below)
- Disadvantages:
  - No long-term results currently known
  - Risk of gastric adaptation (due to distension) with renewed weight gain
- Complications:
  - Gastric perforation (<1%)
  - Excessive gastric constriction (<1%)
  - Slippage
  - Portal or mesenteric thrombosis

Endoscopic Sleeve Gastroplasty "Gastric Plication"

- Restrictive method
- same as laparoscopic gastric plication, but using endoscopy
- lesser results and complications

Mini Gastric Bypass

- Combined method
- Basic principle of surgery: narrow long gastric pouch (close to the gastroesophageal junction); anastomosis of the small intestine (150–200 cm distal from the Treitz ligament; without transection of the small intestine) with the pouch
- Pros:
  - Good weight loss (due to more hypoabsorption)
  - Effective procedure for the therapy of diabetes mellitus type 2
  - Shorter surgery time and anesthesia
- Disadvantages:
  - Dumping Syndrome
  - Hypoglycemia
  - Intestinal obstruction and internal hernia, "afferent-loop syndrome"…
  - Lifelong nutrient substitution (vitamins and minerals)
  - Increased rate of biliary reflux (bile gastritis, bile esophagitis)
  - marginal + gastric ulcers
- Complications:
  - Postoperative ileus (2–4%) due to intestinal obstruction
  - Anastomotic insufficiency (<1%)
  - Bleeding (<1%)
  - Need for conversion to Roux-Y-gastric bypass (5–10% of cases).

Ileal Transposition with/Without Sleeve Gastrectomy

- New method
- Procedural Basis:
  - Transposition of a 100 cm distal segment of the ileum (completely innervated and perfused) to the proximal jejunum
  - Objective = early stimulation of the ileum by nutritional components

Laparoscopic "Jejunal Sleeve" (On Gastric Bypass/Sleeve)

- Combined method
- As a revision procedure after gastric bypass for weight gain or as a primary procedure (in the context of studies)
- Procedural Basis:
  - 40 Fr bougie for stomach/jejunum calibration
  - Lateral resection of the gastric pouch (gastric sleeve)
  - Resection of the blind end of the jejunum

  - Sleeve resection of the jejunum over 15–25 cm
- Pros:
  - Simple rescue method after gastric bypass
  - BMI reduction of 5–10 extra points
- Disadvantages:
  - Currently still within the scope of studies
  - Medium- and long-term results missing
- Complications:
  - Stapler line/anastomosis insufficiency
  - Stenoses

Laparoscopic Single Anastomosis Duodenal Switch (SADI-S)

- Combined method
- Basic principle of the operation: formation of a tubular stomach; transection of the duodenum approx. 3 cm distal from the pylorus; duodenoileostomy approx. 2.5 m from the IC(ileocecal) valve (without transection of the ileum) leads to the absorption of proteins and fats only in the last 2.5 m of the ileum
- Pros:
  - Only one anastomosis (compared to the conventional duodenal switch), lesser operative time
  - Good results in terms of weight loss
  - Effective for reducing cholesterol and triglycerides
  - Effective in the treatment of diabetes mellitus type 2
  - Lesser risk of internal hernias
- Disadvantages:
  - Less weight loss than classic duodenal switch (not studied in detail)
  - No long-term results currently known
  - Possible bile gastritis
- Complications:
  - Intestinal obstruction (2–4%)
  - Anastomotic insufficiency (<1%)
  - Bleeding (<1%)
  - Need for reversion due to excessive hypoabsorption (2–5%) or insufficient weight loss

Myoelectric Gastric Stimulation

- Neurophysiological method
- Principle of action: Influencing the parasympathetic stimulation of the stomach and the intrinsic myoelectric activity of the stomach by means of a pacemaker
- Basic principle of the operation: Stomach stimulation by means of a pacemaker and electrodes in the gastric curvature
- Within the framework of studies

7.7 Metabolic Surgery

- Rapidly increasing importance of metabolic surgery

7.7.1 Definition

- Metabolic surgery (◘ Fig. 7.4 and ◘ Table 7.1) = not clearly defined
- In most cases, concept to denote currently experimental procedures
- Proper definition: shift of the primary focus of surgery to treat weight toward surgery to control metabolic disease (especially diabetes mellitus in those patients **without** severe obesity)

7.7.2 Scientific Basis

- Bariatric surgery = reduction in relative risk (%) for comorbidities in obese patients:
  - Cancer risk (76%)
  - Cardiovascular risk (82%)
  - Endocrinological disease risk (65%; after 10 years: 82.9% treatment of diabetes after bariatric surgery)
  - Infectious disease risk (77%)
  - Musculoskeletal disease risk (59%)
  - Respiratory disease risk (76%)
  - Psychiatric disease risk (47%)
- Bariatric surgery = reduction in direct treatment costs (over 5 years: $8813 in operated patients vs. $11,854 in non-operated patients; SEER registry, USA)

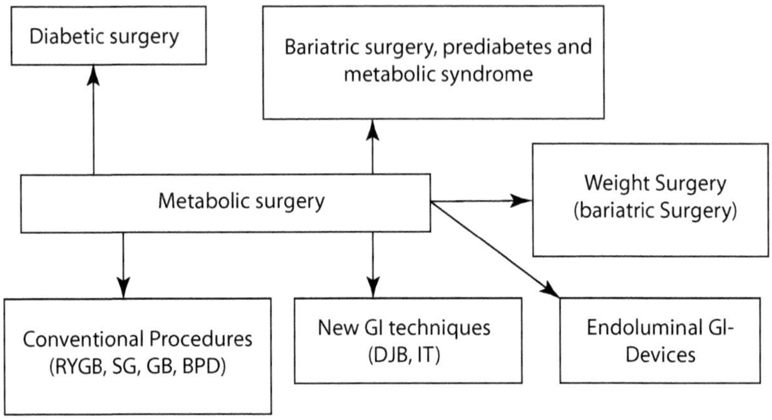

Fig. 7.4 Definition of metabolic surgery based on the goal of surgical therapy. *RYGB* Roux-Y gastric bypass, *SG* sleeve gastrectomy, *GB* gastric banding, *BPD* biliopancreatic diversion, *DJB* duodenojejunal bypass, *IT* ileal transposition. (Mod. according to Rubino et al. 2014)

7

Table 7.1 Bariatric vs. metabolic surgery. (Rubino et al. 2014)

Comparison parameters	Bariatric surgery	Metabolic surgery
Diseases	Severe obesity	"Metabolic" obesity, diabetes mellitus type 2, metabolic syndrome
Primary objective	Weight reduction	Blood glucose and metabolic control, reduction of cardiometabolic risk
Criteria for the surgical indication	Weight-oriented (BMI)	Abdominal circumference, BMI, disease-specific parameters (Hb_{A1c}, C-peptide, insulin and glucose levels), response to alternative therapies, associated conditions that increase CVD risk and can be ameliorated by surgery (hypertension, dyslipidemia, sleep apnea syndrome, etc.)
Procedures	RYGB, sleeve gastrectomy, gastric banding, BPD, BPD/DS	RYGB, sleeve gastrectomy, gastric banding, BPD, BPD/DS, procedures within trials (duodenojejunal bypass, ileal interposition), device-based interventions[a]
Measurement of the treatment success	Overweight reduction >50	Glycemic control, dyslipidemia control, weight loss, CVD risk reduction
Composition of the treatment team	Surgeon, nutritionist, psychologist	Surgeon, endocrinologist, cardiologist, obesity specialist, diabetes consultant, etc.
Possible mechanisms of action	Simple, primarily mechanical[b]	Complex, neuroendocrine and/or metabolic[c]

BMI body mass index, *CVD* cardiovascular disease, *RYGB* Roux-Y gastric bypass, *BPD/DS* biliopancreatic diversion with duodenal switch

[a] Endoluminal liners, electrophysiological devices, etc.

[b] Restriction and/or malabsorption of energy intake

[c] Changes in gastrointestinal hormones, changes in appetite and hunger regulation, changes in nutrient perception, microbiotics, bile acid, etc.

7.8 S3 Guidelines (February 2018)

7.8.1 Quality Assurance

- Bariatric/Metabolic Interventions only in clinics with certification or aiming for certification
- The following procedures only in centers: age < 18 or age > 65, BMI ≥ 60, non-standard procedures (center with special expertise)
- Necessity of suitable equipment; imaging diagnosis + endoscopy available 24 h a day
- Entry of patients in national register; presentation of SOPs (Standard Operating Procedures)

7.8.2 Diagnosis and Evaluation

- Necessity of interdisciplinary opinion before a surgical measure for weight reduction
  - Presentation to a physician experienced in conservative obesity therapy is obligatory (e.g. nutritionist)
  - Further presentations in other disciplines depending on the comorbidities of obese patients (clinical psychology, psychosomatics, psychiatry, endocrinology, nutritional counseling)
- Comprehensive preparation of major abdominal procedures (medical history, documentation of concomitant diseases, current medication, complaints, symptoms, ECG, chest X-ray, routine laboratory, sonography of the abdomen, pulmonary function examination), exercise and behavioural therapy
- Need for an esophagogastroduodenoscopy (EGD) before any bariatric surgery
- Absolute exclusion of secondary causes of obesity (e.g. hypothyroidism)

7.8.3 Indication

- Primary indications for bariatric surgery:
  - BMI > 50 kg/m^2 + conservative weight loss attempt futile (classification of a multidisciplinary team) or in case of severe concomitant secondary disease without possible postponement
  - BMI ≥ 40 kg/m^2 without surgical contraindication after exhaustion of conservative therapy and after comprehensive clarification
  - 35 ≤ BMI < 40 + one or more obesity-associated sequelae/companion diseases (e.g. diabetes mellitus type 2, coronary heart disease) and after exhaustion of conservative therapy
  - Diabetes mellitus type 2 + 30 ≤ BMI < 35, if target levels cannot be met
  - Diabetes mellitus type 2 + BMI < 30, surgery can be offered as part of a study
  - In obese adolescents with significant comorbidities after failure of multimodal conservative therapy
- Age alone (> 65 years) = no contraindication; indication must be particularly justified (aim of the operation = prevention of immobility and need for care)
- Desire to have children = no contraindication to bariatric surgery
- After treatment of contraindication: Reevaluation

7.8.4 Choice of Procedure

- Currently no flat rate procedure for all patients
- Currently effective surgical procedures as first-line therapy:
  - Sleeve Gastrectomy (SM)
  - Roux Y Gastric Bypass (RYGB)
  - Omega Loop Bypass
  - Biliopancreatic diversion with duodenal switch (BPD/DS)
- Further procedures:
  - Biliopancreatic Diversion (BPD)
  - One-anastomosis bypass ("mini-bypass")
  - Vertical Banded Gastroplasty (VBP)
- Choice of procedure depends on:
  - BMI

  - Age
  - Gender
  - Comorbidity
  - Adherence
  - Occupation
- Need for detailed consultation with the patient about:
  - Common procedures
  - Staged concepts (gastric balloon or sleeve gastric resection as first step)
  - Possible treatment alternatives
  - Possible complications (morbidity, mortality)
  - Aftercare (possible lifelong supplementation, plastic follow-up surgery)
- Need to consider patient preference in the absence of contraindication
- Indication + surgery by surgeons with expertise in hospitals with institutional experience

7.8.5 Technical Aspects and Complications

- Gastric balloon:
  - Necessity of the methylene blue sample for early diagnosis of balloon dysfunction
  - Previous gastric operations = contraindication with increased risk of perforation
- Gastric band:
  - Unconditional positioning of the band through pars flaccida of the omentum minus (minimization of the ligament dislocation rate)
  - Always laparoscopic
  - Lowest mortality, but results inferior to other techniques
- Roux-Y gastric bypass:
  - Laparoscopic surgery indicated
  - Target = small stomach pouch
  - Results: approx.—13–14 BMI points up to 5 years postoperatively
  - Length of alimentary limb = approximately 150–200 cm (for adequate weight loss + minor metabolic complications); biliopancreatic limb = 50–80 cm.
  - Position of the alimentary limb = antecolic-antegastric
  - for symptomatic reflux RYGB preferred
- BPD/DS:
  - Laparoscopic surgery indicated
  - Pouch: 200–500 mL
  - Length of the common leg = approx. 100 cm
  - DS with BMI > 50
  - Monitoring/prevention of deficiency symptoms necessary
- Sleeve Gastrectomy:
  - Laparoscopic surgery indicated
  - Calibration for gastric tube formation obligatory
  - For BMI > 60: Sleeve = procedure of choice (first stage of a multistage strategy)
- Simultaneous cholecystectomy
  - Indication in patients with preoperative symptomatic cholelithiasis
  - In asymptomatic cholelithiasis: consider prophylactic cholecystectomy
- Incisional hernia: postponement of surgical treatment until stable weight is reached
- Postbariatric plastic surgery

7.8.6 Aftercare

- Regular aftercare obligatory after bariatric surgery (experienced doctor + nutritionist); if necessary with outpatient cooperation partner
- Need for close monitoring in the first year postoperatively; within the first 3–6 months postop. by an bariatric surgeon
- Laboratory tests recommended for the detection of deficiency symptoms
- Supplementation with vitamins and minerals: obligatory for combination procedures and hypoabsorptive methods, recommended for purely restrictive methods with significant weight loss
- Psychological/psychosomatic/psychiatric care recommended in case of postoperative occurrence of psychological disorders
- Possible recommendation of participation in self-help groups
- In patients of childbearing age: during rapid weight loss Recommendation for contraception
- Consider possible dosage adjustment of medications

7.8.7 Guidelines

AWMF S3 guideline: Surgery for obesity and metabolic diseases. Register No. 088–001. February 2018. ▸ https://www.awmf.org/uploads/tx_szleitlinien/088-001l_S3_Chirurgie-Adipositas-metabolische-Erkrankungen_2018-02.pdf

References

Aminian A, Zajichek A, Arterburn DE, Wolski KE, Brethauer SA, Schauer PR, Kattan MW, Nissen SE (2019) Association of metabolic surgery with major adverse cardiovascular outcomes in patients with type 2 diabetes and obesity. JAMA 322(13):1271–1282. https://doi.org/10.1001/jama.2019.14231

Billmann F, El Shishtawi S, Bruckner T, Spitzner A, Elsheikh M, Müller-Stich BP, Billeter A (2021) Combined non-alcoholic fatty liver disease and type 2 diabetes in severely obese patients—medium term effects of sleeve gastrectomy versus Roux-Y-gastric Bypass on disease markers. Hepatobiliary Surg Nutr; accepted for publication

Chooi YC, Ding C, Magkos F (2019) The epidemiology of obesity. Metabolism 92:6–10

Rubino F, Shukla A, Pomp A, Moreira M, Ahn SM, Dakin G (2014) Bariatric, metabolic, and diabetes surgery. What's in the name? Ann Surg 259: 117–122

Sjöström L (2013) Review of the key results from the Swedish Obese Subjects (SOS) trial—a prospective controlled intervention study of bariatric surgery. J Intern Med 273:219–234

Suggested Reading

Carus T (2014) Operationsatlas Laparoskopische Chirurgie. Springer, Berlin/Heidelberg

Gentileschi P, Kini S, Catarci M, Gagner M (2002) Evidence-based medicine: open and laparoscopic bariatric surgery. Surg Endosc 16:736–744

Inabnet WB, DeMaria EJ, Ikramuddin S (2005) Laparoskopic bariatric surgery. Lippincott Williams & Wilkins, Philadelphia/Baltimore/New York/London

Karcz K, Thomusch O (eds) (2012) Principles of metabolic surgery. Springer, Berlin/Heidelberg/New York

Lucchese M, Scoparino N (eds) (2015) Minimally invasive bariatic and metabolic surgery. Principles and technical aspects. Springer, Berlin/Heidelberg/New York

Migrone G, Panunzi S, De Gaetano A, Guidone C, Iaconelli A, Nanni G, Castagneto M, Bornstein S, Rubino F (2015) Bariatric-metabolic surgery versus conventional medical treatment in obese patients with type 2 diabetes: 5 year follow-up of an open-label, single center, randomised controlled trial. Lancet 386:964–973

Rubino F, Kaplan LM, Schauer PR, Cummings DE (2010b) The diabetes surgery Summit consensus conference: recommendations for the evaluation and use of gastrointestinal surgery to treat type 2 diabetes mellitus. Ann Surg 251:399–405

Rubino F, Nathan DM, Eckel RH, Schauer PR, Alberti KG, Zimmet PZ, Del Prato S, Ji L, Sadikot SM, Herman WH, Amiel SA, Kaplan LM, Taroncher-Oldenburg G, Cummings DE, Delegates of the 2nd Diabetes Surgery Summit (2017) Metabolic surgery in the treatment algorithm of type 2 diabetes: a joint statement by International Diabetes Organizations. Obes Surg 27:2–21

Schauer PR, Bhatt DL, Kirwan JP, Wolski K, Aminian A, Brethauer SA, Navaneethan SD, Singh RP, Pothier CE, Nissen SE, Kashyap SR, Investigators STAMPEDE (2017) Bariatric surgery versus intensive medical therapy for diabetes—5 years outcomes. N Engl J Med 376:641–651

Sundbom M, Näslund E, Vidarsson B, Thorell A, Ottoson J (2020) Low overall mortality during 10 years of bariatric surgery: nationwide study on 63,469 procedures from the Scandinavian Obesity Registry. Surg Obes Relat Dis 16:65–70

White GE, Courcoulas AP, King WC, Flum DR, Yanovski SZ, Pomp A, Wolfe BM, Spaniolas K, Pories W, Belle SH (2019) Mortality after bariatric surgery: findings from a 7-year multicenter cohort study. Surg Obes Relat Dis 15:1755–1765

WHO (2020) Obesity and overweight. https://www.who.int/newsroom/fact-sheets/detail/obesity-and-overweight; Accessed 15 May 2021

Liver, Gallbladder and Bile Ducts

Katrin Hoffmann and Peter Schemmer

Contents

F. Billmann, T. Keck (eds.), *Essentials of Visceral Surgery*,
https://doi.org/10.1007/978-3-662-66735-4_8

8.1 Anatomy and Physiology of the Liver

8.1.1 Definitions

- Liver, gallbladder and bile duct anatomy = variable
- Anatomy of the portal vein branches, the hepatic veins and the hepatic artery = important in liver surgery
- Liver function and liver regeneration = central concepts in understanding the techniques of liver surgery

8.1.2 Macroscopic and Microscopic Anatomy

Macroscopic Anatomy

Ligaments and Ligamentous Attachments

- Lig. coronarium hepatis (Lig. triangulare dextrum + Lig. triangulare sinistrum)/coronary ligament (left and right triangle ligament)
- Lig. falciforme hepatis /falciform ligament (separates segments 4–8 from segments 2 + 3)
- Lig. teres hepatis (obliterated V. umbilicalis)/teres hepatic ligament
- Lig. venosum hepatis (obliterated Ductus venosus)/veneous hepatic ligament
- Lig. hepatogastricum and Lig. hepatoduodenale (part of the omentum minus)/gastrocolic and hepatoduodenal ligament

Functional Subdivision

- In segments (according to Couinaud)
- Oriented to vascular supply
- Subdivision:
  - Right liver lobe (segments 5–8)
  - Left liver lobe (segments 1–4)
  - Caudate lobe (segment 1) + Lobus quadratus
  - Cava-gallbladder line = dividing line between right/left liver lobe

Microscopic Anatomy

- Radial blood flow from portal vein and arterial blood through hepatic sinusoids to central vein
- Intercellular transport of bile into bile ducts
- Glisson's triad = interlobular branches of each portal vein, artery and bile duct

8.1.3 Tasks of the Liver and Functional Liver Volume

Tasks of the Liver

- Liver = central metabolic organ with detoxification and synthesis functions

Blood Formation Site (Embryonic Period)

Protein Biosynthesis and Degradation

- Under hormonal control
- In particular, formation coagulation factors (under the influence of vitamin K)
- Protein degradation with formation of urea (excretion via kidney)

Cleavage of Carbohydrates and Glycogen Storage

- Glycogen storage
- Under the influence of: adrenaline, glucagon

Central Organ of Lipometabolism

- Formation and elimination of lipoproteins

Special Metabolic Services

- Bilirubin transport
- Biosynthesis of bile acids

Detoxification Function (Through Biotransformation)

- Protection of the organism from foreign substances and drugs
- In particular by means of cytochrome P450

Central Organ of the Trace Element Metabolism

- Trace elements: iron, copper, zinc, etc.
- Numerous vitamins: especially vitamin A

Immunological Function

- Phagocytosis of cellular elements (outdated erythrocytes), bacteria
- Elimination of immune complexes and endotoxins

Functional Liver Volume After Resection

Functional Liver Volume After Resection (FLR)

8

- Definition: Proportion (in %) of liver volume that must exist after resection in order to maintain liver function
- Crucial for predicting liver function after liver resection
- Liver disease (Nonalcoholic steatohepatitis-NASH) or pre-damage of the liver (chemotherapy associated steatohepatitis-CASH) = influence on functional liver volume after resection

FLR Targets

- With normal liver function: FLR ≥20%
- After chemotherapy: FLR ≥30%
- In cirrhosis: FLR ≥40%

Measurement of FLR

- Mostly by 3D-CT volumetry: direct measurement of total liver volume (TLV)
- Calculation of the standardized FLR (sFLR): taking into account the portion to be resected

8.1.4 Location

Position Projection

- Hepatic superior border: medioclavicular = fourth intercostal space (ICS); medioaxillary = sixth ICR; paravertebral = eighth ICS
- Liver inferior border: medioclavicular = eighth rib; medioaxillary = tenth rib; paravertebral = tenth ICS
- Topographical relationship: to the inferior pleural space + base of the lung
- Variable with inspiration/expiration

8.1.5 Measured Values

Weight

- General liver = 2.5% of body weight
- Adult man = approx. 1600 g
- Adult woman = approx. 1400 g
- Volume and weight increased during digestion (blood inflow approx. 500 g)

Linear Readings

- Cross diameter (right-left) = 28 cm (20–40 cm)
- Sagittal diameter (ventral-dorsal) = 8 cm (5–12 cm)
- Height (cranial-caudal) = 10 cm (up to 27 cm)

8.1.6 Blood Supply and Drainage

Blood Supply and Drainage of the Liver

Arterial Inflow = Hepatic Artery

- Common hepatic artery: direct outlet from truncus coeliacus
- Hepatic artery proper: after delivery A. gastroduodenalis and A. gastrica dextra
- Division into right abd kifte hepatic artery
- Cystic artery: usually from right hepatic artery
- Numerous position variations

Numerous variants of arterial inflow
- Aberrant outflow from superior mesenteric artery possible (complete or right hepatic artery)
- Left hepatic artery partly from left gastric artery or from coeliac trunc directly
- Variants with accessory vessels e.g. separate branch to supply segment 4 from the hepatica propria artery

Portal Venous Inflow = portal vein

- Liver side of the confluence of splenic vein + superior mesenteric vein, if necessary inferior mesenteric vein (position variants)

- Collaterals: V. coronarian vein + cystic vein, as well as branches to the pancreatic head
- Division pattern in liver hilum:
  - Right portal venous branch (segments 5–8); subdivision into:
    - Anterior pedicle (segments 5 + 8 + parts of 4 if necessary) +
    - Posterior pedicle (segments 6 + 7)
  - Left portal venous branch (segments 2–4)
  - Rare trifurcation

Venous Outflow

- Hepatic veins:
  - Right hepatic vein (segments 6 + 7)
  - Middle hepatic vein (segments 4, 5 + 8)
  - Left hepatic vein (segments 2 + 3)
  - Norm variant accessory right inferior hepatic vein (segments 6 + 7)
- The hepatic veins open directly subdiaphragmally into the inferior vena cava

Different variants

- Common orifice of middle + left hepatic vein
- Direct orifice of segmental veins into inferior vena cava (segment 1)
- Sonographically distinguishable from portal venous branches by the absence of a connective tissue sheath

- Blood supply to the liver: 25% hepatic artery, 75% portal vein
- Proportion of oxygenation of liver blood: 40–50% hepatic artery, 60% portal vein
- Autoregulation: low portal venous flow leads to increased arterial flow - hepatic arterial buffer response

8.1.7 Terminology of Liver Resections (◘ Fig. 8.1)

- Consensus Terminology: International Conference (Belghiti et al. 2000)

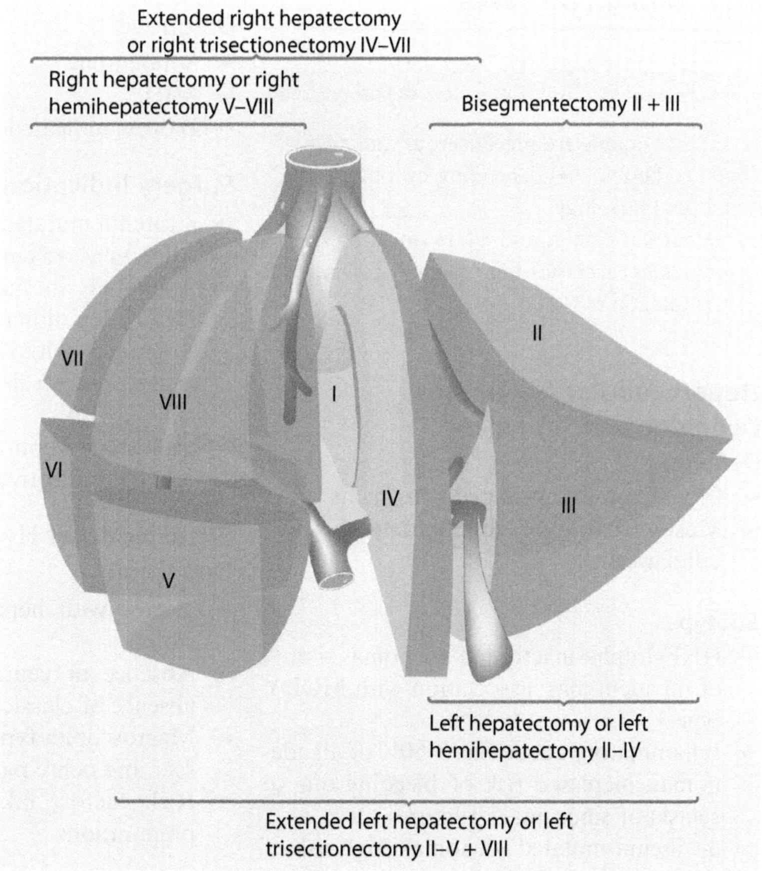

◘ **Fig. 8.1** Functional subdivision of the liver and terminology of liver resections. (Mod. according to Scott-Conner 2002)

Anatomical (= Typical) Liver Resections

- Right hemihepatectomy = right hepatectomy: resection of segments V–VIII
- Left hemihepatectomy = left hepatectomy: resection of segments II–IV
- Left-lateral sectorectomy = Bisegmentectomy II + III: Resection of segments II–III
- Extended right hepatectomy = right trisectorectomy: resection of segments IV–VIII
- Extended left hepatectomy = left trisectorectomy: resection of segments II–IV + V + VIII

Atypical Liver Resections

- Resections outside the anatomical landmarks (regardless of the resected liver volume)

8

8.2 Diseases of the Liver

8.2.1 Benign Diseases

Key Points

- Adenomas are precancerous and need to be resected depending on both size and histology
- Hemangiomas and FNH (focal nodular hyperplasia) are resected if symptomatic

Hepatocellular Adenomas

Definition and Subtypes

Definition

- Clonal non-encapsulated neoplasms
- Mostly from highly differentiated hepatocellular cells

Subtypes

- HNF-1alpha-inactivated adenomas = 40% of all adenomas; association with MODY type 3
- Inflammatory adenomas = 50% of all adenomas, increased risk of bleeding due to ectasia of sinusoidal structures
- β-Catenin-mutated adenomas, high risk of malignant transformation (approx. 40%)
- Unclassified adenomas = approx. 10% of all adenomas
- Adenomatosis ≥10 adenomas

Epidemiology and Risk Factors

Epidemiology

- Incidence = 3–4/100.000 in Europe

Risk Factors

- Taking oral contraceptives
- Anabolic Abuse
- Glycogen storage disorders, galactosemia
- perfusion disturbances of the liver

Symptoms and Complications

- Often diagnosed incidentially in asymptomatic patients
- Possible complications:
  - Sponaneous rupture and hemorrhage
  - Malignant transformation into HCC (hepatocellular carcinoma), risk 8–13% in β-Catenin-mutated adenomas

Diagnosis

- Sonography
- MRI
- Biopsy: indicated for all adenomas

Surgery Indication

- β-catenin mutated adenomas
- Adenomas >5 cm
- Adenomas in men—differentiation from HCC often difficult
- Adenomas with risk of rupture (in case of acute bleeding first embolization, surgery two-sided)
- Size progression after discontinuation of oral contraceptives

Focal Nodular Hyperplasia (FNH)

Definition

- Tumor with hepatocellular origin, polyclonal
- Absence of central and portal veins (= absence of classical hepatic architecture)
- Macroscopic: typical picture with central scar and ochre parenchyma
- Risk factor: taking estrogen-containing preparations

Epidemiology
- Second most common benign liver tumor

Diagnosis
- Sonography
- MRI
- Biopsy: not indicated with clear imaging

Complications
- Progressive growth
- Rupture
- Portal hypertension
- Bleeding: rare
- Necrosis: rare
- Malignant degeneration: not described

Therapy

Conservative Approach: Generally

Surgical Therapy
- Indications:
  - Symptomatic patients
  - Large displacing-growing FNH
  - Cholestasis
  - Vascular compression

Hemangiomas
Definition
- haemangioma of mesenchymal origin

Epidemiology
- Most frequent benign lesions = 0.5–7% of all patients
- Women three times more often affected than men

Clinical Presentation and Complications
Clinical Presentation
- Mostly incidental findings and often asymptomatic

Complications
- No malignant transformation risk
- Kasabach-Merritt syndrome:
  - Hemangioma bleeding, thrombocytopenia and consumption coagulopathy
  - Rare complication of generalized giant hemangiomas
  - Mortality risk in case of hemorrhage 30–40%

Diagnosis
- Sonography (also contrast medium supported ultrasound)
- CT
- Biopsy: not indicated

Therapy

Conservative Therapy
- Whenever there is no indication for surgery

Surgical Therapy
- Surgery indication:
  - Symptomatic patients
  - Lesion >5 cm
  - Significant hemorrhage, location near the capsule with risk of rupture
  - Acute bleeding without the possibility of control by interventional radiology

Echinococcosis
Definition
- Tapeworm zoonosis
- Human = intermediate host
- Tapeworm species:
  - Echinococcus granulosus = Echinococcus cysticus = dog tapeworm
  - Echinococcus multilocularis = Echinococcus alveolaris = fox tapeworm

Clinical Presentation
E. granulosus (Cysticus, Unilocularis), Dog Tapeworm
- Displacing growth
- Infestation of lung and pericardium also possible
- Pericyst partly calcified as membrane around cystic hydatid
- Often asymptomatic
- Due to size non-specific upper abdominal complaints or infection symptoms

E. multilocularis (alveolaris), Fox Tapeworm

- Infiltrative (tumor-like) growth with formation of small cysts
- Recognised occupational disease in hunters and foresters
- Often asymptomatic
- Due to size non-specific upper abdominal complaints or infection symptoms

Diagnosis

- Incidental finding on imaging
- Serological: Detection of antibodies
- Puncture: Contraindicated!

Therapy

Surgical Therapy

- Whenever possible
- Only under perioperative medication with mebendazole or albendazole
- Treatment only in cooperation with infectiologists

Surgical Procedure

Surgery for Echinococcosis Cyst

- Rupture of the cyst and/or extravasation of cyst fluid must be avoided at all costs, otherwise contamination of the situs with the development of disseminated intra-abdominal disease
- Endocystectomy (procedure of choice for E. granulosus (Kniepeiss et al. 2020)):
  - Repositioning of the liver and the cyst with cloths soaked in 20% saline solution
  - Puncture of the cyst with a disposable trocar + aspiration of the cyst fluid while filling with physiological saline solution
  - Uncapping of the cyst
  - Exclusion of connection to the bile duct system = e.g. White test (white fat emulsion approved for i.v. infusion, e.g. lipofundin®, intralipid® via ductus cysticus)
  - Installation of compresses soaked in 20% saline solution for 20 min = **Caution:** If bile ducts are opened, bile duct necrosis!—rule out beforehand and over sew bile leaks if necessary
  - Suturing of the caspel edge or bipolar coagulation
- Pericystectomy: Resection of the entire cyst plus surrounding liver tissue—technically more difficult, risk of rupture!
- Typical/anatomical liver resection according to oncological criteria in E. multilocularis

8.2.2 Malignant Diseases of the Liver

Key Points

- Distinguish primary—such as CCC (cholangiocarcinoma), HCC (hepatocellular carcinoma)—and secondary malignant findings (metastases)

Primary Tumors

Hepatocellular Carcinoma (HCC)

Epidemiology and Risk Factors

- Incidence
  - Incidence = 10/100.000 in Germany
- Risk factors
  - Cirrhosis of the liver of any etiology (alcohol, hepatitis, hemochromatosis, etc.)
  - Chronic hepatitis B/C virus infection
- Cumulative 5-year risk of developing HCC in patients with HCV(hepatitis C virus)-associated liver cirrhosis in Europe = about 17%
  - Non-alcoholic fatty liver hepatitis (NASH) as a consequence of diabetes mellitus and the metabolic syndrome—number 1 rising risk factor world wide
  - Aflatoxin exposure

Early Detection

- Screening program for all patients with:
  - Liver cirrhosis
  - Chronic hepatitis B/C
  - Fatty liver disease,
  - Steatohepatitis
- Sonography every 6 months

Special Forms

- Fibrolamellar HCC—young patients often better prognosis
- Mixed differentiated tumors (combined HCC/intrahepatic cholangiocarcinoma)
- Early HCC—transition from regenerated node to HCC

Clinical presentation and Classification

- Clinical presentation
  - Mostly asymptomatic
  - Conspicuous in routine examinations of cirrhotic patients
- TNM classification (HCC)
  - T (tumor)
    - T1 Solitary tumor without vascular invasion
    - T2 Solitary tumor with vascular invasion or multiple tumors all <5 cm
    - T3a Multiple tumors >5 cm
    - T3b Multiple tumors involving a major branch of the V. portae or Vv. hepaticae
    - T4 Tumor with invasion of adjacent organs or perforation of the visceral peritoneum
  - N (lymph nodes)
    - N0 No locoregional lymph nodes
    - N1 Locoregional lymph nodes
  - M (metastases)
    - M0 No distant metastases
    - M1 Distant metastases
    - UICC stages according to the TNM classification (eighth edition, January 2018)

I	T1 N0 M0	II	T2 N0 M0
IIIA	T3 N0 M0	IIIB	T4 N0 M0
IVA	Any T N1 M0	IVB	Each T Each N M1

Diagnosis

- Diagnostic imaging
  - CM Sonography
  - Primovist MRI
  - CT
  - Characteristic signs in imaging
  - Arterial hypervascularization with rapid washout of the contrast medium and relative contrast reversal to the surrounding liver parenchyma
- Biopsy
  - Only if unclear imaging or therapeutic consequence
- Tumor marker
  - AFP only suitable for assessment of progression, not for diagnosis

Surgical Therapy

- Liver resection (Lin et al. 2012; de Santibañes et al. 2017)
  - Indications:
    - Patients with potentially resectable HCC without cirrhosis
    - Patients with potentially resectable HCC and Child A/B cirrhosis
    - Presence of portal hypertension (ascites, platelets <100.000, splenomegaly) = not a sole exclusion criterion for resection, but significantly increases the surgical risk
    - Atypical resections = leaving as much functional liver tissue as possible
    - 5-year survival = 30–50%, but high recurrence rates due to de novo tumors in cirrhosis or micrometastases
- Liver transplantation (Lin et al. 2012)
  - Indications depending on local/national legal regulations and/or guidelines
  - Treatment of HCC + underlying liver cirrhosis
  - Prioritization and organ distribution according to local/national legal regulations and/or guidelines (Eurotransplant region—MELD (Model for End-Stage Liver Disease) score based:
    - Patients receive extra points with increasing waiting time)
    - Transarterial chemoembolisation (TACE), local thermal ablation (up to 3 cm diameter), liver resection: allows

bridging during waiting period = recommended to avoid progression
- Other local ablation procedures (RFA (radiofrequency ablation), PEI (percutaneous ethanol injection), SIRT (selective internal radiotherapy), IRE (irreversible electroporation), cryotherapy)
- 5-year survival rates = up to 70%; local recurrence rate < 15%

Intrahepatic Cholangiocarcinoma: CCC

Definition

- Originating in the liver from the bile ducts

8

Epidemiology

- Incidence
  - Incidence = 1–2/100.000 in Germany
- Risk factors
  - Cholelithiasis
  - Cirrhosis on the basis of chronic hepatitis C infection, alcoholic and non-alcoholic hepatitis
  - Uptake of carcinogens (nitrosamines, aflatoxins, anabolic steroids, etc.)
  - Congenital anomalies of the bile ducts
  - Concomitant diseases (e.g. primary sclerosing cholangitis, ulcerative colitis, α-antitrypsin deficiency)

Symptoms and Classification

- Symptoms
  - Abdominal pain
  - B-symptomatics
  - Icterus
- TNM classification (CCC)
  - T (tumor)
    - Tis carcinoma in situ intraductal tumor
    - T1 Solitary tumor without vascular infiltration
    - T2a Solitary tumor with vascular infiltration
    - T2b Multiple tumors with or without vascular infiltration
    - T3 tumors with infiltration of the peritoneum or direct invasion of extrahepatic structures
    - T4 tumors with periductal invasion
  - N (lymph nodes)
    - N0 No lymph node metastases
    - N1 Lymph node metastases
  - M (metastases)
    - M0 No distant metastases
    - M1 Distant metastases
  - UICC stages according to the TNM classification

0	Tis	N0	M0
I	T1	N0	M0
II	T2	N0	M0
III	T3	N0	M0
IVa	T4	N0	M0
	Each T	N1	M0
IVb	Each T	Each N	M1

Diagnosis

- Imaging
  - Sonography
  - CT
  - MRI with MRCP (with Primovist)
  - ERCP (endoscopic retrograde cholangiopancreaticography)
- Tumor marker
  - CA 19-9 = progress assessment
  - **Caution:** Also elevated in cholangitis and jaundice

Therapy

- Surgical therapy
  - Resection = only curative option
  - Anatomical resection + lymphadenectomy in the hepatoduodenal ligamentrecommended
  - Contraindications:
    - Satellite nodules and or bilobar manifestation
    - Remote metastases
    - Peritoneal carcinomatosis
    - 5-year survival rates = 23–42% after R0 resection without lymph node metastases
- Adjuvant therapy:
  - according to local guide lines, preferably within the context of clinical trials

CCC of the Common Hepatic Duct Bifurcation: Klatskin Tumors

Definition

- First described by Gerald Klatskin in 1965 (hence the synonym Klatskin tumor).
- Perihilar cholangiocellular carcinoma in the region of the common hepatic duct bifurcation

Epidemiology

- Incidence 1/100.000 in Germany

Symptoms and Classification

- Symptoms
  - Icterus
  - Pruritus
  - Abdominal pain
  - B-symptomatics
- Differential diagnosis
  - HCC
  - Liver metastases
  - Pancreatic cancer
  - Cholangitis
  - Cholecystitis, choledocholithiasis
  - Biliary strictures, bile duct cysts
- Classification according to Bismuth-Corlette in type I-IV
  - I Distal common hepatic duct to the confluence of the right and left bile duct
  - II Common hepatic duct bifurcation
  - IIIa Common hepatic duct bifurcation and right hepatic duct
  - IIIb Common hepatic duct bifurcation and left hepatic duct
  - IV Common hepatic duct bifurcation and both hepatic ducts or multifocal
- TNM classification (Klatskin tumours)
  - T (tumor)
    - Tis carcinoma in situ, intraductal tumor
    - T1 Tumor limited to bile duct with spread to muscularis
    - T2a Tumor infiltrates periductal fat tissue
    - T2b Tumor infiltrates surrounding liver tissue
    - T3 Tumor with infiltration of the equilateral portal vein or hepatic artery
    - T4 Tumor infiltrates main trunk of portal vein or bilateral portal vein branches or common hepatic artery or secondary bile ducts bilaterally or secondary bile ducts unilaterally with invasion of contralateral portal vein or hepatic artery
  - N (lymph nodes)
    - N0 No lymph node metastases
    - N1 Regional lymph node metastases (incl. metastases along the cystic duct, choledochal duct, portal vein and hepatic artery)
    - N2 Lymph node metastases periaortic, pericaval, along the superior mesenteric artery and or truncus coeliacus
  - M (metastases)
    - M0 No distant metastases
    - M1 Distant metastases
  - UICC stages according to the TNM classification

0	Tis	N0	M0
I	T1	N0	M0
II	T2	N0	M0
III	T3	N0	M0
IVa	T4	N0	M0
	Each T	N1	M0
IVb	Each T	Each N	M1

Prognosis

- Prognostic factors:
  - Lymphnode metastases
  - Tumor differentiation
  - Perineural invasion
  - R1 resection status

Therapy

- Surgical therapy
  - Resection = only curative option
  - Indications:
    - Type 1 Extrahepatic bile duct resection possibly with duodenopancreatectomy
    - Type 2–4 Extrahepatic bile duct resection + liver resection

Surgical Procedure

Klatskin Tumors

- Depending on the type (extended) hemihepatectomy right or left + creation of biliodigestive anastomosis + lymphadenectomy in the hepatoduodenal ligament
- if necessary in combination with resection of the equilateral portal vein and hepatic artery in case of infiltration
- General portal vein resection without oncological advantage
- Intraoperative frozen sections from the proximal and distal resectional margins; **caution:** discontinuous growth
- If bilirubin is highly elevated = preoperative PTCD (cholangiodrainage) or ERCP + stent = relief of cholestasis = better liver function and less morbidity postoperatively
- In preparation for augmentation procedures to increase functional liver reserve prior to resection (portal vein embolization)

- Contraindication:
  - Secondary bile ducts infiltrated on both sides
  - Invasion of the portal vein or hepatic artery of the opposite side
  - Bilateral vascular infiltration
  - Remote metastases
  - Liver cirrhosis or pronounced fibrosis (functional liver reserve)
- Chemotherapy/radiochemotherapy:
  - according to local guide lines, preferably within the context of clinical trials

Liver Metastases

Indications

- Resection of metastases of colorectal cancers = standard therapy
- Resection of metastases from non-colorectal cancers:
  - Increasing frequency
  - Individual tumor biology and the possibility of R0 resection are decisive here
  - Recurrent resections as well as two-stage resections possible

Therapy

- All resection techniques and circumferences possible
- Decisive = possibility of extrahepatic tumor freedom
- Prognosis-limiting factor = R0 resection
- If necessary, combination with multimodal concepts—neoadjuvant chemotherapy and/or interventional radiological procedures such as RFA
- **Caution:** Chemotherapy-pretreated liver = reduced regenerative capacity, at least 45% residual volume required

8.2.3 Technique of Liver Resection

Planning of the Resection

Technical Conditions

- Review of vascular anatomy—inflow (hepatic artery and portal vein), outflow (hepatic veins) and bile ducts; normative variants (aberrant or accessory vessels)
- Exclusion infiltration of structures

Parenchyma Conditions

- Normal tissue, steatosis, steatohepatitis (after chemotherapy), fibrosis, cirrhosis
- Liver function
- Planned extent of resection vs. volume of future liver remnant = functional liver reserve

Caution

- Normal tissue 25% residual volume sufficient
- After chemotherapy at least 45% residual volume
- In cirrhosis only if hyper-Child-Pugh A or A and bilirubin <2—otherwise high mortality after conventional (open) resection; laparoscopic parenchymal-sparing minor resection also acceptable in Child C patients, the minimal invasive robotic approach has similar complication rates as open or laparoscopic procedures (Murtha-Lemekhova et al. 2022)

Strategy of Resection

- Limited resections only
- Anatomical resections along the segment boundaries
- Always choose the most parenchyma-sparing procedure if possible
- if necessary, two-stage resections or multimodal combination with ablation

Resection Type

Minor Resection (<3 Segments)

- Monosegmentectomy
- Bisegmentectomy
- Anterior (segments V + VIII) or posterior (segments VI + VII) sectorectomy
- Wedge resection = for superficial findings
- Atypical resection = incision after marking and sonography of vascular structures which must be spared

Major Resection

- Right hemihepatectomy (segments V, VI, VII, VIII)
- Left hemihepatectomy (segments II, III, IVa, IVb)
- Extended right hemihepatectomy (segments IVa, IVb, V, VI, VII, VIII)
- Extended left hemihepatectomy (segments II, III, IVa, IVb, V, VIII)
- Mesohepatectomy (segment IVa, IVb, V, VIII)

Surgical Procedure

Liver Resection (Conventional/Open)

- Supine position
- Reversed L shape incision for right/left or extended right/left resections; median laparotomy for left lateral resections
- Inspection and palpation of the liver, the hepatoduodenal ligament and the entire abdomen
- Complete mobilization of the liver: use of the falciform ligament to pull on the liver, transection of the triangular ligaments and the teres hepatis ligament to obtain enough mobility for sonography and resection
- Dissection along the vena cava:
  - **Caution:** Makuuchi ligament between segment 8 dorsal to v. cava often includes veins draining into v. caval vein (to be divided for right hemihepatectomy)
  - **Caution:** Mobilize the whole liver and not only the liver lobe that will be resected!
- Intraoperative ultrasound to check vascular anatomy, extent of findings and positional relationship of lesions to vascular structures obligatory
- Complete lymphadenectomy in the hepatoduodenal ligament only indicated for cholangiocarcinoma and gallbladder cancer; for liver metastases of CRC in studies
- Cholecystectomy with long-left ductus cysticus—temporary closure with Bulldog clamp for later white test (Lipofundin®, Intralipid®, or similar) for visualization of the bile ducts at the resection area
- For all major resections:
  - Intravascular control: exposure and tightening of the artery and portal vein of the half of the liver to be resected (right pedicle in the area of the Gans fissure)
  - Outflow control: visualization and tightening of the hepatic vein to be resected
- Before parenchymal transection a CVP <5 is obligatory = less bleeding! (Anti-Trendelenburg positioning, low volume supply, if necessary vasodilators i.v.)
  - Control of the arterial inflow by dividing the feeding artery by means of clips or hemostatic suturing
  - Dividing the portal vein and hepatic vein by means of a vascular stapler or hemostatic suturing after clamping
- Parenchymal transection:
  - Ultrasonic dissection (CUSA = Cavitron Ultrasonic Surgical Aspirator) in combination with bipolar coagulation, clipping and ligation = advantage: precise transection; disadvantage: time-consuming

- Endovascular staplers (= stapler hepatectomy (Schemmer et al. 2006)) = crush clamp of the liver parenchyma with a straight clamp with subsequent stapling = advantage: time-saving; disadvantage: not applicable for all anatomical resections (e.g. isolated segment VIII)
- Water jet dissection = similar to ultrasonic method
- Ultrasonic scissors = especially for atypical resections, less precise than ultrasonic dissector
- Advanced coagulation technology = e.g. LigaSure®, Ultracision®/ Sonicision™, bipolar scissors, Habib-Sealer (thermoablative)
- Finger fracture = crushing of liver tissue between fingers, supply of vessels by means of clips or stitches

Technology

- It is essential to ensure that the vascular and bile duct structures of the remaining liver areas are protected, irrespective of the resection procedure used
- Pringle maneuver:
  - Targeted short-term clamping of the portal vein + hepatic artery during the transection phase using silicone reins in order to reduce the tendency to bleed
  - Rarely used with modern open resection techniques as ischemia-reperfusion damage in the remaining liver tissue as well as a higher tumor recurrence rate can be detected
  - No differences between intermittent and continuous Pringle manoeuvre
  - If necessary, maximum 20 min recommended
- Post-resection phase:
  - Achiving haemostasis with argon beamer, bipolar electrocoagulation, etc.; if necessary over sawing of vessels
  - Retrograde control for bile leakage with White-Test (alternatively diluted blue staining = lower detection rate) via cystic duct under manual compression of the Ductus choledochus (**Caution:** Dislodging of the Ductus choledochus with clamp or bulldog may lead to necrosis) = if necessary re-positioning of bile ducts at the resection area
  - Optional application of haemostyptics or sealants
- If necessary, reconstruction of the bile duct by means of biliodigestive anastomosis according to Y-Roux

Possible Complications

- Postoperative (postheoatectomy) liver failure PHLF—insufficient residual volume—definition according ISGLS (Rahbari et al. 2011)
- Protein deficiency—edema, ascites
- Hepatorenal syndrome
- Postoperative bleeding
- Biliary leakage and bilioma formation—definition according ISGLS (Koch et al. 2011):
- Low "sweating out" of bilirubin = usually suspended
- High volume leakage: indicates bile leakage = revise early + oversaw
- Superinfected fluid collection/abscess = interventional CT-guided drainage
- Biliopleural fistula = rare, especially after simultaneous diaphragmatic resection
- Atelectasis + pleural effusion on the right = respiratory training and drainage if necessary

8.3 Liver Transplantation

8.3.1 General and Legal Basis

(National) Legal Basis

Definition

- Regulated by:
  - Local official regulations and guidelines

Indication and Listing

Indication for Liver Transplantation

- Based on the local official regulations and guidelines
- Set in the interdisciplinary transplant conference in consensus between the departments involved and legal guidelines

Listing

- Potentially all patients with rapidly progressing or already far advanced irreversible chronic liver diseases, for which no conservative-internistic or surgical treatment alternative with equal chances of success exists
- Listing for transplantation (waiting list), if probability of survival appears to be greater with a liver transplant
- Listing based on assessment of liver function and tumor stage (HCC and others (Talakic et al. 2021) as well as disease-specific complications (dominant stenosis PSC)

Organ Allocation

Eurotransplant

- Organization for organ allocation based on national guidelines
- Coordinates the allocation of organs subject to transfer such as heart, kidney, liver, lung, pancreas and intestine (§ 8 TPG)
- In Austria, Belgium, Croatia, Hungary, Luxembourg, the Netherlands, Slovenia and Germany

Principles of Organ Allocation

- Allocation of organs to individual patients or centres by Eurotransplant on the basis of national regulations
- Patients' listing on the Eurotransplant wait list for transplantation as soon as the treating transplant centre has made the indication and all necessary examinations are available

8.3.2 Evaluation and Follow-Up of Liver Function

Clinical Follow-Up

- Basic parameters:
  - Progressive physical weakness, fatigue, muscular deficits
  - Hepatic encephalopathy
  - Therapy refractory ascites
  - Spontaneous bacterial peritonitis
  - Hepatorenal syndrome
  - Gastrointestinal bleeding/variceal bleeding
  - Hepatopulmonary syndrome
  - Progressive osteopathy
  - Recurrent biliary sepsis
  - Occurrence of hepatocellular carcinoma

Laboratory Parameters of Liver Synthesis and Excretion

- Only limited suitability for risk assessment

Hepatocellular Integrity

- GOT
- GPT
- LDH

Biliary Integrity

- alkaline phosphatase
- γ-GT

Synthesis Performance of the Liver

- Albumin
- Cholinesterase (CHE)
- PT
- INR
- Fibrinogen

Excretory Capacity of the Liver

- Bilirubin (direct, indirect)
- Bile acids

Scoring Systems for Liver Function and Prognosis

- For the assessment of patient survival and mortality risk (limited possible)

Child-Pugh Score (◘ Table 8.1)

- Disadvantages:
  - Subjective assessment of the therapeutic response of ascites and encephalopathy
  - Continuous deterioration of the patient's condition is often not reflected in a change in child classification

MELD Score

- MELD Criteria:
  - Bilirubin
  - Creatinine

Table 8.1 Child-Pugh score[a]

	1 point	2 points	3 points
Encephalopathy	None		
Ascites, therapy	No ascites	Moderate, controlled by therapy	Pronounced despite therapy
Bilirubin	<35 μmol/L	–35 to 50 μmol/L	>50 μmol/L
Albumin	>3.5 g/dL	–2.8 to 3.5 g/dL	<2.8 g/dL
INR	<1.7	–1.7 to 2.3	>2.3

INR International Normalized Ratio
[a]Child A = 5–6 points; Child B = 7–9 points; Child C = >10 points

- Coagulation: INR (International Normalized Ratio; Prothrombin Ratio)
- Formula:
  - MELD score = 10 × (0.957 × log(creati nine) + 0.378 log(bilirubin) + 1.12 log(INR) + 0.643)

8.3.3 Indications for Liver Transplantation: Relevant Underlying Diseases in Adults

Chronic Liver Disease

Underlying Disease for Liver Cirrhosis

- Hepatitis B, C, D
- Autoimmune hepatitis
- Alcololic liver disease
- Cryptogenic

Cholestatic Liver Disease

- Primary sclerosing cholangitis (PSC)
- Primary biliary cirrhosis (PBC)
- Secondary sclerosing cholangitis
- Familial cholestasis syndromes
- Biliary atresia

Chronic Drug Toxicity

Metabolic Diseases/Genetic Diseases

- α_1-antitrypsin deficiency
- Wilson's disease
- Hemochromatosis
- Glycogen storage diseases
- Galactosemia
- Tyrosinemia
- β-Thalassemia
- TTR (transthyretin) amyloidosis
- Cystic Fibrosis
- Hypercholesterolemia (LDL receptor deficiency, Crigler-Najjar syndrome type 1)
- Erythropoietic protoporphyria
- Primary amyloidosis
- Urea Cycle Defects

Other Diseases

- Congenital cystic liver
- Echinococcosis of the liver
- Chronic Budd-Chiari syndrome

Acute Liver Disease

- Fulminant liver failure
  - Etiologies:
    - Poisoning
    - Hepatitis
    - Budd-Chiari Syndrome
    - Drug toxicity, etc.
  - Definition: Acute liver failure based on Kings College score, Clichy criteria, or BiLE score
- Pregnancy-associated liver diseases
- Extensive liver trauma
- Postoperative liver failure after liver resection or transplantation

Malignant Diseases of the Liver

Hepatocellular Carcinoma (HCC)

- Based on national german guidelines indication only if within MILAN criteria for the entire period prior to liver transplantation = singular HCC <5 cm or up to 3 foci

<3 cm (international scientific based guidelines i.e. MILAN citeria (with possible downstaging), UCSF criteria, Up-to-5 criteria, Kyoto criteria, AASLD, EASL) (Bento de Sousa et al. 2021; Cusi et al. 2022; European Association for the Study of the Liver. Electronic address: easloffice@easloffice.eu; European Association for the Study of the Liver 2018)
- 5 year survival up to 85%

Cholangiocarcinoma (CCC)

- Should be performed within prospective randomized clinical trials only

Epithelioid Hemangioendothelioma

Caution
- Indication for liver transplantation in the case of malignant primary disease
- Transplantation only in patients who have a significantly better chance for recovery and long-term survival with transplantation than without transplantation or with the use of alternative therapies
- Liver metastases in other primary tumors (e.g. colorectal tumors) = currently (at least outside of studies) no indication for liver transplantation

8.3.4 Contraindications for Liver Transplantation

Lack of Patient Adherence/ Psychosocial Problems

- Adherence = beyond consent to transplantation, willingness and ability to cooperate in the treatments and examinations required before and after transplantation
- Reliable intake of immunosuppressants + regular outpatient follow-up examinations = absolute prerequisites for successful transplantation
- Psychological consultation before transplantation = obligatory
- Continued alcohol or drug abuse = clear contraindication until completion of consistent withdrawal and addiction treatment

High Age

- Probability of presence of concomitant diseases that speak against transplantation (such as cardiovascular problems) increases with age
- Above 65 years of age Clarify indication individually
- The decisive factor is the biological age of the patient

Cardiovascular and Pulmonary Concomitant Diseases

- To be excluded:
  - Severe valvular heart disease
  - Severe pulmonary hypertension
  - (Alcohol Toxic) Cardiomyopathy
  - Coronary vascular disease and myocardial infarction

Caution
Cardiovascular and pulmonary concomitant diseases = risk during transplantation or longer-term transplant success.

- General fitness for anaesthesia must always be checked

Infections

- Chronic suppurative infections (e.g. osteomyelitis, sinusitis, abscesses):
  - Need to be treated before transplantation
  - So is spontaneous bacterial peritonitis
- In active tuberculosis:
  - No liver transplant
  - Tuberculostatic therapy required for at least 3 months (if possible for 1 year)
- HIV infection = no contraindication
- AIDS = contraindication

Extrahepatic Metastases

- Extrahepatic tumor manifestation = absolute contraindication

8.3.5 Surgical Principles

Patient Positioning

- Supine position
- Both arms alongside the body

Laparotomy

- "Reversed L-shape incision" in the right upper quadrant of the abdominal wall (reversed angle incision to the right)
- Alternatively, transverse upper abdominal laparotomy (costal margin incision) without or with median extension to the xyphoid (bilateral rooftop incision with vertical extension)

Recipient Hepatectomy

- Severing of the falciform ligament between ligatures
- Mobilization of the diseased liver from the hepatoligamentous structures
- Ductus hepatocholedochus, hepatic artery and portal vein separated after close-to-life preparation—corresponds to the beginning of the anhepatic phase of the recipient
- Completely mobilized liver is dissected from the recipient vena cava while supplying (clipping/LigaSure) numerous small hepatic veins (Houben et al. 2014; Kniepeiss et al. 2020)
- 3 large hepatic veins are transected with the help of two endo-vascular stackers
- Stop bleeding
- Inferior vena cava is partially clamped tangentially with a Satinski clamp

Machine Perfusion of the liver

- Novel method for organ preservation + reconditioning (van Rijn et al. 2021; Karangwa et al. 2020; Martins et al. 2020; Ceresa et al. 2022; Sousa Da Silva et al. 2022)
- Considering shortage of donor livers suitable for transplantation, this technique may help avoid needless wastage of organs
- Goals: (1) improvement of quality of marginal livers, (2) extension of time for which liver can be preserved, (3) enabling an objective assessment of liver quality/viability
- Hypothermic vs. normothermic machine perfusion

Implantation

- Donor organ placed in the right upper abdomen of the recipient

Vena Cava Anastomosis

- In modified piggy-back technique side-to-side cavocaval anastomosis between donor and recipient
- Front and back wall each separately continuous with Prolene threads of strength 4-0

Portal Vein Anastomosis

- if necessary, shortening of the portal vein to avoid kinking
- End-to-end portal vein anastomosis
- Separately for the front and back wall in continuous technique with Prolene threads of strength 5-0

Reperfusion

- With the reperfusion of the liver the anhepatic phase is finished

Portal vein

- Portal venous reperfusion is widely considered as standard in adults
- Subsequently, completion of the portal venous anastomosis and closure of the caudal opening of the donor's vena cava; the cranial portion of the donor's vena cava was already closed during backtable surgery

Hepatic artery

- Artery is usually anastomosed with Prolene sutures of different thicknesses (5-0 to 7-0) in continuous or single button suture technique.
- Here, the back wall can be sewn continuously; front wall in single button technique
- To avoid anastomotic stenosis, the branch-patch technique is used so that the anastomosis is located between the bifurcation of the gastroduodenal artery (which is usually blocked) and the hepatic artery on the recipient side and the bifurcation between the gastroduodenal artery and the hepatic propriocele artery on the donor side.

After reperfusion, arterial and portal venous blood flow is determined in mL/min.

Bile Duct

- Bile duct anastomosis:
  - Usually as end-to-end anastomosis with 5-0 PDS (polydioxanon)
  - Either single knots or running suture
  - In selected cases (e.g. PSC of the recipient), a biliodigestive anastomosis with Roux-Y reconstruction is indicated
- 2 percutaneously inserted easy-flow drains, one subphrenic, the other subhepatic

Postoperative Phase

- Interdisciplinary intensive care unit
- Interdisciplinary treatment (e.g. gastroenterologists/hepatologists, nephrologists, infectiologists, etc.)

8.4 Anatomy and Physiology of the Gallbladder and Bile Ducts

8.4.1 Gallbladder (Vesica Biliaris)

- Lateral under lobus quadratus of liver segments IVb/V
- Positional relationship to right colonic flexure, duodenum and V. portae
- Consisting of:
  - Fundus
  - Corpus
  - Infundibulum
  - Collum (= transition to the cystic duct)

8.4.2 Bile Ducts

- Outflow into left (segments I–IV) and right hepatic duct (segments V–VIII)
- Ductus hepaticus communis = union of right + left ductus hepaticus
- Ductus choledochus = Ductus hepaticus after inflow of the Ductus cysticus
- Common orifice of the ductus choledochus with ductus pancreaticus Orifice in papilla Vateri of the duodenum, pars inferior
- Calot's triangle = bounded by cystic duct, hepatic duct and hepatic subsurface

Variants:
- Course of the right posterior bile duct
- Crossing over/under the common bile duct, accessory bile duct of seg. IV
- Ostium of choledochal duct: common excretory duct with confluence, common ostium without confluence, separate ostia of both ducts

8.4.3 Blood Supply and Drainage of the Gallbladder and Bile Ducts

Blood Supply of the Extrahepatic Bile Ducts + Gallbladder

- Right hepatic artery, gastroduodenal and retroduodenal arteries
- Cystic artery from right hepatic artery (numerous variants, rarely cystic artery directly from main hepatic artery)

Blood Supply of the Intrahepatic Bile Ducts

- Common hepatic artery from Coeliac trunc
- After delivery of the gastroduodenal and right gastric arteries as the proper hepatic artery
- Branching into the right and left hepatic artery (variable anatomy)
- Venous outflow via the hepatic veins

8.5 Diseases of the Gallbladder and Bile Ducts

8.5.1 Benign Diseases of the Gallbladder

Key Points

- Gallstones in 10–15% of population (m:f = 1:1.8)
- 75% are asymptomatic at diagnosis
- 20%Of those turn symptomatic within 15–20 years
- Indication for surgery in symptomatic cholecystolithiasis with and without complications, porcelain gallbladder and stones >3 cm

- Laparoscopic cholecystectomy is the standard procedure
- Acute cholecystitis = most frequent complication of cholecystolithiasis; if detected = immediate indication for surgery
- Gallbladder polyps rare overall, but if gallbladder polyps ≥1 cm or symptomatic = indication for surgery

8

Cholecystolithiasis

Definition

- Inability to ensure the solubility of the bile component (cholesterol, calcium, pigments)
- Precipitation and formation of concrements (gallstones)

Epidemiology

- Gallstone carriers = 15–20% of the population
- Risk factors:
  - Overweight
  - Rapid weight loss
  - Pregnancy
  - Multiparity
  - Female gender
  - First degree family history
  - Medications: Ceftriaxone, postmenopausal estrogens, parenteral nutrition.
  - Geographical origin (Scandinavia, American Indians)
  - Ileal diseases, secondary to resection or bypass of the small intestine
  - Age (risk increased from 40 years)
- Symptomatic cholecystolithiasis: approx. 30% of carriers
- Hereditary component in the development of gallbladder stones about 25%
- More than 190,000 cholecystectomies/year in Germany

Classification

- Asymptomatic cholecystolithiasis
- Symptomatic uncomplicated cholecystolithiasis
- Symptomatic complicated cholecystolithiasis with complications
  - Due to trapped concrement
  - Acute cholecystitis = most frequent complication

Symptoms

- Colicky attacks of pain
  - Of more than 15 min duration in the epigastrium/right upper abdomen
  - Radiation into the back and right shoulder
- Nausea, occasionally bilious vomiting
- Possibly intolerance for fat, alcohol
- Dyspepsia and flatulence
- Additionally in case of complicated form:
  - Fever
  - Chills
  - Painful jaundice (due to stone entrapment in the choledochal duct)
  - Defensive tension in the upper abdomen (in acute cholecystitis, gallbladder empyema or perforation)
  - Possibly signs of purulent cholangitis or biliary pancreatitis, liver abscesses

Complications

- Stone impaction in the choledochal duct
- Acute cholecystitis
- Gall bladder empyema/perforation
- Purulent cholangitis
- Liver abscesses
- Biliary pancreatitis
- Mirizzi's syndrome: larger trapped stone in the cystic duct compresses the common hepatic duct or the choledochal duct:
  - Penetration into the duodenum—gallstone ileus
  - Development of biliodigestive fistulas possible
- Shrinking gallbladder: after recurrent inflammation and scarring
- Porcelain Bubble:
  - Chronic calcifying cholecystitis
  - Increased risk of carcinoma

Annual complication rate
- After first colic = 1–3%
- In asymptomatic stone carriers = 0.1–0.3%

Diagnosis

Clinical Presentation

- Pressure pain right upper abdomen
- possibly palpable tumor
- Murphy's sign (focal pain under direct pressure) on inspiration
- possibly sclerenicterus

Lab Chemistry

- Bilirubin, AP, γ-GT, if necessary GOT, GPT, lipase, amylase, blood count, CRP

Imaging Non-Invasive Procedures

- Sonography:
  - Sensitivity >95
  - Standardized transcutaneous B-mode sonography
  - Complete visualization of the gallbladder in variable sectional planes (in at least 2 patient positioning variants, offset by 90° to each other)
  - Assessment of: Gallbladder stones, sludge, wall composition, caliber ductus hepaticocholedochus (up to 7 mm normal), free fluid, cholestasis intrahepatic, liver abscesses, pancreatic head, multilayered wall (cholecystitis)
- CT:
  - For poor sound conditions
  - In the case of complicated courses in individual cases
  - In case of suspected tumor for differential diagnosis
- MRI/MRCP:
  - In case of suspected tumor for differential diagnosis
- Oral/i.v. cholangiography:
  - Almost no longer used for the diagnosis of gallstones

Imaging Invasive Procedures

- ERCP (endoscopic retrograde cholangiopancreaticography):
  - For choledocholithiasis
  - If necessary in combination with papillotomy
  - In biliary pancreatitis with cholestasis/icterus and/or signs of cholangitis: as soon as possible
  - For cholangitis within 2 h after admission
- Therapeutic splitting: Bile duct repair by ERCP before cholecystectomy (CCE)
- PCT (percutaneous transhepatic cholangiography):
  - Only rarely, if ERCP is not possible

Further Etiological Clarification

- In case of unusual clinical constellation (e.g. family history, occurrence in childhood and adolescence, intrahepatic microstones, association with diarrhoea)
- Possible etiologies: e.g., hemolytic anemias, bile acidosis syndrome, drug history, infections

Therapy

Conservative Therapy

- Serious complications: only 2% of gallstone carriers
- If asymptomatic cholecystolithiasis = monitoring, no indication for therapy

Surgical Therapy

- Surgery indications
  - Symptomatic uncomplicated or complicated cholecystolithiasis
  - Asymptomatic patients with porcelain gallbladder: due to increased risk of carcinoma
  - Asymptomatic patients with gallbladder stones >3 cm in diameter: Because of increased risk of carcinoma (in men nine- to ten-fold)
  - In major abdominal surgery: simultaneous cholecystectomy even for asymptomatic stones
  - Surgery may be considered in
    - patients with *chronic hemolytic diseases* due to increased risk of biliary symptoms
    - *undergoing solid organ Tx* due to increase risk of developing symptoms post-Tx
    - *bariatric surgery patients*

Caution

- No indication in asymptomatic cholecystolithiasis with gallbladder stones <3 cm in diameter
- In the first and second trimester of pregnancy only in case of urgent indication (laparoscopic, intraabdominal pressure below 12 mmHg, intraoperative fetal monitoring), otherwise post partum
- OP procedure

- Laparoscopic/robotic cholecystectomy:
  - Worldwide standard procedure (more than 93% of all cholecystectomies started laparoscopically)
  - Conversion rate to open cholecystectomy = 4–7%
  - Identical complication rates with shorter hospital stay and shorter convalescence (fewer wound infections)
  - Contraindication laparoscopic: Manifest portal hypertension (relative), liver cirrhosis MELD score >8, gallbladder carcinoma, severe pulmonary obstruction, gravidity third trimester
- Open cholecystectomy:
  - Well suited for unclear conditions
  - In case of suspected tumor or strong bleeding tendency
- Mini-laparotomy cholecystectomy:
  - Laparotomy <8 cm
  - No differences to laparoscopic cholecystectomy with regard to complication rates, length of hospital stay and convalescence times
- NOTES cholecystectomy ("natural orifice transluminal endoscopic surgery"):
  - Transvaginal or transgastric
  - Elective surgery only
  - Complication rate = 3.1%, conversion rate = 4.9% (German NOTES registry)

Surgical Procedure

Laparoscopic Cholecystectomy

- Supine position with legs apart or flat supine position
- Surgeon between legs or left
- Access pneumoperitoneum at 12 mmHg, (Veress needle) or mini-laparotomy via subumbilical skin incision approx. 1.5 cm
- Insertion camera trocar + 10 mm working trocar + 1–2 × 5 mm working trocars
- Elevating the gallbladder and pulling the infundibulum to the right
- Representing the Calot Triangle
- Dissection of the cystic duct and cystic artery, including visualization of the opening into the choledochal duct.
- Clip supply—2 each to central, 1 to peripheral
- Subserosal release of the gall bladder and transfer to salvage bag
- Hemostasis
- Moving the camera in 10 mm trocar
- Removal of the gallbladder via a subumbilical skin incision, if necessary with a spreading instrument (using a salvage bag)

Inspection of the surgical area, removal of the trocars under visual control, fascial closure, skin suture.

Surgical Procedure

Open Cholecystectomy

- Rib-arch margin incision or transrectal incision
- Antegrade subserosal extirpation of the gallbladder
- Settling of the cystic duct + cystic artery in Calot's triangle near the gallbladder
- Clip supply of these structures—2 each to central, 1 to peripheral

- Complications
  - Recurrent cholelithiasis = 2% of cases
  - Bile leak (mostly liver bed) = 0.4–1.5%
  - Wound infection = 1.3–1.8%
  - Pancreatitis = 0.3
  - Bleeding = 0.2–1.4
  - Bile duct injury rate = 0.2–0.4%
  - Subhepatic abscess
  - Infected bilioma/hematoma
  - Occlusive icterus due to remaining concrements

- Post surgical care
  - Clinical control first post-op day
  - Blood count, CRP and bilirubin on post-op day 2
  - Discharge when symptom-free + laboratory inconspicuous
  - In case of bilirubin elevation: sonography to exclude cholestasis

Gallbladder Polyps

Definition

- Benign tumors of the gallbladder wall
- Subdivision into 2 groups:
  - Benign pseudotumors (e.g. cholesterol polyps or adenomatosis)
  - Adenomas

Epidemiology

- Prevalence of gallbladder polyps = between 1 and 7%
- Polyps ≥1 cm in diameter = significantly increased probability of neoplastic genesis (adenomas) = risk of carcinoma in up to 50%
- Risk factors for adenoma development:
  - Age > 50 years
  - Solitary polyps
  - Gallstones
- Presence of more than one polyp = speaks against an adenoma and for the presence of cholesterol polyps
- Risk factors for malignancy:
  - Age > 60 years
  - Coexistence gallstones
  - Size increase
  - Size >10 mm

Clinical Presentation

- Mostly asymptomatic
- Otherwise see Cholecystolithiasis

Diagnosis

- Sonography
  - No change in position when repositioning the patient
- If necessary endosonography and CT

Therapy

Surgical Therapy

- Surgery indication
  - Gallbladder polyps ≥1 cm: Independent of symptoms
  - For polyps >18–20 mm: Because of the significant risk of malignancy, primarily consider open cholecystectomy
- Laparoscopic vs. open cholecystectomy

Conservative Therapy

- For polyps <1 cm
- Sonographic control:
  - Initially every 6 months
  - Later annually, if no increase in size

Acute Cholecystitis

Definition

- The most frequent complication of cholecystolithiasis
- Acute inflammation of the gallbladder wall

Pathophysiology

Course

- Stone entrapment with passive or permanent occlusion of the cystic duct
- Gallbladder hydrops with abacterial infection
- Secondary colonization by ascension from duodenum or hematogenous/lymphogenous dissemination
- possibly gallbladder empyema and ulcerophlegmonous course

Other Risk Factors

- Diabetes mellitus
- Atrial fibrillation
- Terminal renal failure
- Severe liver dysfunction

Symptoms

Symptoms

- Colicky upper abdominal pain
- Fever + possibly chills
- Nausea + vomiting

Complications of Acute Cholecystitis

- Gallbladder gangrene
- Gall bladder empyema or perforation
- Rare formation of biliodigestive fistula (60% to the duodenum)
- Gallstone ileus

Diagnosis

Clinical Presentation

- Positive Murphy sign
- Defensive tension right upper quadrant in peritonitis

Lab

- AP, γ-GT, transaminases, bilirubin, lipase, coagulation parameters (INR, PTT), CRP and blood count
- Clear signs of infection: leukocytes plus CRP elevated
- Cholangitis: AP, γ-GT elevated

Sonography

- Sensitivity = 94%; Specificity = 78%
- Wall thickening (>4 mm) with possibly triple stratification of the gallbladder
- Pericholecystitis with free fluid
- Dense internal pattern: with empyema
- Evidence of covered or open perforation, if applicable

Therapy

- Always operative

Indication

- If acute cholecystitis is detected, surgery is indicated immediately
- In patients on anticoagulants:
  - If necessary, adjustment of coagulation or start of fluid substitution
  - Antibiotic administration and electrolyte balance
  - Subsequent early selective surgery within 1–3 days
- If patient cannot be operated early (diagnosis too late, other medical reasons (= too high risk of surgery): Cholecystectomy in interval only after 6 weeks
- ACDC ("acute cholecystitis: early versus delayed cholecystectomy") study (Gutt et al. 2013): early selective laparoscopic cholecystectomy vs. interval cholecystectomy after primary conservative antibiotic therapy:
  - Reduction of morbidity and mortality
  - Total in hospital time significantly lower
  - Significantly reduced hospital costs
  - Comparable numbers of bile duct injuries and bile leakages

OP Procedure

- Laparoscopic cholecystectomy:
  - Standard procedure
  - Conversion rate 2–7% (some series up to 20%)
- Primary open surgery:
  - In case of expected complications
  - In case of multiple previous operations
  - For "intensive gallbladder"

Acute cholecystitis in patients requiring intensive care (acute acalculous cholecystitis):

- Incidence = 0.2–0.4% in patients who were in an intensive care unit for more than 2 days
- Often associated with high morbidity and mortality
- Surgical rehabilitation obligatory as long as no clinical contraindications are present
- Open procedure justified with similar peri- and postoperative complication rates
- No operability given:
  - Interventional percutaneous cholecystostomy or endoscopic transpapillary bile duct drainage
  - Secondary cholecystectomy after re-evaluation and stabilization of the patient (early or late elective = no clear recommendations)

8.5.2 Benign Diseases of the Bile Ducts

Key Points

- Choledocholithiasis in up to 15% of patients with cholecystolithiasis
- Hyperbilirubinemia + sonographically dilated bile duct suspicious

- Therapeutic splitting ERC (endoscopic retrograde cholangiography) and CCE (cholecystectomy) recommended
- Choledochal cysts very rare overall

Choledocholithiasis

Definition

- Concrement in the common bile duct (Ductus choledochus)
- Most frequently: formation of the calculus in the gallbladder and migration into the choledochal duct; rarely formation directly in the choledochus

Epidemiology

- Prevalence of gallstones in patients with cholecystolithiasis = age-dependent: 5–15%
- High probability of simultaneous choledocholithiasis in:
  - Sonographically dilated bile duct (>7–10 mm) + hyperbilirubinemia + elevated γ-GT/GPT
  - Bile duct >10 mm + gallbladder stones + colic
  - Direct sonographic detection of stones in the bile duct

Clinical Presentation

- Strong evidence of choledocholithiasis
  - Cholangitis
  - Stone visible in ultrasound
  - Icterus
  - Hyperbilirubinemia + sonographically dilated bile duct

Therapy

Indication

- Patients with gallbladder + bile duct stones = therapeutic splitting recommended
- Preoperative ERC = primary procedure in combination with papillotomy
- In case of cholangitis or severe biliary pancreatitis within 24 h
  - Cholecystectomy only after pancreatitis has subsided
  - In case of cholecystolithiasis under risk assessment = cholecystectomy within 6 weeks if possible
- Symptomatic bile duct stones in gravidity: primary endoscopic papillotomy + stone extraction
- If ERCP is not possible:
  - Laparoscopic cholecystectomy + simultaneous surgical bile duct revision (transcystic bile duct exploration or laparoscopic choledochotomy, cholangiography and extraction via grasping forceps, basket, Fogarty catheter if necessary with bougienage of the papilla), if expertise available
  - Insertion of a T-drainage possible

Choledochal Cysts

Definition

- Cystic dilatation of the choledochus
- Affects extra- and/or intrahepatic bile ducts
- Mostly indication for surgical therapy

Epidemiology

- Rare clinical picture: incidence = 1/100.000 to 1/150.000 in western countries
- More common in Japan
- Women: Men = 7–8: 1
- Genetic predisposition

Pathogenesis

- Abnormal connection between the choledochus and the pancreatic duct
- Reflux of pancreatic juice into distal choledochus = chronic inflammation = slackening of the choledochal wall
- Classification according to Todani/Alonso-Lej

Clinical Presentation

- Classic triad (only 10% of patients):
  - Pain in the right upper abdomen
  - Icterus
  - Abdominal mass
- Complications (if left long term without surgical treatment)
  - Portal hypertension
  - Cirrhosis of the liver
  - Biliary obstruction
  - Malignant degeneration = 2.5–26%

Diagnosis

- Lab
  - Liver dysfunction (60% of cases)
- Sonography
- CT/MRI abdomen
- ERCP/percutaneous transhepatic cholangiography (PTC)

Therapy

- Targets
  - Symptom relief
  - Preventing complications
- Technique = cholecystectomy + resection of the extrahepatic cyst-bearing bile ducts if necessary biliodigestive anastomosis

8.5.3 Gallbladder Carcinoma

Epidemiology

- Incidental finding in 0.2–0.4% of cholecystectomies
- Proportion of potentially resectable gallbladder carcinomas at the time of diagnosis = 10–30%
- Risk factors:
  - Disposition due to cholecystolithiasis (1–3%)
  - Porcelain gallbladder (–20%) = indication for surgery even without tumor evidence in imaging
  - Gallbladder polyps = metaplasia-dysplasia pathway and adenoma-carcinoma sequence identified

Symptoms

- Often asymptomatic
- History of cholecystolithiasis
- Courvoisier sign = painless palpable enlargement of the gallbladder, if applicable
- Later: Icterus, B-symptomatics

Diagnosis

Sonography

- Mural tumor
- Expansion in the liver bed
- Metastases intrahepatic

CT Abdomen and Thorax

- Environment diagnosis
- Exclusion of metastases intrahepatic
- OP planning

Alternative MRI with Magnetic Resonance Cholangiopancreatography (MRCP)

- Exclusion of intrahepatic metastases
- OP planning
- Assessment of the intra- and extrahepatic bile ducts
- If necessary ERCP for the evaluation of the intra- and extrahepatic bile ducts

TNM Classification and Staging (UICC 2010)

TNM Classification

- T (tumor)
  - T1 Tumor infiltrates lamina propria or musculature
  - T1a Tumor infiltrates mucosa
  - T1b Tumor infiltrates bile duct muscles
  - T2 Tumour infiltrates perimuscular connective tissue, but no spread via serosa or liver
  - T3 Infiltration of serosa or infiltration of liver and/or other organ such as stomach, colon, pancreas, extrahepatic bile ducts or other organs
  - T4 infiltration of portal vein or hepatic artery or multiple extrahepatic organs
- N (lymph nodes)
  - N0 No regional lymph nodes affected
  - N1 Regional lymph nodes affected
- M (metastases)
  - M0 No distant metastases
  - M1 distant metastases

UICC Stages According to the TNM Classification (2010)

Stage Ia	T1	N0	M0
Stage Ib	T2	N0	M0
Stage IIa	T3	N0	M0
Stage IIb	T1, T2, T3	N1	M0
Stage III	T4	Each N	M0
Stage IV	Each T	Each N	M1

Therapy

Surgical Therapy

- Complete resection = only curative approach

OP Indication/Strategy

- Extent of surgery depends on TNM stage (see above):
  - T1a cholecystectomy
  - T1b Radical cholecystectomy—resection in the liver bed 3 cm hem apical + lymphadenectomy
  - T2 en bloc resection Couinaud segments IVb and V + lymphadenectomy; 5-year survival 40% vs. 90%
  - T3 Extended right hemihepatectomy + lymphadenectomy
  - T3 with infiltration of an extrahepatic organ or T4 individual decision only; 5-year survival <10%
- If incidental finding after cholecystectomy:
  - Early resection within 2 to max. 4 weeks
  - Goal = Avoid lymphogenic and peritoneal metastasis according to recommendations
- If incidental finding during cholecystectomy:
  - Switch to open procedure
  - Resection according to recommendations
  - If no expertise for liver resection available = early presentation to liver center within 2 to max. 4 weeks
- If gallbladder carcinoma suspected in diagnosis:
  - Either diagnostic laparoscopy in case of frequent early peritoneal metastasis and open resection according to recommendations
  - If no expertise for liver resection available = immediate presentation to liver center
- Early lymphogenic metastasis = extensive lymphadenectomy, ligamentum hepatoduodenale to the truncus coeliacus
- Always excise trocar injection channels to avoid cutaneous metastases

Adjuvant Therapy

- According to current guidelines
- Preferably inclusion of patients in randomized controlled trials

Malignant diseases of the bile ducts are discussed in the chapter on malignant diseases of the liver with Klatskin tumours (► Sect. 8.2.2).

References

Belghiti J et al (2000) The Brisbane terminology of liver anatomy and resections. HPB 2:333–339

Bento de Sousa JH, Calil IL, Tustumi F, da Cunha KD, Felga GEG, de Arruda Pecora RA, de Almeida MD (2021) Comparison between Milan and UCSF criteria for liver transplantation in patients with hepatocellular carcinoma: a systematic review and meta-analysis. Transl Gastroenterol Hepatol 5(6):11

Ceresa CDL, Nasralla D, Pollok JM, Friend PJ (2022) Machine perfusion of the liver: applications in transplantation and beyond. Nat Rev Gastroenterol Hepatol 19(3):199–209

Cusi K, Isaacs S, Barb D, Basu R, Caprio S, Garvey WT, Kashyap S, Mechanick JI, Mouzaki M, Nadolsky K, Rinella ME, Vos MB, Younossi Z (2022) American Association of Clinical Endocrinology Clinical Practice Guideline for the diagnosis and management of nonalcoholic fatty liver disease in primary care and endocrinology clinical settings: co-sponsored by the American Association for the Study of Liver Diseases (AASLD). Endocr Pract 28(5):528–562

de Santibañes E, Ardiles V, Alvarez FA, Busnelli VC, de Santibañes M (2017) Extreme hepatic surgery and other strategies. Springer, Heidelberg

European Association for the Study of the Liver. Electronic address: easloffice@easloffice.eu; European Association for the Study of the Liver (2018) EASL clinical practice guidelines: management of hepatocellular carcinoma. J Hepatol 69(1):182–236

Gutt CN, Encke J, Köninger J, Harnoss JC, Weigand K, Kipfmüller K, Schunter O, Götze T, Golling MT, Menges M, Klar E, Feilhauer K, Zoller WG, Ridwelski K, Ackmann S, Baron A, Schön MR, Seitz HK, Daniel D, Stremmel W, Büchler MW (2013) Acute cholecystitis: early versus delayed cholecystectomy, a multicenter randomized trial (ACDC study, NCT00447304). Ann Surg 258:385–393

Houben P, Büchler MW, Schemmer P (2014) Use of an electrothermal bipolar vessel sealing device during recipient hepatectomy for liver transplantation. J Am Coll Surg 219(5):e59–e63

Karangwa S, Panayotova G, Dutkowski P, Porte RJ, Guarrera JV, Schlegel A (2020) Hypothermic machine perfusion in liver transplantation. Int J Surg 82S:44–51

Kniepeiss D, Stiegler P, Talakic E, Schemmer P (2020) Anterior approach for hepatectomy before piggyback liver transplantation in giant polycystic liver disease. Liver Transpl 26(12):1662–1664. https://doi.org/10.1002/lt.25824. Epub ahead of print

Koch M, Garden OJ, Padbury R, Rahbari NN, Adam R, Capussotti L, Tat Fan S, Yokoyama Y, Crawford M, Makuuchi M, Christophi C, Banting S, Brooke-Smith M, Usatoff V, Nagino M, Maddern G, Hugh TJ, Vauthey JN, Greig P, Rees M, Nimura Y, Figueras J, DeMatteo RP, Büchler MW, Weitz J (2011) Bile leakage after hepatobiliary and pancreatic surgery: a definition and grading of severity by the International Study Group of Liver Surgery. Surgery 149(5):680–688

Lin S, Hoffmann K, Schemmer P (2012) Treatment of hepatocellular carcinoma: a systematic review. Liver Cancer 1(3–4):144–158

Martins PN, Buchwald JE, Mergental H, Vargas L, Quintini C (2020) The role of normothermic machine perfusion in liver transplantation. Int J Surg 82S:52–60

Murtha-Lemekhova A, Fuchs J, Hoffmann K (2022) Innovation for the sake of innovation? How does robotic hepatectomy compare to laparoscopic or open resection for HCC—A systematic review and meta-analysis. Cancers (Basel) 14(14):3359

Rahbari NN, Garden OJ, Padbury R, Brooke-Smith M, Crawford M, Adam R, Koch M, Makuuchi M, Dematteo RP, Christophi C, Banting S, Usatoff V, Nagino M, Maddern G, Hugh TJ, Vauthey JN, Greig P, Rees M, Yokoyama Y, Tat Fan S, Weitz J (2011) Posthepatectomy liver failure: a definition and grading by the International Study Group of Liver Surgery (ISGLS). Surgery 149(5):713–724

Schemmer P, Friess H, Hinz U, Mehrabi A, Kraus TW, Z'graggen K, Schmidt J, Uhl W, Büchler MW (2006) Stapler hepatectomy is a safe dissection technique: analysis of 300 patients. World J Surg 30(3):419–430

Scott-Conner CEH (2002) Chassin's operative strategy in general surgery. An expositive atlas, 3. Aufl. Springer, New York

Sousa Da Silva RX, Weber A, Dutkowski P, Clavien PA (2022) Machine perfusion in liver transplantation. Hepatology 76(5):1531–1549

van Rijn R, Schurink IJ, de Vries Y, van den Berg AP, Cortes Cerisuelo M, Darwish Murad S, Erdmann JI, Gilbo N, de Haas RJ, Heaton N, van Hoek B, Huurman VAL, Jochmans I, van Leeuwen OB, de Meijer VE, Monbaliu D, Polak WG, Slangen JJG, Troisi RI, Vanlander A, de Jonge J, Porte RJ, DHOPE-DCD Trial Investigators (2021) Hypothermic machine perfusion in liver transplantation—a randomized Trial. N Engl J Med 384(15):1391–1401

8

Further Reading

Adam R, Kitano Y, Abdelrafee A, Allard MA, Baba H (2020) Debulking surgery for colorectal liver metastases: foolish or chance? Surg Oncol 33:266–269

Arroyo V, Moreau R, Jalan R (2020) Acute-on-chronic liver failure. N Engl J Med 382:2137–2145

Asencio JM, Sabrido JLG, Olmedilla L (2014) How to expand the safe limits in hepatic resections? J Hepatobiliary Pancreat Sci 21:399–404

Baili E, Tsilimigras DI, Moris D, Sahara K, Pawlik TM (2020) Technical modifications and outcomes after associating liver partition and portal vein ligation for staged hepatectomy (ALPPS) for primary liver malignancies: a systematic review. Surg Oncol 33:70–80

Banales JM, Marin JJG, Lamarca A, Rodrigues PM, Khan SA, Roberts LR, Cardinale V, Carpino G, Andersen JB, Braconi C, Calvisi DF, Perugorria MJ, Fabris L, Boulter L, Macias RIR, Gaudio E, Alvaro D, Gradilone SA, Strazzabosco M, Marzioni M, Coulouarn C, Fouassier L, Raggi C, Invernizzi P, Mertens JC, Moncsek A, Rizvi S, Heimbach J, Koerkamp BG, Bruix J, Forner A, Bridgewater J, Valle JW, Gores GJ (2020) Nat Rev Gastroenterol Hepatol. https://doi.org/10.1038/s41575-020-0310

Best LM, Leung J, Freeman SC, Sutton AJ, Cooper NJ, Milne EJ, Cowlin M, Payne A, Walshaw D, Thorburn D, Pavlov CS, Davidson BR, Tsochatzis E, Williams NR, Gurusamy KS (2020) Induction immunosuppression in adult undergoing liver transplantation: a network meta-analysis. Cochrane Database Syst Rev 1:CD013203

Cai W, Liu Z, Xiao Y, Zhang W, Tang D, Cheng B, Li Q (2019) Comparison of clinical outcomes of laparoscopic versus open surgery for recurrent hepatocellular carcinoma: a meta-analysis. Surg Endosc 33:3550–3557

Caruso S, O'Brien DR, Cleary SP, Roberts LR, Zucman-Rossi J (2020) Genetics of HCC: novel approaches to explore molecular diversity. Hepatology https://doi.org/10.1002/hep.31394

Castaing D, Azoulay D, Adam R (2006) Chirurgie du foie et de l'hypertension portale. Elsevier, Masson Paris

Cho HD, Samstein B, Chaundry S, Kim KH (2020) Minimally invasive donor hepatectomy, systemic review. Int J Surg 82S:187–191. https://doi.org/10.1016/j.ijsu.2020.06.023

Chu KK, Wong KH, Chok KS (2021) Expanding indications for liver transplant: tumor and patient factors. Gut Liver 15(1):19–30. https://doi.org/10.5009/gnl19265

de'Angelis N, Baldini C, Brustia R, Pessaux P, Sommacale D, Laurent A, Le Roy B, Tacher V, Kobeiter H, Luciani A, Paillaud E, Aparicio T, Canuï-Poitrine F, Liuu E (2020) Surgical and regional treatments for colorectal cancer metastases in older patients: a systematic review and meta-analysis. PLoS One 15(4):e0230914. https://doi.org/10.1371/journal.pone.0230914

Di Martino M, Rompianesi G, Mora-Guzmán I, Martín-Pérez E, Montati R, Troisi RI (2020) Systematic review and meta-analysis of local ablative therapies for resectable colorectal liver metastases. Eur J Surg Oncol 46:772–781

Dufour JF, Caussy C, Loomba R (2020) Combination therapy for non-alcoholic steatohepatitis: ratinale, opportunities and challenges. Gut 69(10):1877–1884. https://doi.org/10.1136/gutjnl-2019-319104
Edgar L, Pu T, Porter B, Aziz JM, La Pointe C, Asthana A, Orlando G (2020) Regenerative medicine, organ bioengenering and transplantation. Br J Surg 107:793–800
Fatourou EM, Tsochatzis EA (2019) Management of metabolic syndrome and cardiovascular risk after liver transplantation. Lancet Gastroenterol Hepatol 4:731–741
Gangi A, Howe JR (2020) The landmark series: neuroendocrine tumor liver metastases. Ann Surg Oncol 27(9):3270–3280. https://doi.org/10.1245/s10434-020-08787
Gavriilidis P, Roberts KJ, Aldrighetti L, Sutcliffe RP (2020) A comparison between robotic, laparoscopic and open hepatectomy: a systematic review and network meta-analysis. Eur J Surg Oncol 46:1214–1224
Gentile D, Donadon M, Lleo A, Aghemo A, Roncalli M, di Tommaso L, Torzilli G (2020) Surgical treatment of hepatocholangiocarcinoma: a systematic review. Liver Cancer 9:15–27
Guglielmi A, Ruzzenente A, Conci S, Valdegamberi A, Iacono C (2012) How much remnant is enough in liver resection? Dig Surg 29:6–17
Im GY, Neuberger J (2020) Debate on selection criteria for liver transplantation for alcoholic hepatitis: tighten or loosen? Liver Transpl 26:916–921
Jarnagin WR (2012) Blumgart's surgery of the liver, biliary tract and pancreas, 5. Aufl. Elsevier, Philadelphia
Jung KW, Kang J, Kwon HM, Moon YJ, Jun IG, Song JG, Hwang GS (2019) Effects of remote ischemic preconditioning conducted in living liver donors on postoperative liver function in donors and recipients following liver transplantation: a randomized clinical trial. Ann Surg 271:646–653
Jung KW, Kang J, Kwon HM, Moon YJ, Jun IG, Song JG, Hwang GS (2020) Effect of remote ischemic preconditioning conducted in living liver donors on postoperative liver function in donors and recipients following liver transplantation: a randomized clinical trial. Ann Surg 271:646–653
Ke Q, Lin N, Deng M, Wang L, Zeng Y, Liu J (2020) The effect of adjuvant therapy for patients with intrahepatic cholangiocarcinoma after surgical resection: a systematic review and meta-analysis. PLoS One 15:e0229292
Kniepeiss D, Talakic E, Schemmer P (2020a) Echinococcus granulosus: a novel parenchymal sparing surgical treatment. Hepatobiliary Pancreat Dis Int 19(4):390–393
Kniepeiss D, Rosenkranz AR, Fickert P, Schemmer P (2020b) Update Immunsuppression bei Organtransplantation. Allgemein Viszeralchirurgie up2date 14:223–235
Kniepeiss D, Talakic E, Schemmer P (2020c) Interventionelle und chirurgische Therapie non-kolorektaler Lebermetastasen. Allgemein Viszeralchirurgie up2date 14:379–395
Kohut TJ, Barandiaran JF, Keating BJ (2020) Genomics and liver transplantation: genomic biomarkers for the diagnosis of acute cellular rejection. Liver Transpl 26(10):1337–1350. https://doi.org/10.1002/lt.25812
Kokudo T, Hasegawa K, Shirata C, Tanimoto M, Ishizawa T, Kaneko J, Akamatsu N, Arita J, Demartines N, Uldry E, Kokudo N, Halkic N (2019) Assessment of preoperative liver function for surgical resection in patients with hepatocellular carcinoma. Liver Cancer 8:447–456
Kremer M, Manzini G, Hristov B, Polychronidis G, Mokry T, Sommer CM, Mehrabi A, Weitz J, Büchler MW, Schemmer P (2015) Impact of neoadjuvant chemotherapy on hypertrophy of the future liver remnant after associating liver partition and portal vein ligation for staged hepatectomy. J Am Coll Surg 221(3):717–728
Kvietkauskas M, Zitkute V, Leber B, Strupas K, Stiegler P, Schemmer P (2020) The role of metabolomics in current concepts of organ preservation. Int J Mol Sci 21(18):E6607
Lafaro KJ, Stewart C, Fong A, Fong Y (2020) Robotic liver resection. Surg Clin North Am 100:265–281
Lang H, Huber T (2020) Virtual and augmented reality in liver surgery. Ann Surg 271:e8
Lee TC, Kaiser TE, Alloway R, Woodle ES, Edwards MJ, Shah SA (2019) Telemedicine based remote home monitoring after liver transplantation: results of a randomized prospective trial. Ann Surg 270:564–572
Lin XJ, Yang J, Chen XB, Zhang M, Xu MQ (2014) The critical value of remnant liver volume-to-body weight ratio to estimate posthepatectomy liver failure in cirrhotic patients. J Surg Res 188:489–495
Lingiah VA, Niazi M, Olivo R, Paterno F, Guarrera JV, Pyrsopoulos NT (2020) Liver transplantation beyond Milan criteria. J Clin Transl Hepatol 8:69–75
Massironi S, Pilla L, Elvevi A, Longarini R, Rossi RE, Bidoli P, Invernizzi P (2020) New emerging systemic therapeutic options for advanced cholangiocarcinoma. Cell 9:688
Mathurin P, Lucey MR (2020) Liver transplantation in patients with alcohol-related liver disease: current status and future directions. Lancet Gastroenterol Hepatol 5:507–514
Mayer P, Grözinger M, Mokry T, Schemmer P, Waldburger N, Kauczor HU, Klauss M, Sommer CM (2019) Semi-automated computed tomography volumetry can predict hemihepatectomy specimens' volumes in patients with hepatic malignancy. BMC Med Imaging 19(1):20
Mejia JC, Pasko J (2020) Primary liver cancers: intrahepatic cholangiocarcinoma and hepatocellular carcinoma. Surg Clin North Am 100:535–549
Michal K, Sau M, Tamara GMH, Long JR (2020) A better route to ALPPS: minimally invasive vs open ALPPS. Surg Endosc 34:2379–2389
Moris D, Kostakis ID, Machairas N, Prodromidou A, Tsilimigras DI, Ravindra KV, Sudan DL, Knechtle SJ, Barbas AS (2019) Comparison between liver transplantation and resection for hilar

cholangiocarcinoma: a systematic review and meta-analysis. PLoS One 14:e0220527
Nickkholgh A, Nikdad M, Shafie S, Abbasi Dezfoui S, Mehrabi A, Eason JD, Mas VR, Maluf DG (2019) Ex situ liver machine perfusion as an emerging graft protective strategy in clinical liver transplantation: the Dawn of a new era. Transplantation 103: 2003–2011
Nikkholgh A, Nikdad M, Shafie S, Abbasi Dezfouli S, Mehrabi A, Eason JD, Mas VR, Maluf DG (2019) Ex situ machine perfusion as an emerging graft protective strategy in clinical liver transplantation: the Dawn of an era. Transplantation 103:2003–2011
Panayotova GG, Paterno F, Guarrera JV, Lunsford KE (2020) Liver transplantation for cholangiocarcinoma: insights into the prognosis and the evolving indications. Curr Oncol Rep 22:49
Rashidian N, Alseidi A, Kirks RC (2020) Cancers metastatic to the liver. Surg Clin N Am 100:551–563
Rauber A, Kopsch F (1987) Lehrbuch und Atlas der Anatomie des Menschen, Bd 2: Innere Organe. Thieme, Stuttgart
Ren L, Zhu D, Benson AB 3rd, Nordlinger B, Koehne CH, Delaney CP, Kerr D, Lenz HJ, Fan J, Wang J, Gu J, Li J, Shen L, Tsarkov P, Tejpar S, Zheng S, Zhang S, Gruenberger T, Qin X, Wang X, Zhang Z, Poston GJ, Xu J, SINCE Group (2020) Shangai international consensus on diagnosis and comprehensive treatment of colorectal liver metastases (version 2019). Eur J Surg Oncol 46:955–966
Sakon M, Kobayashi S, Wada H, Eguchi H, Marubashi S, Takahashi H, Akita H, Gotoh K, Yamada D, Asukai K, Hasegawa S, Ohue M, Yano M, Nagano H (2020) "Logic-based Medicine" is more feasible than "evidence-based medicine" in the local treatment for hepatocellular carcinoma. Oncology 98: 259–266
Schoening WN, Denecke T, Neumann UP (2015) Präoperative Bildgebung/Operationsplanung für die Leberchirurgie. Chirurg 86:1167–1182
Sheka AC, Adeyi O, Thompson J, Hameed B, Crawford PA, Ikramuddin S (2020) Nonalcoholic steatohepatitis: a review. JAMA 323:1175–1183
Singh N, Winston DJ, Razonable RR, Lyon GM, Silveira FP, Wagener MM, Stevens-Ayers T, Edminson B, Boeckh M, Limaye AP (2020) Effect of preemptive therapy vs antiviral prophylaxis on cytomegalovirus disease in seronegative liver transplant recipients with seropositive donors: a randomized clinical trial. JAMA 323:1378–1387
Standring S (2009) Gray's anatomy. The anatomical basis of clinical practice, 40. Aufl. Churchill Livingstone, Elsevier, London
Stravitz RT, Lee WM (2019) Acute liver failure. Lancet 394:869–881
Talakic E, Janek E, Mikalauskas S, Schemmer P. Liver transplantation in malignancies: a comprehensive and systematic review on oncological outcome. Visc Med 2021;37:302–14
Trebicka J, Sundaram V, Moreau R, Jalan R, Arroyo V (2020) Liver transplantation for acute-on-chronic liver failure: science or fiction? Liver Transpl 26: 906–915
Troisi RI, Pegoraro F, Giglio MC, Rompianesi G, Berardi G, Tomassini F, De Simone G, Aprea G, Montalti R, De Palma GD (2020) Robotic approach to the liver: open surgery in a closed abdomen laparoscopic surgery with technical constraints? Surg Oncol 33: 239–248
Vierling JM, Kerkar N, Czaja AJ, Mack CL, Adams D, Assis D, Manns M, Mayo M, Nayfeh T, Majzoub AMM, Alzuabi MA, Ding J, Haffar S, Murad MH, Alsawas M (2020) Immunosuppressive treatment regiments in autoimmune hepatitis: systematic reviews and meta-analysis supporting AASLD guidelines. Hepatology 72(2):753–769. https://doi.org/10.1002/hep.31407
von Lanz T, Wachsmuth W (2004) Praktische Anatomie, Bauch. Springer, Berlin/Heidelberg
Weisenbacher A, Vrakas G, Nasralla D, Ceresa CDL (2019) The future of organ perfusion and reconditioning. Transpl Int 32:586–597
Zhou J, Chen J, Wie Q, Saeb-Parsy K, Xu X (2020) The role of ischemia-reperfusion injury in early hepatic allograft dysfunction. Liver Transpl 26(8):1034–1048. https://doi.org/10.1002/lt.25779
Zilles K, Tillmann BN (2010) Anatomie. Springer, Berlin/Heidelberg

8

Suggested reading

Kniepeiss D, Schemmer P (2020) Transplantation bei Lebermetastasen neuroendokriner Tumoren—Heilung oder Palliation? J Klein Endokrinol Stoffw 13:54–58

Pancreas

Kim C. Honselmann and Tobias Keck

Contents

F. Billmann, T. Keck (eds.), *Essentials of Visceral Surgery*,
https://doi.org/10.1007/978-3-662-66735-4_9

9.1 Anatomy and Physiology

9.1.1 Definition, Location and Structure

- Endocrine (increment) and exocrine (excretion) gland
- Retroperitoneal position at the level of lumbar vertebrae I–II
- Structure in four parts:
  - Pancreatic head (= Caput pancreatis)
  - Pancreatic isthmus (= Collum pancreatis)
  - Pancreatic body (= Corpus pancreatis)
  - Pancreatic tail (= Cauda pancreatis)

9.1.2 Anatomy and Embryology

Embryology (◘ Fig. 9.1)

- Development from endoderm (= into 2 opposite epithelial buds at caudal end of foregut; at end of fourth week of development):
  - Ventral pancreas: In the angle of the intestine and bile duct, with connection to the choledochal duct
  - Dorsal pancreas: larger, in connection with the foregut (= later duodenum)
- Formation of the pancreatic head (caput pancreatis; ◘ Fig. 9.1):
  - Due to right rotation of the intestine + growth of the duodenum
  - Ventral pancreas origin is located caudal to the dorsal pancreas + fusion of the bile ducts (Ductus Wirsungianus) + excrete together in Papilla duodeni major (Papilla Vateri)-in case of fusion disorder Pancreas divisum
- Formation of the pancreatic corpus + tail
  - Dorsal pancreas alone forms the corpus and cauda pancreatis,
  - Ductus Santorini: Original excretory duct of this origin, opens further proximally in the duodenum at the papilla duodeni minor; frequent obliteration (Cano et al. 2007)

Anatomy

- Localization and size
  - Approx. 16 cm × 3 cm × 2 cm (L × W × D), 60–80 g weight
  - Retroperitoneal at the level of lumbar vertebrae 1–3
  - Pancreatic head in duodenal C; pancreatic tail to splenic hilum
  - Pancreatic body = dorsal border of the bursa omentalis (ventral to the abdominal aorta, inferior vena cava and left adrenal gland)
- Arterial blood supply (◘ Fig. 9.2):
  - Celiac trunc: Superior posterior and anterior pancreaticoduodenal artery and from superior mesenteric artery: anastomosis to gastroduodenal artery (Arcade described by Rio-Branco) + dorsal pancreatic artery from the splenic artery
  - Superior mesenteric artery: inferior pancreaticduodenal artery (forms arcade with superior pancreaticoduodenal artery and connection to gastroduodenal artery, see above)
- Venous outflow via:
  - Pancreaticoduodenal veins (via pancreatic head) into superior mesenteric vein and portal vein
  - Pancreatic veins (multiple veins) flow into the splenic vein (pancreatic tail area)

9.1.3 Physiology

- Two functions: Exocrine and endocrine

Exocrine Function

- External secretion (i.e., in this case, into the intestinal lumen)
- 1.5–3 L secretion daily
- Secretion stimulants: secretin and cholecystokinin
- Pancreatic exocrine tissue (98% of pancreatic tissue) =
  - Acinar cells + ductal epithelial cells
  - Arrangement in acini (=cell groups) around excretory ducts

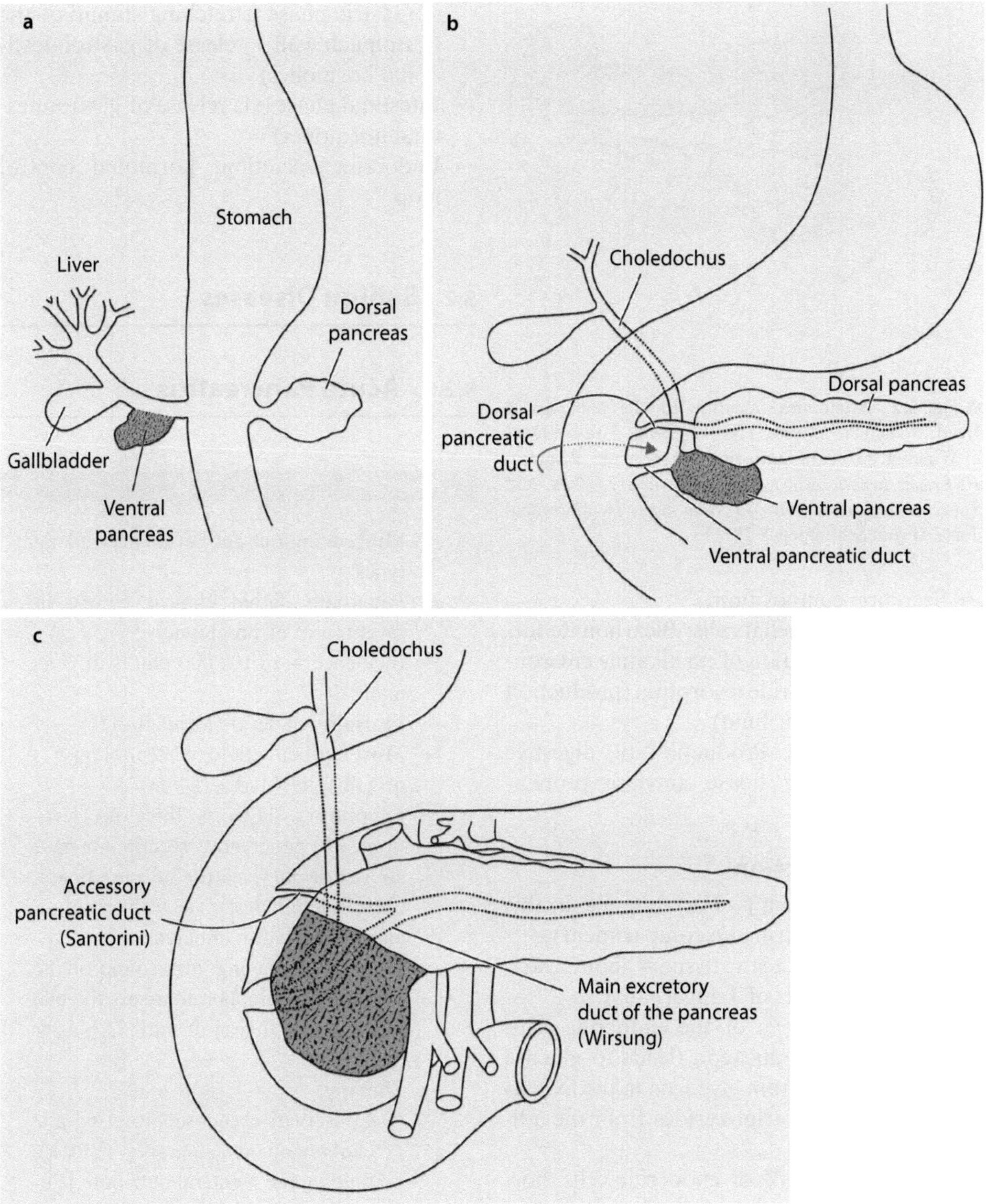

Fig. 9.1 **a–c** Development of the pancreatic origin (embryology). (Mod. according to Schumpelick 2011)

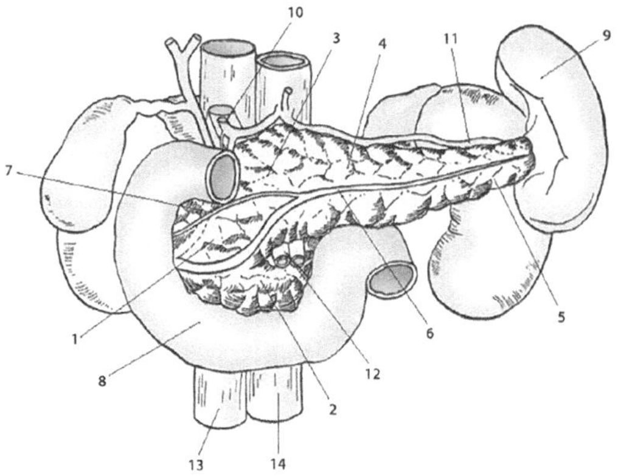

Fig. 9.2 Anatomical location of the pancreas. *1* Head, *2* Uncinate process, *3* Neck, *4* Body, *5* Tail, *6* Duct of Wirsung, *7* Duct of Santorini, *8* Duodenum, *9* Spleen, *10 Proper hepatic artery*, *11 Splenic artery*, *12* A. and Superior mesenteric vein, *13* Vena cava, *14* abdominal aorta. (From Schumpelick 2011)

9

- Secretion composition:
  - Ductal epithelial cells: Bicarbonate formation (creation of an alkaline environment) + chloride resorption (production of an isotonic fluid)
  - Acinar cells: Production of digestive enzymes (e.g. lipase, amylase, proteinases)

Endocrine Function

- Internal secretion (= hormone; i.e. in this case into the plasmatic compartment)
- Endocrine pancreatic tissue = about 2% of the cells (= islets of Langerhans)
  - A(α)-cells: 10% of the endocrine cells, hormone = glucagon (leads to glucose production from glycogen in the liver as well as from triglycerides from the adipocytes)
  - B(β)-cells: 80% of endocrine cells, hormone = insulin (stimulates glucose absorption in liver, fat cells and muscle cells)
  - D(δ)-cells: 10%, hormone = somatostatin (inhibits the secretion of pancreatic enzymes, gastrin and pepsin)

Control of the Functions

- Exocrine secretion:
  - Cephalic phase (olfactory, gustatory, visual stimuli)
  - Gastric phase (stretching stimuli of the stomach wall + release of gastrointestinal hormones)
- Intestinal phase (via release of gastrointestinal hormones)
- Endocrine secretion: hormonal control loop

9.2 Benign Diseases

9.2.1 Acute Pancreatitis

Key Points

- Mild edematous and severe necrotizing types
- Potentially lethal clinical course in severe form of progression
- Incidence = 18/100,000 adults in Germany
- Mortality of severe form: 10–15%
- Most frequent etiology: alcohol (m > f) or gallstones/sludge (f > m)
- Laboratory diagnosis: threefold elevation of pancreatic serum amylase above normal levels (definition), lipase, liver function tests, electrolyte imbalance, coagulation imbalance
- Diagnostic imaging: ultrasound of the abdomen within 24 h to assess the bile ducts, if CT, then wait until 72 h after admission
- Therapy:
  - Conservative: endoscopic retrograde cholangiopancreatography (ERCP), fluid intake + enteral nutrition (jejunal feeding tube if necessary), antibiotics only therapeutically (if microbiology cultures are positive), not prophylactically
  - Operative/Interventional: As late as possible (>4 weeks), only in case of complications such as necrosis or abscess, infection, pseudocyst (step-up approach: drainage → minimally invasive necrosectomy → open necrosectomy)

Definition

- Upper abdominal pain and serum amylase three times above normal
- Temporal inflammatory process
- Autodigestion of the pancreas gland (usually only partial)

Forms

Acute Edematous Pancreatitis

- Self-limiting
- Mild progressive form (80%)

Acute Necrotizing Pancreatitis

- Formation of necrosis (20%)
- Risk = secondary infection of necroses

Epidemiology

Incidence

- 40 new cases per 100,000 population (USA)
- 73 per 100,000 (Finland)
- 18 per 100,000 (Germany)
- Women:Men = 1:1 (different aetiology see above)
- Age = 38–70 years

Etiology

- Biliary (about 40%): Originating from stones in the common bile duct and secondary obstruction of the duct of Wirsung
- Alcohol-induced (approx. 40%)
- Hypertriglyceridemia (approx. 10%)
- After abdominal trauma
- Side effects from medication: Azathioprine, sulfonamides, tetracyclines, valproate, methyldopa, estrogens, 6-mercaptopurine, 5-aminosalicylic acid (5-ASA), corticosteroids, octreotide, furosemide.
- Hereditary
- Viral (children: mumps)
- Hypercalcemia
- Mechanical obstruction (tumor, pancreas divisum, papillary stenosis)
- Tropical pancreatitis

Symptoms

- Severe epigastric pain with belt-like radiation into the back
- Abdomen is taut and elastic: “rubber belly”
- Meteorism
- Fever
- Paralytic (sub)ileus
- Vomiting
- Hypocalcemia
- Skin signs (rare) as a sign of coagulation disorder and as a result of fat tissue necrosis (severe course):
  - Cullen’s sign (periumbilical)
  - Grey Turner sign (flank)
  - Fox sign (inguinal)
- Sepsis
- Septic shock

Diagnosis

Laboratory Diagnosis

- In the serum:
  - Amylase (threefold above normal)
  - More specific (at more than 48 h after symptom onset) = lipase and pancreatic amylase (as distinct from salivary amylase)
  - Coagulation: Onset of *systemic inflammatory response syndrome* (SIRS)
  - Urea (elevation indicative of severe course)
  - Cholestasis parameters: Bilirubin, γ-GT, alkaline phosphatase (AP): Biliary etiology
  - C-reactive protein (for differentiation between edematous and necrotizing pancreatitis) (>120 mg/L); highly sensitive, correlation with progression/development of necrosis, also procalcitonin (PCT)
  - Blood sugar (low is indicative of a severe course)
  - Hematocrit (increase indicative of a severe course)
- In urine: amylase (rare)

Caution
No correlation between level of pancreatic enzymes and severity of pancreatitis, but correlation present for CRP, urea and hematocrit.

Diagnostic Imaging

- Chest and abdominal X-rays:
  - To exclude free abdominal air
  - Detection of pleural effusion, calcifications due to pancreatic secretion, air-fluid level formation
- Contrast-enhanced CT
  - In the presence of necrosis (necroses do not absorb contrast media)
  - Significance for disease course only after 72 h

Risk Assessment (◘ Table 9.1)

9

- Ranson criteria:
  - For mortality estimation
  - For risk assessment of necrotizing pancreatitis: (1 point per item)

◘ **Table 9.1** Ranson criteria for acute pancreatitis

Time	Criterion
On admission (1 point each)	– Age >55 years – WBC >16 G/L – AST >250 U/L – LDH >350 U/L – Glucose >200 mg/dL
After 48 h (1 point each)	– Volume deficit >6 L – BUN increase by >5 mg/dL – Base deficit >4 mmol/L – Drop in P_aO_2 to 60 mmHg – Drop in serum calcium <2 mmol/L
Point total after 48 h	*Mortality*
0–2 points	<1%
3–4 points	15%
5–6 points	40%
>6 points	100%

WBC White blood cell count, *AST* Aspartate Aminotransferase, *LDH* lactate dehydrogenase, *BUN* Blood urea nitrogen, P_aO_2 arterial oxygen partial pressure

Differential Diagnosis

- Acute cholecystitis/cholecystolithiasis
- Mesenteric ischemia/venous thrombosis
- Abdominal aortic aneurysm (AAA)
- Mechanical bowel obstruction
- Perforated gastric ulcer
- Colonic diverticulitis

Therapy

Etiology-Oriented Therapy

- Goal = Elimination of cause, if possible
- Biliary pancreatitis:
  - ERCP + papillotomy (within 24 h)
  - Laparoscopic cholecystectomy: after approx. 5–7 days (during the same inpatient stay for mild pancreatitis); Rationale: Biliary pancreatitis = high recurrence rate at 30%, early (<48 h) laparoscopic cholecystectomy possible for mild pancreatitis (Ranson score <3)
- Alcohol-induced pancreatitis: secondary alcohol withdrawal therapy in the interval
- Hypertriglyceridemia-induced pancreatitis: lower blood lipids
- Medication pancreatitis: discontinue medication

Conservative Therapy

- In edematous pancreatitis:
  - Inpatient admission and monitoring of vital parameters
  - Analgesia: paracetamol, metamizol, tramadol or buprenorphine (use opiates with restraint due to papillary spasm, but not as strictly as in the past)
  - Fluid intake (target = urine output >0.5 mL/kg bw/h)
  - Aim for early enteral feeding (but often gastric emptying disorder)
  - Propulsive medication
  - Gastric tube to prevent vomiting
  - Ulcer prophylaxis
  - Compensation for electrolyte deficiency, calcium only from corr. Calcium level of 0.9 mmol/L [corr. Ca^{2+} = measured Ca^{2+} (mmol/L) × (0.025 × albumin (g/L)) + 1]
- In acute necrotizing pancreatitis:
  - Edema to edematous pancreatitis

- Volume-controlled therapy (PICCO, CVC, pulmonary catheter)
- Intensive care unit with invasive monitoring
- No prophylactic antibiotic administration
- Antibiotics for positive microbiology cultures after diagnostic puncture of fluid accumulation or FNA
- Early enteral nutrition, if necessary via jejunal tube

Step-Up Approach

- In necrotizing pancreatitis with infected necrosis
- First CT-guided drain insertion percutaneously/endoscopically
- In the absence of improvement after 72 h (= improved function of at least 2 organ systems or at least 10% improvement of 2 out of 3 parameters, white blood cell count/CRP and temperature):
  - Retroperitoneoscopic necrosectomy or
  - Transgastric necrosectomy or
  - Open procedure

Operative Therapy Principles

- (Laparoscopic)/Open transabdominal retroperitoneal necrosectomy (disadvantage = elimination of compartmentation)
  - Indication: in the event of ineffective or unsuccessful drainage
  - Wait until the findings are consolidated (if at all possible wait more than 4 weeks until the operation)
  - Imaging of the pancreas
  - Relief from fluid retention
  - Removal of the clay-like necrosis areas in digital preparation—Beware of venous bleeding!

Surgical Procedure

Retroperitoneoscopic Necrosectomy

- CT-guided drainage of the retentive cavity with target drain
- General anesthesia
- Supine position with elevation of the punctured side
- Indwelling urinary catheter
- Access: Five circular incision around the inserted retroperitoneal drainage
- Digital exploration: drainage of the fluid accumulation
- Digital opening of the fluid collection, then insertion of a retroperitoneoscope, necrosectomy above (with grasping forceps/laparoscopic suction/via retroperitoneoscope as optical channel)
- Alternatively, insertion of a long 10-mm trocar + long 10-mm 0° optic via incision into the retroperitoneum
- Inspection of the retroperitoneal cavity + removal of the remaining loose areas with forceps (**caution**: venous bleeding from the splenic vein, if necessary tamponade with tamponade strips and revision after 24 h)
- Final placement of 2 large luminal drains
- Extensive rinsing, if necessary continuous rinsing via drains (disadvantage: rinsing lanes)

Surgical Procedure

Open Retroperitoneal Necrosectomy

- General anesthesia
- Supine position, indwelling urinary catheter
- Approach: Large bilateral subcostal incision
- Opening of the omental bursa
- Mobilization of both colonic flexures
- Removal of necrotic areas by blunt dissection with fingers: paracolic, around the mesenteric root and in the lesser sac (omental bursa) (**caution**: high risk of bleeding). Carefully remove necrotic tissue
- Extensive rinsing
- Insertion of several drains with relaparotomy on demand or
- Insertion of e.g. an ABthera vacuum dressing (3M, St. Paul, MN 55144-1000, USA) (= continuous irrigation of the necrosis area and permanent suction) (**caution**: intestinal fistulas) with

repeated relaparotomies (**caution**: irrigation lanes)
- Postoperative treatment
  - Intensive monitoring
  - SIRS/sepsis therapy

Prognosis
- Lethality (acute edematous pancreatitis) = 1%
- Lethality (acute necrotizing pancreatitis with infected necrosis) >20%

9.2.2 Chronic Pancreatitis

Key Points

- Recurrent episodes of pain
- Alcohol = most common cause
- Pain + complications = surgically treatable
- Alcohol abstinence + nicotine abstinence (progression effect) should be recommended
- Imaging diagnosis: In case of chronic recurrent course = detection of complications + localization before planned pseudocyst removal

Definition
- German Society for Gastroenterology, Digestive and Metabolic Diseases (guideline):
  - Pancreatic disease
  - Recurrent inflammatory episodes and pain
  - Gradual fibrotic remodeling of the gland
  - Progressive loss of exocrine + endocrine pancreatic function

Forms
- Chronic pancreatitis with focal fibrosis
- Chronic pancreatitis with segmental/diffuse fibrosis
- Chronic pancreatitis with or without calcifications (inflammatory pancreatic head pseudotumor)
- Special form:
  - Obstructive chronic pancreatitis (duodenal diverticulum, pancreas divisum, tumors, papillary stenosis)
  - Hereditary chronic pancreatitis
  - Idiopathic chronic pancreatitis: when no cause is found

Complications
- Pseudocysts: cyst-like pancreatic structure without epithelial lining
- Pancreatic duct stenosis: inflammation-induced narrowing of the pancreatic duct (pearl cord-like duct)
- Duodenal stenosis: inflammation-related narrowing of the duodenum
- Vascular complications: Arterial hemorrhage, aneurysm rupture, portal vein stenosis and thrombosis
- Compression or scarring stenosis of the bile ducts, with obstructive jaundice
- Duct rupture with pancreatogenic ascites or pancreato-pleural fistula

Epidemiology
- Prevalence: 25–30 cases/1 million inhabitants
- Incidence: 23 new cases/100,000 inhabitants (increases with age)
- m > f
- Average age: 3rd–4th decade of life (social problems, disability)
- 10-year survival rate: 70%
- Overall lethality: 30–35%
- Risk increase for pancreatic cancer (tenfold)

Etiology
- Mostly unclear

Alcohol Abuse (75–90%)
- Most important factor
- For women, >40 g alcohol/day for 6–12 years is considered as threshold.
- For men, >80 g alcohol/day is considered as threshold

- Time between onset of alcohol abuse and onset of chronic pancreatitis: on average 18 ± 11 years

Nicotine Abuse

- Leads to progression of the disease

Hyperparathyroidism (with Ca^{2+} Elevation)

Hereditary

- Prevalence 1/300,000
- Mutation in the cationic trypsinogen gene (PRSS1): approx. 67% of patients with hereditary pancreatitis
- Other responsible genes: SPINK1 gene, CFTR gene

Autoimmunological (IgG-4 and Lymphoplasmocytic Infiltrates)

- Plasma cellular infiltrates in the pancreas
- IgG-4 elevation in serum
- CT morphologically bulky pancreas often without visible ductal changes

Symptoms

Abdominal Pain

- Main symptom
- Mechanism = infiltration of the parenchyma, nerve myelin sheaths + pressure increase in the pancreatic duct (obstruction)
- Neuropathic pain

Symptoms Associated with Loss of Function

- Malnutrition
- Steatorrhea (lipase secretion reduced by more than 90%): Greasy stools
- Weight loss
- Vitamin deficiencies (fat-soluble vitamins A, D, E, K)
- Pancreatogenic (type III) diabetes mellitus
- Chronic pain syndrome

Diagnosis

Genetic Examination

- Indications for mutation analysis of the PRSS1 gene:
  - Positive family history (one or two first-degree relatives with idiopathic chronic pancreatitis)
  - Two or more episodes of acute pancreatitis without identifiable cause before the age of 25 years
  - Idiopathic chronic pancreatitis with first symptoms before the age of 25

Laboratory Diagnosis (◘ Table 9.2)

Diagnostic Imaging

- Only to be used in case of insufficient correlation of clinical, morphological and functional parameters or for the assessment of complications

Sonography

- Inhomogeneous organ with normal pancreatic duct, possibly calcifications = uncertain sign

Endosonography

- Highest sensitivity
- Endosonographically assisted fine needle aspiration (not percutaneous!):
  - To confirm the histological diagnosis (often false negative in cancer and chronic pancreatitis)
  - To confirm autoimmune pancreatitis (plasma cells, IgG-4)

CT/MRI/Magnetic Resonance Cholangiopancreaticography (MRCP)

- Supplementary for unclear pancreatic changes
- MRCP helpful for pancreatic duct assessment

ERCP

- Disadvantages of ERCP (vs MRCP):

Table 9.2 Non-invasive pancreatic function tests[a]

Test	Mild exocrine insufficiency sensitivity (%)	Moderate exocrine insufficiency sensitivity (%)	Severe exocrine insufficiency sensitivity (%)	Specificity (%)
Stool Elastase	54%	75%	95%	85%
Qualitative stool fat determination	0%	0%	78%[b]	70%[b]
Chymotrypsin activity	<50%	Approx. 60%	80–90%	80–90%
^{13}C-breath test (mixed triglycerides)	62–100%		90–100%	80–90%

[a] The direct invasive pancreatic function tests (secretin or secretin-pancreazymin test) were used as reference procedures

[b] Related to the quantitative stool fat determination

9

- Increased morbidity (5–10% overall; 3.47% post-ERCP pancreatitis)
  - Increased mortality (3.3‰)
  - Therefore, diagnostic endoscopic retrograde cholangiopancreaticography (ERCP) should be omitted in favor of MRCP for purely diagnostic indications
- Evaluation criteria of ERCP (according to Cambridge classification)
- Cambridge classification (for different examination procedures; Table 9.3)

Differential Diagnosis

- Cystic Fibrosis
- Cystic pancreatic neoplasms (especially main duct IPMN)
- Schwachmann-Diamond syndrome (autosomal recessive bone marrow disease)
- Johansen-Blizzard-Syndrome (disturbed development pancreas, nose and galea)
- Congenital enzyme defects (trypsinogen, α_1-antitrypsin deficiency)
- Divisive pancreas

Therapy

Treatment Strategy

Indications for Conservative Therapy

- For nicotine abuse: nicotine abstinence
- Pain medication according to WHO guidelines (Table 9.4)
- Enzyme substitution
  - Indication: steatorrhea, pathological pancreatic function tests, weight loss
  - Start with 20,000–40,000 units per meal, 10,000–20,000 units for small snacks, doubling or tripling of dose possible if insufficient effect

Indications for Interventional or Surgical Therapy

- Sustained pain requiring analgesics (new guideline: over 3 months: consider surgical therapy)
- Complications:
  - Strictures of the common bile duct, cholestasis, jaundice, cholangitis
  - Inflammatory or unclear malignant suspicious masses
  - Pancreatic pseudocysts
  - Pancreatic duct stones

30–60% of patients with chronic pancreatitis develop pain or a complication.

- Strategy:
  - Endoscopic procedures: Possibility of short-term pain reduction (66% of cases/few years)
  - Mid-term/long-term pain control: significant superiority of surgery vs. endoscopic therapy
  - Symptomatic pancreatic duct stones, stenoses in the pancreatic head and

Table 9.3 Evaluation criteria according to the Cambridge Classification

Endoscopic retrograde cholangiopancreaticography (ERCP)	
Cambridge 0	No pathological changes on complete visualization of the pancreatic duct
Cambridge 1	<3 pathological side branches, main duct regular
Cambridge 2	>3 pathological side branches, main duct regular
Cambridge 3	Pathological side branches plus pathological main duct
Cambridge 4	Like 3 plus cyst, duct stones, strictures, involvement, adjacent orifices
Transabdominal ultrasound	
Cambridge 0	Normal organ, duct <2 mm, smooth contour
Cambridge 1	Echo dense organ contour, organ enlarged, duct <3 mm, lobulated texture with echo dense segments
Cambridge 2	Irregular contour, irregular echo-enhanced main duct >3 mm, lobulated texture with echo-dense septa
Cambridge 3	Like 2 and cysts, focal calcifications
Cambridge 4	Like 3 and ductal stones, ductal obstruction, tumorous distention of the organ >2-fold, splenic vein thrombosis
Endosonography (EUS)	
Cambridge 0	None
Cambridge 1	Honeycomb texture, honeycomb-like, aisle <3 mm
Cambridge 2	Hyperechogenic duct, hyperechogenic foci, echo-dense contour, duct <3 mm
Cambridge 3	Lobulated, septate, hyperechogenic foci, duct >3 mm, irregular duct, no duct stones
Cambridge 4	Like 3 and calcifications, duct stones, cysts
Computed tomography (CT)/Magnetic resonance cholangiopancreaticography (MRCP)	
Cambridge 0	None
Cambridge 1	Not delineable with current methods in CT/MRCP
Cambridge 2	Two or more of the following changes: – Pancreatic duct >2 and <4 mm in the corpus pancreatis – Mild pancreatic duct enlargement – Heterogeneous parenchyma structure – Small cystic changes (<10 mm) – Duct irregularities – >3 pathological secondary ducts
Cambridge 3	All changes mentioned in 2 plus pathological main duct (>4 mm)
Cambridge 4	One of the changes listed at 2 and 3 plus one or more of the following: – Cystic structures >10 mm – Parenchymal calcifications – Intraductal filling defects (limestones) – Duct obstructions (strictures) – Severe duct irregularities
Cambridge 0: No chronic pancreatitis (CP), Cambridge 1: Possible CP, Cambridge 2: Low CP, Cambridge 3: Moderate CP, Cambridge 4: Heavy CP	

Table 9.4 WHO guidelines for pain medication in chronic pancreatitis

Active substance	Dosage	Analgesics effect
Paracetamol	2–3 times 500–1000 mg	Peripheral
Metamizole	1–4 times 500–1000 mg	Peripheral
Tramadol	4 times 100 mg, 2–3 times 200 mg retard	Low potent central
Tilidine	3 times 50–200 mg	Low potent central
Buprenorphine	3–4 times 0.2–0.4 mg	Highly potent central
Morphine	Individual according to effect	Highly potent central
Levopromazine	3–5 times 10 mg	tricyclic antidepressant
Clompramine	1 time 50–100 mg	tricyclic antidepressant

pseudocysts: according to the guideline, endoscopic or surgical therapy (▶ Sect. 9.2.3)
- In the case of suspected pancreatic cancer (unclear mass): Surgical therapy (oncological pancreatic head resection)
- For symptomatic pseudocysts + complication (e.g. gastric outlet stenosis, bleeding, cholestasis, vascular stenosis): Higher success rate for surgical procedures (vs. endoscopic pseudocyst drainage into duodenum or stomach), use according to expertise
- Asymptomatic pancreatic pseudocysts >5 cm in diameter without regression after 6 weeks: Individual treatment possible (41% of cases lead to complications)

Operative Therapy: Principles

Division: Resecting/Draining Procedures

- Resecting procedures:
  - Surgery according to Kausch-Whipple
  - Pylorus-preserving pancreatic head resection according to Longmire and Traverso (PPPD)
  - Surgery according to Beger, Frey or Bern Modification: Duodenum-preserving pancreatic head resection (DPPHR)
  - Rarely distal pancreatic resection (inflammatory pancreatic head tumor remains)
- Draining procedures
  - Partington-Rochelle or Puestow procedure
  - V-shape excision (Hamburg modification of the Frey procedure for so-called small duct disease)
- Total pancreatectomy and autologous islet cell transplantation (TPIAT)—so far not relevantly used in Europe

Surgical Strategy

- Inflammatory pseudotumor of the pancreatic head:
  - Standard = pancreatic head resection (classic Whipple operation/pylorus-preserving pancreatoduodenectomy/duodenum-preserving pancreatic head resection)
  - Duodenum-preserving therapy: better perioperative quality of life/results in some studies, long-term results equal to PPPD
- Indication for draining procedures:
  - Congested pancreatic duct >7 mm without inflammatory pseudotumor in the pancreatic head
  - Obstruction of the pancreatic duct system in risk constellations (portal hypertension with occlusion of the mesentericoportal axis)
  - Long-term inferiority of draining procedures compared to resecting procedures with regard to freedom from pain

Poor long-term results of draining procedures compared to resecting procedures with regard to freedom from pain.

- Surgery according to Kausch-Whipple or PPPD (► Sect. 9.3.1)
- Surgery according to Beger
  - Indications:
    - Segmental chronic pancreatitis with pain syndrome
    - Expression of an inflammatory pancreatic head tumor
  - Summary: Duodenum-preserving pancreatic head resection with subtotal resection of the pancreatic head (a very small margin of pancreatic tissue remains for blood supply to the duodenum) followed by anastomoses to the duodenal C, bile duct, and pancreatic remnant (corpus).

Surgical Procedure

Operation According to Beger

- General anesthesia
- Approach: Transverse laparotomy of the upper abdomen or median laparotomy
- Opening of the omental bursa
- Limited Cooker Maneuver
- Identification of the superior mesenteric vein at the lower edge of the pancreas and careful undermining of the pancreas (difficult step)
- At the upper edge of the pancreas identification of the portal vein + detachment from their adhesions
- Looping of the common bile duct and the common hepatic artery
- Transection of the pancreas after undermining, if necessary gradual transection without undermining (risky step)
- Subtle hemostasis of the pancreas after transection with single sutures (5-0 PDS)
- Free preparation at the upper edge of the pancreatic head up to the common bile duct
- For visualization of the intrapancreatic bile duct, insertion of a probe via the cystic duct
- Subtotal pancreatic head resection and uncinate process along the wall of the intrapancreatic bile duct segment (◘ Fig. 9.3)
- Extensive hemostasis on remaining pancreatic head margin (5–8 mm) at the duodenum with single sutures (preservation of gastroduodenal artery branches)
- For reconstruction: pull up a retrocolic jejunum;
- Two anastomoses as an interposition with the distal pancreas (end-to-side or end-to-end pancreato-pancreaticojejunostomy) and the head of the pancreas (side-to-side) connected with a biliodigestive anastomosis to the intrapancreatic bile duct (◘ Fig. 9.3)
- Connection of the inflow and outflow jejunum loop via a Y-Roux reconstruction
- Drainage of the anastomoses
- **Surgery according to Partington-Rochelle (pancreaticojejunostomy)**
  - Indication: only in case of massive ductal dilatation (≥7 mm) without pancreatic head pseudotumor
  - Modification of the Puestow operation, in which only a distal pancreaticojejunostomy is performed via the mesentericoportal axis to the head of the pancreas
    - Summary: Longitudinal opening of the pancreatic duct from the tail of the pancreas to the prepapillary segment; the duct of the Santorini towards the papilla should also be opened longitudinally; drainage of the opened duct via a deactivated jejunum loop side-to-side anastomosis according to Roux-Y.
  - Results:
    - Primary pain resolution 61–90%
    - Long-term success = only in 50% of cases (with complete freedom from pain)
- Surgery according to Frey (laterolateral pancreaticojejunostomy with

duodenum-preserving pancreatic head resection (extensive excavation of the pancreatic head))
  - Indication:
    - As in Partington-Rochelle, but with inflammatory pancreatic head tumor.
    - Proximal or long pancreatic duct stricture + inflammatory pancreatic head tumor
  - Synopsis:
    - Hybrid procedure = combination of a longitudinal pancreaticojejunostomy (ductal drainage) according to Partington-Rochelle + an extensive but careful local pancreatic head excision (in the case of inflammatory pancreatic head tumor, the extent of the removed pancreatic head tissue is decisive)
- Hamburg modification (Izbicki procedure or V-shape excision): in advanced disease with large inflammatory pancreatic head tumor and small duct disease (without obstructed pancreatic duct) = V-shaped excision in pancreatic corpus and tail

Surgical Procedure

Operation According to Partington-Rochelle

- General anesthesia
- Supine
- Approach: Transverse laparotomy of the upper abdomen or median laparotomy
- In case of uncertain localisation of the duct (not palpable) = small incision with removal of an elliptical shaped tissue part in the pancreatic body or tail (if necessary palpation and pre-puncture with a thin needle or intraoperative ultrasound)
- Longitudinal opening of the pancreatic duct over an overholt (curved clamp) in a small segment and then in full length
- Dissection of a V-shaped tissue block over the pancreatic duct
- If necessary, removal of pancreatic duct stones
- Pulling up an aboral jejunal loop retrocolically
- Creation of a side-to-side anastomosis
- Drainage of the pancreatic anastomosis

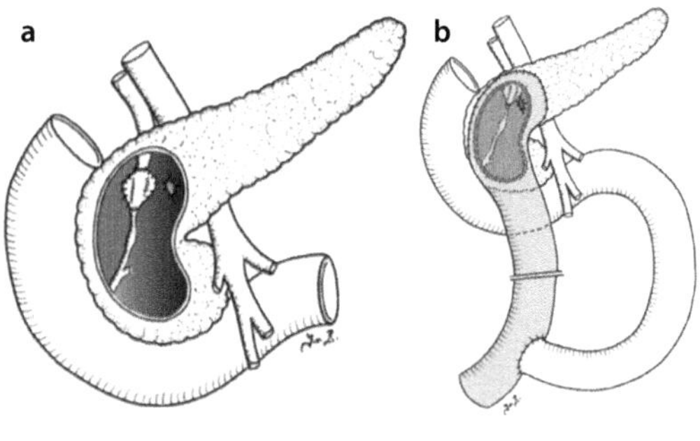

Fig. 9.3 **a**, **b** Operation according to Beger. (Mod. after Strobel et al. 2009)

Surgical Procedure

OP According to Frey (Fig. 9.4)

- General anesthesia
- Supine
- Transverse laparotomy of the upper abdomen or median laparotomy
- Access to the omental bursa through dissection of the gastrocolic ligament
- Identification of the superior mesenteric vein at the lower edge of the pancreatic neck

- Identification of the portal vein at the upper edge of the pancreatic neck + release from their adhesions
- Undertunneling of the pancreatic body on the mesentericoportal axis not necessary (advantage in portal hypertension or severe adhesions)
- Identification of the pancreatic duct with 20G needle + aspiration of pancreatic juice
- Wide opening of the pancreatic duct from the pancreatic tail to the neck and further to the pancreatic head
- Probing of the duct of Wirsung with Overholt (curved clamp)
- Placement of prophylactic haemostatic sutures at the pancreatic head to the duodenum (4-0 or 3-0 Prolene)
- Generous sharp peeling of the pancreatic head up to the pancreatic duct with scalpel (sufficient extent is important for the surgical result). Some pancreatic tissue must remain caudally
- Hemostasis and manual compression
- If bile duct stricture due to compression (inflammatory, fibrotic tissue in the pancreatic head) excision pancreatic head up to the common bile duct with subsequent door-wing-like anastomosis of the common bile duct in the pancreatic head (Bern modification)
- Pulling up the aboral jejunum loop retrocolic and creation of a side-to-side pancreaticojejunostomy, Roux-Y reconstruction
- Postoperative treatment
  - Blood glucose daily profile
  - Drainage analysis: amylase and bilirubin
  - Bleeding control (caution bleeding into the anastomosed jejunal small bowel)
  - Enteral nutrition: from the first postoperative day (water + tea), from the third postoperative day: liquid diet

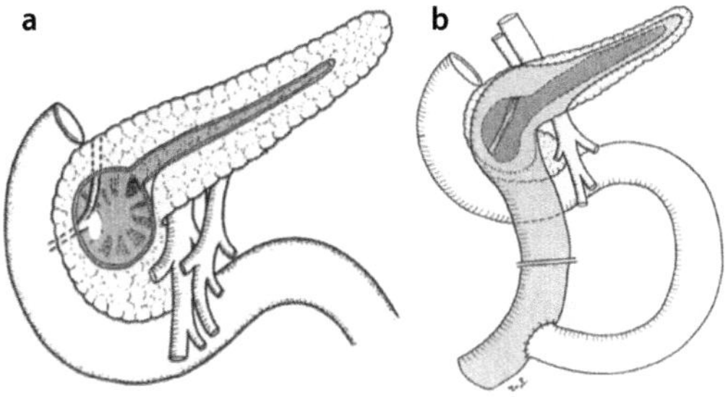

Fig. 9.4 Operation according to Frey. (**a**) Situs after resection of pancreatic head and tail. (**b**) Situs after reconstruction by latero-lateral pancreatico-jejunostomy. (Mod. after Strobel et al. 2009)

Monitoring and Follow-Up

- Rationale: mortality 20 years after initial diagnosis (ED) increased by 38% = need for follow-up, exocrine and endocrine dysfunction.
- Possible recurrence of pain after limited surgical procedures (drainage)
- Annual inspection:
  - Clinical examination
  - Transabdominal ultrasound
  - Laboratory with HbA_{1C}

9.2.3 Guidelines

German S3 guideline for chronic pancreatitis. Definition, etiology, diagnosis, conservative, interventional, endoscopic and surgical therapy of chronic pancreatitis. DGVS guideline 2012 Renewed version 2021.

9.3 Malignant Diseases

9.3.1 Pancreatic Carcinoma

Key Points

- Fourth leading cause of cancer death (incidence = mortality)
- Ductal adenocarcinoma: Histologically leading (>95%)
- 5-year survival = 10%
- Mostly asymptomatic for a long time

- So far the only curative treatment = radical removal of the tumour + regional lymph node removal

Definition

- Pancreatic carcinoma = malignant tumour of the pancreas

Epidemiology

- Incidence: 14.4 new cases/100,000 in men; 10.9/100,000 in women (Robert Koch Institute)
- Women:Men = 1:1.5
- Age peak: 65–75 years of age
- Localization: approx. 65% of all pancreatic tumors = in the pancreatic head, uncinate process or pancreatic neck
- Risk factors:
  - Age (>80-year-olds: 40-fold increase in risk compared to 40-year-olds)
  - Nicotine abuse (relative risk = 1.5-fold increased)
  - Diabetes mellitus type 2
  - Obesity
  - Hereditary syndromes

9

Etiology

- Malignant degeneration of the exocrine part of the pancreas
- Precursor stages = pancreatic intraepithelial neoplasia (PanIn; ◘ Fig. 9.5) or cystic neoplasia

Underlying Genetic Defects

- KRAS mutation (most common mutation)
- Inactivation of the tumor suppressor genes p16, p53 and Smad/DPC4

Hereditary Syndromes

- Increased risk of pancreatic cancer: Oncology guideline programme (German Cancer Society 2013, ▶ Sect. 9.3.2)
- Familial atypical multiple mole melanoma syndrome (FAMMM syndrome)
- Hereditary pancreatitis
- HNPCC ("hereditary non-polyposis colorectal cancer")
- Familial breast cancer (BRCA 1 and BRCA 2)
- Peutz-Jeghers Syndrome
- Familial adenomatous polyposis
- Li-Fraumeni Syndrome
- Fanconi anemia
- Von Hippel-Lindau Syndrome

Forms

- Ductal adenocarcinoma (very common)
- Serous cystadenocarcinoma (very rare)
- Mucinous cystadenocarcinoma
- Intraductal papillary mucinous carcinoma
- Pancreatoblastoma
- Solid-pseudopapillary carcinoma
- Acinar cell carcinoma
- Adenosquamous carcinoma

Symptoms

- Initially asymptomatic

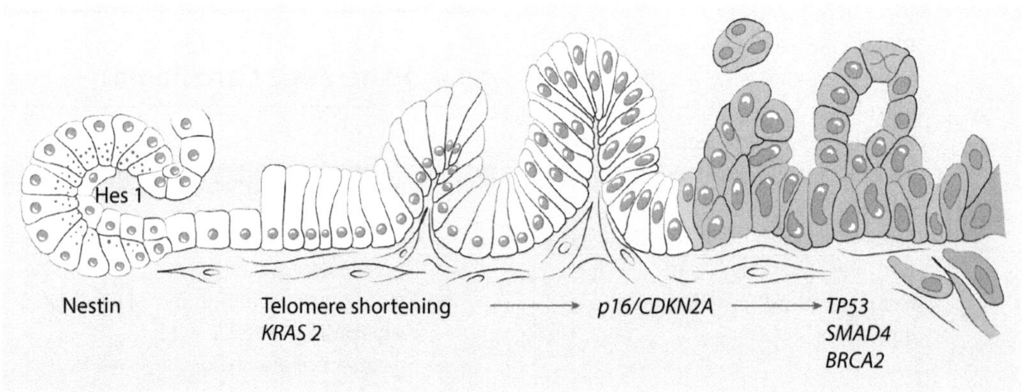

◘ **Fig. 9.5** Adenoma-carcinoma sequence in pancreatic cancer

- Often unspecific
- Symptoms
  - Weight loss
  - Painless jaundice in bile duct obstruction (leading symptom)
  - New-onset diabetes mellitus over the age of 50 (**caution**!)
  - Upper abdominal or back pain

Diagnosis (◘ Fig. 9.6)

Patient History + Clinical Examination

Imaging Techniques

- Preoperative assessment of resectability
- Preferred modalities:
  - Multidetector computed tomography (thin-slice angio-CT) or MRCP
  - Endosonography
- Criteria studied (of resectability):
  - Resectable (R) and borderline resectable (BR) tumors:
    - No distant metastases
    - No infiltration of the superior mesenteric vein or portal vein (R)
    - No complete encasement of the superior mesenteric vein or portal vein (R)
    - No long-distance venous occlusion not allowing reconstruction (BR)
    - No encasement of the gastroduodenal artery up to the hepatic artery (BR)
    - No walled superior mesenteric artery or cealiac trunc >180° of circumference (BR)

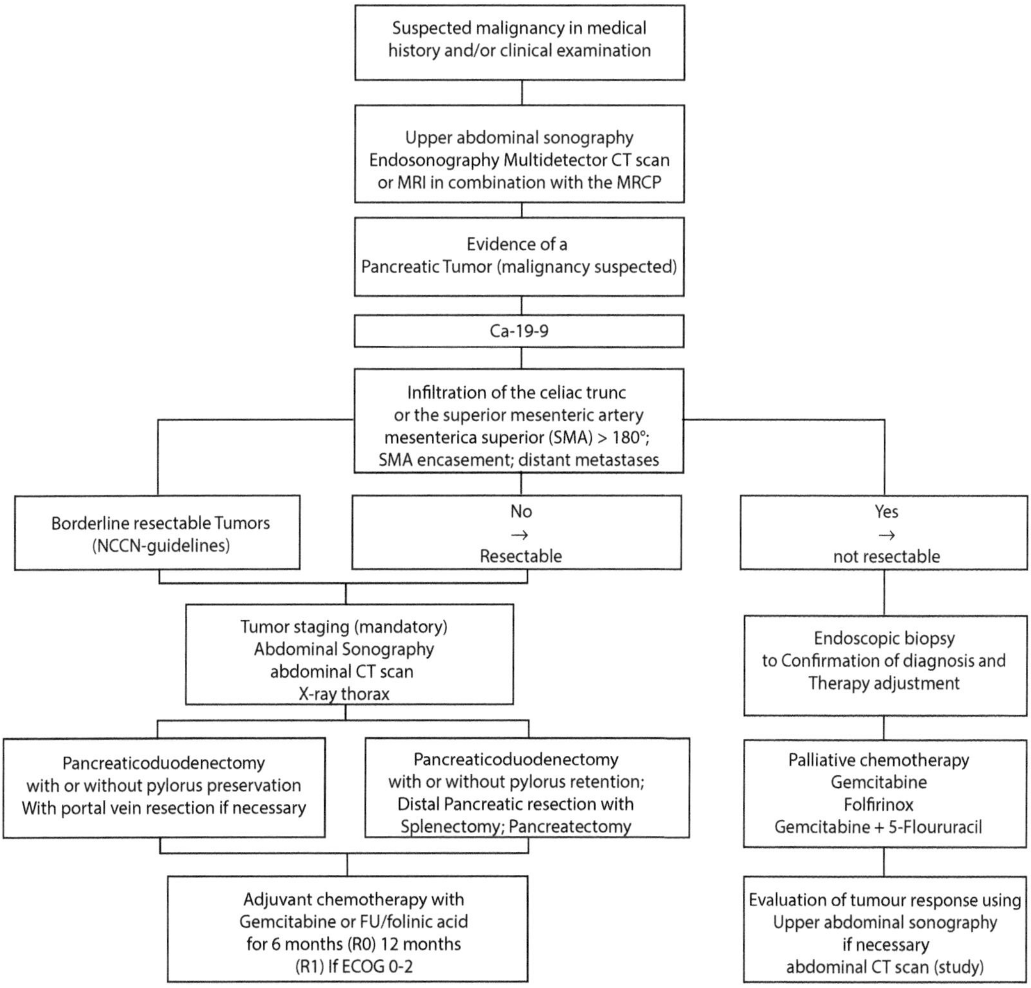

◘ **Fig. 9.6** Treatment tree according to German S3 guideline of exocrine pancreatic cancer 2013

Therapy

Curative Therapy

Preoperative Therapy

- Preoperative biliary drainage using a stent: indications:
  - Cholangitis
  - If surgery cannot be performed promptly. Avoid if possible, as significant increase in infectious complications
- Neoadjuvant chemotherapy: Already used in trials for borderline resectable and locally advanced tumours, aim for inclusion in trials

Operation

- If surgery is possible: increase of 5-year survival rate to over 20% (with adjuvant FOLFIRINOX up to 55%)
- Partial duodenopancreatectomy with or without pylorus preservation
- Depending on the location, distal pancreatic resection or pancreatectomy (RAMPS, Strasberg)
- In case of infiltration of the neighbouring organs = corresponding extension of the resection (adrenal gland, portal vein, mesocolon, colon)
- Removal of at least 10 locoregional lymph nodes

9

Surgical Procedure

Pylorus-Preserving/Classical Pancreatoduodenectomy (PPPD/Kausch-Whipple Operation; ◘ Fig. 9.7)

- Supine position (left arm resting, right arm extended)
- Right transverse laparotomy/longitudinal laparotomy
- Exploration of the abdominal cavity, exclusion of metastases
- Opening of the omental sac while sparing the gastroepiploic vessels with transection of the gastrocolic ligament
- Mobilization of the right colonic flexure
- Triggering of duodenal C from its retroperitoneal connections: Kocher maneuver
- Mobilization of the pancreatic head up to the mesentericoportal axis
- Open cholecystectomy
- Opening of the lesser omentum and exposure of the common hepatic artery at the upper edge of the pancreas
- Lymphadenectomy in the area of the hepatoduodenal ligament, visualization of all structures
- Ligation of the gastric and gastroduodenal arteries
- Slinging of the common bile duct and dissection proximal to the cystic duct
- Exposure of the portal vein at the upper edge of the pancreas
- Presentation of the superior mesenteric vein at the lower edge of the pancreas and ligation of the outlet of the right gastroepiploic vein
- Tunelling of the pancreas and placement of hemostatic stay sutures at the upper and lower parenchymal border
- Transsection of the duodenum post pylorus, with the GIA stapler or distal 2/3 gastric resection (classic Whipple operation)
- Transection of the pancreas at the level of the mesentericoportal axis
- Transection of the jejunum approx. 30 cm from Treitz
- Raising the proximal jejunum retrocolically
- Detachment of the uncinate process along the superior mesenteric artery
- Completion of the dissection of the mesopancreas along the superior mesenteric artery and removal of the specimen
- Marking of the incision margins with ink or sutures, intraoperative quick incision
- Start of the reconstruction phase
- Reconstruction by means of hepaticojejunostomy and either pancreaticojejunostomy and end-to-side gastrojejunostomy or pylorojejunostomy or pancreatogastrostomy with

Y-Roux reconstruction or omega loop with or without Braun anastomosis (◘ Fig. 9.7)

- Warren-Catell pancreaticojejunostomy: End-to-side anastomosis with duct-to-mucosa anastomosis (◘ Fig. 9.8)
  - Posterior wall suture: pancreatic parenchyma to jejunal serosa made in single button technique (4-0 PDS). The sutures are presented
  - After tie knotting, the anterior wall of the pancreatic duct is presented with double-armored sutures (5-0 or 6-0 PDS)
  - Punctual opening of the jejunum opposite of the pancreatic duct and single sutures of the posterior wall (duct-to-mucosa, 5-0 PDS); if necessary splinting of the pancreatic duct and completion of the anterior wall (duct-to-mucosa)
  - The external anterior wall suture is performed using a single suture technique (4-0 PDS) so that the jejunum covers the anastomosis
- **Pancreatogastrostomy** (◘ Fig. 9.9): between pancreatic parenchyma and stomach
  - A larger (7 cm) anterior gastrotomy and a small (depending on the cross-sectional size of the organ) (2 cm) dorsal gastrotomy are performed as the approach.
  - The mobilized pancreatic tail is invaginated into the stomach via the dorsal gastrotomy (posterior wall of the stomach) and fixed by means of a circular tabac pouch suture in the stomach wall and several parenchyma to serosa sutures
- Bilioenteric anastomosis: Hepaticojejunostomy
  - Length of the small intestine loop approx. 60 cm (Y-Roux)
  - Rear and front wall: single layer, interrupted, PDS 5-0/6-0
  - In case of narrow duct, if necessary, extension plastic according to Gütgemann
  - In case of high hilar anastomosis hepaticojejunostomy according to Hepp-Couinaud may be necessary
  - Enterotomy in the size of the hepatic duct
- Roux-Y reconstruction (2 loops), Omega reconstruction (1 loop) or 3-loop reconstruction (one isolated Roux-Y loop each to the pancreas and the bile duct as well as to the postpyloric duodenal remnant (PPPD)/stomach (Whipple))
- At the end of the reconstruction: rinsing and insertion of 4 easy-flow drains ventrally and dorsally of the pancreatic and biliodigestive anastomosis respectively (according to pancreatic fistula score possibly omitting drains all together)

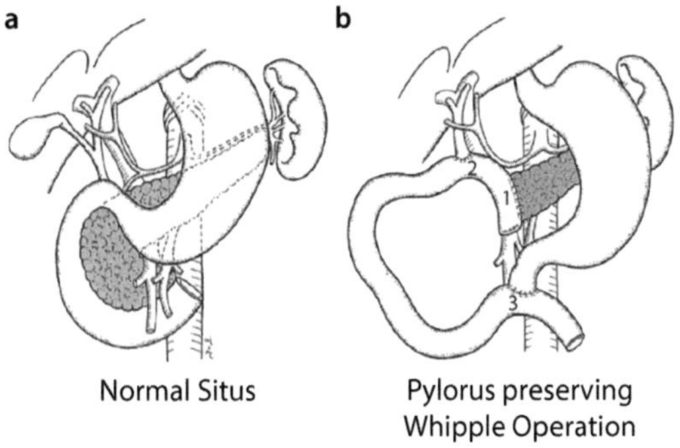

◘ **Fig. 9.7** Pylorus-preserving or classic pancreaticoduodenectomy according to Whipple, (**a**) normal situs, (**b**) after Whipple operation. *1* pancreatic anastomosis, *2* bile duct anastomosis, *3* gastroenterostomy. (Mod. according to Künzli et al. 2004)

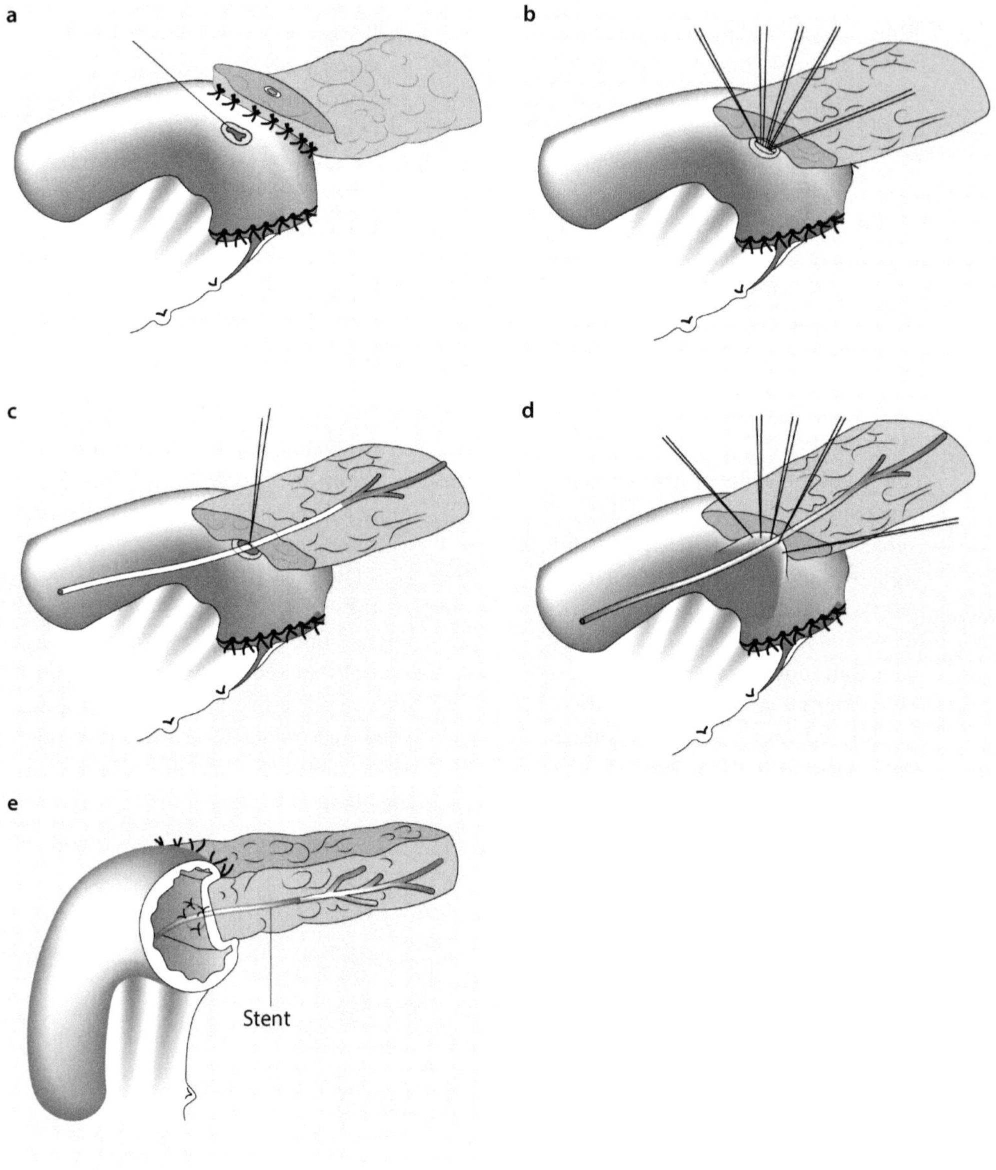

Fig. 9.8 **a–e** Pancreaticojejunostomy

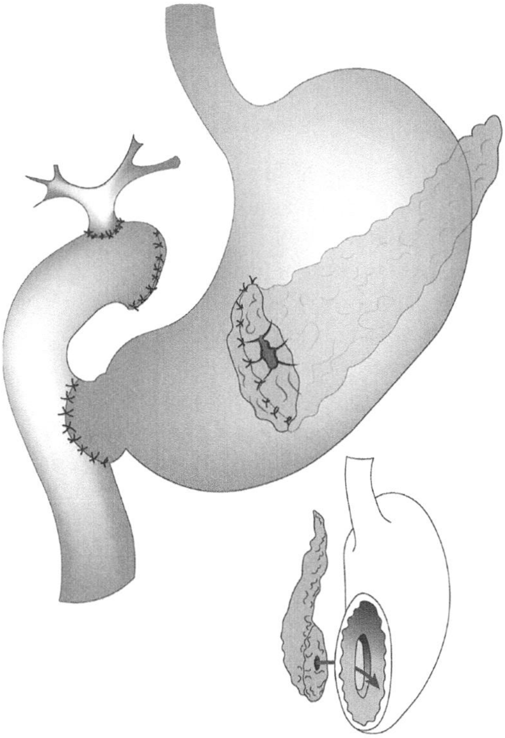

Fig. 9.9 Pancreatogastrostomy

Pathology

- R0-narrow, if circumferential resection margin (CRM) ≤1 mm
- R0-wide or CRM negative if CRM >1 mm
- With stringent pathological workup (Leeds protocol) high R1 resection rate (up to 60%)
- N0 (0 pos. LK), N1 (1–3 pos. LK), N2 (>3 pos. LK) (8th version of AJCC)

Postoperative Complications

- Post-pancreatectomy hemorrhage (gastroduodenal artery arterial hemorrhage and pancreatic sedimentation marginal hemorrhage), late post-pancreatectomy hemorrhage (late PPH)

> **Caution**
> Mortality of the arrosion hemorrhage up to 50%.

- Pancreatic fistula (type A-C) = 20%
- Gastric emptying disorders (higher with pancreatogastrostomy) = 20%.
- Bile leakage/bilioma
- Anastomosis insufficiency
- Residual pancreatitis (postoperative pancreatitis)
- Diabetes mellitus requiring insulin
- Endocrine and exocrine pancreatic insufficiency
- Wound infection = 10% (for open surgery)

Postoperative Treatment: Adjuvant Chemotherapy

- Adjuvant chemotherapy in UICC stages I-III
- Contraindications to adjuvant chemotherapy:
  - Eastern Cooperative Oncology Group (ECOG): Performance Status >2
  - Uncontrolled infection
  - Liver cirrhosis Child B and C
  - Severe coronary artery disease; heart failure (NYHA III and IV)
  - Preterminal and terminal renal failure
  - Impaired bone marrow function
  - Inability to attend regular check-ups
- Adjuvant therapy = improvement of 5-year survival after curative resection from 10% to 20% (with mFOLFIRINOX to 55%)
- 5-Fluorouracil plus gemcitabine for 6 months
- mFOLFIRINOX for 6 months (PRODIGE-Group)

Palliative Therapy

Indications

- For locally advanced or metastatic pancreatic cancer
- ECOG 0–2 (Table 9.5)

Therapy Regime

- First-line therapy: Gemcitabine (1000 mg/m^2) (to be discussed)
- 5-FU with or without folinic acid: not as sole first-line therapy
- Alternative to monotherapy with gemcitabine: combination with the EGF (epidermal growth factor) receptor tyrosine kinase inhibitor erlotinib depending on the development of skin exanthema

Table 9.5 Eastern Cooperative Oncology Group (ECOG)[a] (according to Oken et al. 1982)

Points	ECOG performance status
0	Normal, unrestricted activity, as before the disease
1	Restricted during physical exertion, able to walk, light physical work possible
2	Able to walk, self-care possible but not able to work, can stand up more than 50% of waking time
3	Limited self-care possible; confined to bed or chair for 50% or more of waking hours
4	Completely dependent, self-care not possible, completely confined to bed or chair
5	Death

[a] Performance status describes the physical condition of cancer patients and is used to quantify general well-being and limitations in activities of daily living

- In healthier patients (ECOG 0–1, age ≤75 years and a bilirubin level below 1.5 times the normal level): Combination of 5-FU/folinic acid, irinotecan and oxaliplatin (FOLFIRINOX protocol)
- Nab-paclitaxel plus gemcitabine

9.3.2 Guidelines

Oncology guideline program (German Cancer Society, German Cancer Aid, AWMF): S3 guideline Exocrine pancreatic cancer, long version 1.0, 2013, AWMF register number: 032-010OL, ▶ http://leitlinienprogramm--onkologie.de/Leitlinien.7.0.html, Renewed 2022.

9.4 Cystic Neoplasms

Key Points

- Increasing incidence and detection of cystic neoplasms in the last two decades
- About 90% of pancreatic cystic neoplasms are classified into four entities:
  - Intraductal papillary mucinous neoplasia (IPMN)
  - Serous cystic neoplasia (SCN)
  - Mucinous cystic neoplasia (MCN)
  - Solid pseudopapillary neoplasia (SPN)
  - Frequently incidental findings
- Malignant progression of mucinous cystic lesions in 10–50% of cases

9.4.1 Intraductal Papillary Mucinous Neoplasia (IPMN)

Definition

- Macroscopically visible, mucin-producing epithelial tumors arising from pancreatic duct epithelium (papillary)
- Precursor lesion of IPMN carcinoma
- WHO classification: inclusion of IPMN in this classification in 1996
- Breakdown:
  - Main-duct-IPMN
  - Branch-duct-IPMN
  - Mixed-type IPMN
  - IPMN with low, intermediate or high grade dysplasia or with invasive cancer
- Histologically prognostically relevant subclassification:
  - Gastric
  - Intestinal

- Pancreatobiliary
- Oncocytic

Epidemiology (◘ Table 9.6)

- Estimated incidence = 1/280,000 patients
- Women:Men = 1:1
- Frequency peak: 60–70 years of age
- Often incidental findings
- 5-year survival from MD ("main-duct")-IPMN = 31–54%
  - Intestinal IPMN (20%): Roughly correspond to villous neoplasms of the colon; if invasive, 5-year survival rate = 50%
  - Pancreatobiliary IPMN (8–10%): "High-grade tumors"; in >50% presence of an invasive component; a 5-year survival = like ductal adenocarcinoma of the pancreas
  - Oncocytic IPMN: Extremely rare; frequently "high-grade carcinomas"

Etiology

- Unclear
- Association with extrapancreatic primary tumors (colorectal, breast, and prostate cancer)

Symptoms

- Most frequently due to pancreatic duct obstruction
- Nausea
- Vomiting
- Abdominal discomfort (59%)

◘ **Table 9.6** Clinical and imaging features of cystic neoplasms of the pancreas. (According to Grützmann et al. 2011; Tanaka et al. 2012)

	IPMN	MCN	SCN	SPN
Age (average)	64 years	47 years	70 years	30 years
Male (%)	60%	5%	30%	13%
Symptoms	Frequently	50%	Rarely	Rarely
Localization	Mainly pancreatic head	Almost always pancreas tail	Variable	Mainly pancreatic head
Main course	Dilated ("main duct type") Non-dilated ("branch duct type")	Normal	Normal	Normal
Calcifications	No	Rarely	Central scar (30–40%)	
Main aisle connection	Always	Sometimes	No	No
Muzin	Yes	Yes	No	No
Appearance	"Grape-like"	"Orange-like"	"Honeycomb-like"	
Malignancy	Frequently (Sendai Criteria)	Very often >70%	Very rarely <5%	Up to 10%
Special features	Main and side aisle Type	Ovarian stroma	Microcystic and oligocystic	Young women
Therapy	MD: Operation always, BD: ◘ Fig. 9.10	Operation	Watch	Operation

IPMN intraductal papillary-mucinous neoplasia, *MCN* mucinous-cystic neoplasia, *SCN* serous-cystic neoplasia, *SPN* solid pseudopapillary neoplasia, *MD* main duct, *BD* branch duct

- Back pain
- Weight loss (29%)
- Jaundice (biliary obstruction) (16%)
- Previous episodes of pancreatitis (14%)
- Diabetes mellitus (IDDM)

Diagnosis

CT or MRI

- MRI (MRCP) = better method in centers with experience (duct association and main duct connection)

Imaging Signs

- Endosonography (ductal association and worrying nodules)
- Dilated pancreatic duct
- BD-IPMN = "Grape-like configuration"

Therapy (◘ Fig. 9.10)

Surgical Therapy of MD-IPMN

Indication for Surgery

- All MD-IPMN with main duct diameter >1 cm
- Since 62% of all MD-IPMN = malignant and 43% of all MD-IPMN = invasive

Aim of the Operation

- Removal of the lesion ideally before malignant transition

Principle

- Resection according to localization: R0 resection to be aimed at (oncologic radical operation)

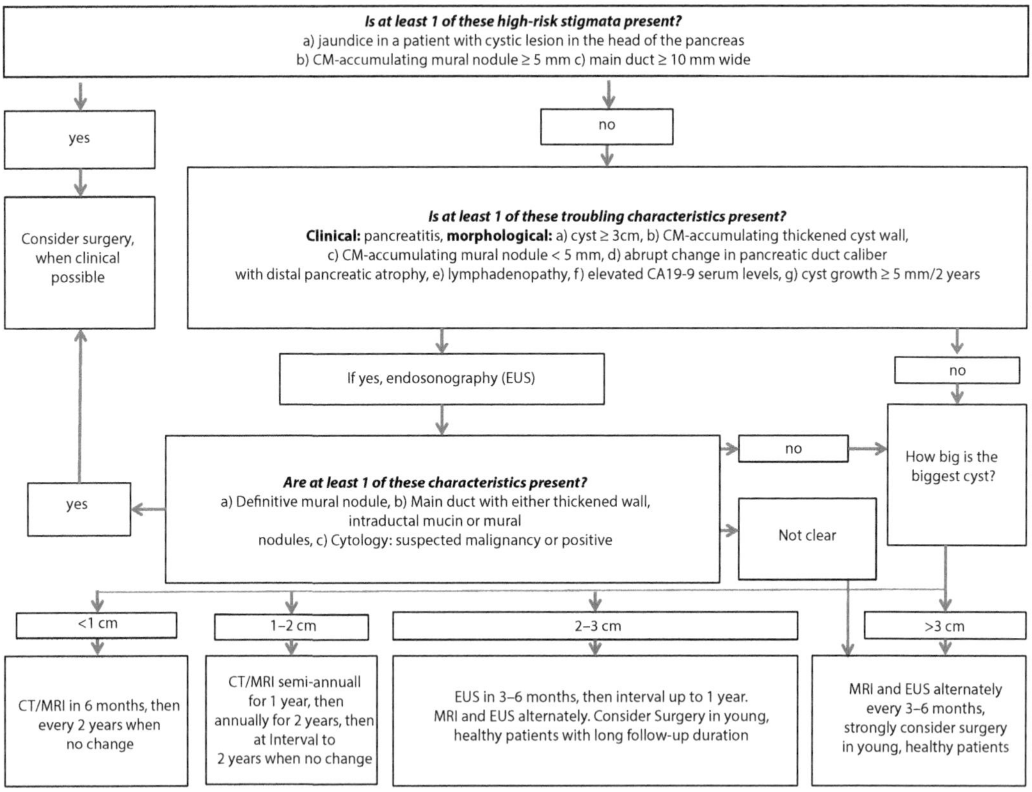

◘ **Fig. 9.10** Flowchart for the treatment of cystic neoplasms. (After Tanaka et al. 2017)

- Frequent PPPD vs. classical pancreatic head resection vs. pancreatectomy for multifocal type
- If necessary, total pancreatectomy in multifocal IPMN, decision according to histology of leading lesion
- Operate main finding, if frozen section shows high-grade dysplasia at the sedimentation margin, resect further until total pancreatectomy. If low-grade dysplasia, no further resection and organ-preserving procedure

Further Indications for Total Pancreatec tomy
- Positive margins at the pancreatic incision margin in pancreatic head carcinoma as isolated positive margin
- Multifocal metastases of renal cell cancer (urological consultation)
- Multifocal advanced neuroendocrine tumors
- Refractory pain syndrome in chronic pancreatitis (TPIAT (see above)—very controversial!)
- Resection margin:
  - In case of high-grade dysplasia = extension of the resection
  - In moderate and low-grade dysplasia = no further additional resection necessary
  - If the main duct diameter is <1 cm = further evaluation (◘ Fig. 9.10)

Preoperative for planned splenectomy: vaccination against Pneumococcus, Haemophilus influenzae group B and Meningococcus group C 2 weeks before planned surgery.

Surgical Procedure
Total Pancreatectomy with Splenectomy
- Supine position (left arm supported, right arm extended)
- Transverse upper abdominal laparotomy, right and left extended
- exploration of the abdominal cavity
- Opening of the omental sac while sparing the gastroepiploic vessels with transection of the gastrocolic ligament
- Mobilization of the right colonic flexure
- Release of duodenal C from its retroperitoneal connections (Kocher maneuver)
- Lifting of the duodenum and pancreas from the inferior vena cava up to the left renal vein
- Extension of the Kocher maneuver by mobilization of the pars horizontalis duodeni up to the superior mesenteric vein, presentation of the same from caudal right in the region of the mesenteric root
- Elevation of the pancreatic neck = view of the avascular plane dorsal to the pancreas, here preparation up to the sinus confluens venosum, exposure of the superior mesenteric artery just to the left of the vein in this area (mesenteric artery first approach)
- Open antegrade cholecystectomy, opening of the hepatoduodenal ligament with exposure of the choledochal duct and the common hepatic artery. **Caution**: Expose the right hepatic artery with intersection of the bile duct (often variable course)
- Dissection and ligation of the gastroduodenal artery and the right gastric artery
- Dissection and ligation of the splenic artery and confluent placement and suturing of the splenic vein
- In spleen-preserving pancreatectomy, visualization of the pancreatic tail from caudal and cranial and stepwise visualization of the individual branches from the splenic artery and into the splenicvein
- Separation of the splenorenal ligament and medial elevation of the spleen together with the pancreatic tail, so that the retroperitoneal layer is exposed
- Mobilization of the distal stomach and the duodenojejunal flexure

- Approx. 10–15 cm aboral of the ligament of Treitz = deposition of the jejunum
- Removal of the specimen en bloc after stepwise separation of the pancreatic head from the mesentericoportal axis (pancreas, distal stomach, duodenum, spleen)
- Reconstruction with end-to-side hepaticojejunostomy and end-to-side duodenojejunostomy if pylorus-preserving, otherwise gastrojejunostomy (◘ Fig. 9.10)

Postoperative Management After Pancreatectomy

- Screening/prophylaxis/therapy of weight loss (80% of patients loose >10% of their weight)
- Enzyme substitution (median 8 capsules/day, taken regularly with each meal)
- Insulin administration in pancreatogenic (type III) diabetes (median 25 IU/day)
- In total pancreatectomy, sugar control is more difficult with reduced hypoglycemia sensitivity

Surgical Therapy of BD ("Branch-Duct")-IPMN

- Indication:
  - Consider surgical therapy, ideally before transition to carcinoma; in selected series, up to 26% of all BD-IPMN are malignant and up to 18% are invasive carcinomas
  - Patients <65 years and cyst size >2 cm = resection (due to cumulative malignancy rate)
- Patients with "worrisome features" (nodules, wall thickening) or symptoms (pain, new-onset diabetes mellitus, etc.)

Conservative therapy for BD-IPMN (see below)

- Only in Sendai (Fukuoka)-negative tumors: i.e. <2 cm without symptoms or "worrisome features"
- Annual malignancy rate of only 2–3%
- Patients with BD-IPMN = significantly older
- Conservative therapy + check-ups

Postoperative Follow-Up

- Recurrence rate after 5 years = 0–20% (disease of the entire pancreas!)
- 5-year survival in resected non-invasive IPMN = 80–100%
- 5-year survival in resected invasive IPMN = 40–60%
- 5-year survival rate for IPMN carcinoma = 20% (like adenocarcinoma—thus avoid transition to carcinoma by prophylactic surgery in high-risk constellations)
- Control examinations after 2 and 5 years due to general risk of development of IPMN at further sites in the pancreas (R0-situation)

Conservative Therapy of MD-IPMN (5–9 mm Main Duct) and BD-IPMN

(**Caution!**) 5 mm might still be dangerous as far as development of IPMN cancer

- ◘ Figure 9.10

9.4.2 Serous Cystic Neoplasms (SCN)

Definition

- Benign tumors consisting of numerous cysts
- 10–20% of cystic pancreatic lesions
- Honeycomb structure
- Star-shaped scar in 20% of patients
- Virtually never degenerate malignant
- Localization: Pancreatic corpus and tail (70%)

Epidemiology (◘ Table 9.6)

- Women > Men = 5:1
- Frequency peak: >60 years of age
- 18–39% of all cystic neoplasms

Symptoms

- Mostly asymptomatic
- Nausea
- Vomiting
- Abdominal discomfort
- Back pain
- Weight loss

Diagnosis
- Multi-slice CT
- MRI
- Endosonography

Therapy

Surgical Therapy
- From a size of >4 cm, due to increased growth and all with symptoms

Conservative Therapy + Monitoring
- In all other cases

9.4.3 Mucinous Cystic Neoplasia (MCN)

Definition
- Solitary, round tumors with uni- or multilocular cysts
- Cysts lined by mucin-forming cells
- Ovarian stroma (probably scattered ovarian cells)
- Approx. 10% of cystic tumors of the pancreas
- Mostly in the body-tail area
- Potential precursor for pancreatic cancer

Epidemiology (◘ Table 9.6)
- 95% women
- Frequency peak: 40–60 years of age
- Malignancy rate = 30–50%
- Prevalence of invasive cancer = up to 15%
- 5-year survival rate of invasive MCN = 57%
- 5-year survival rate of MCN adenocarcinoma = 20%

Symptoms
- 20% = asymptomatic
- Non-specific abdominal complaints

Diagnosis
- Multi-slice CT
- MRI

Therapy
- Always surgical therapy
- Principles:
  - MCN <4 cm without mural nodules = parenchyma-sparing or laparoscopic (central or distal) pancreatectomy
  - Otherwise, classic pancreatic resection with lymphadenectomy (LAD) and (often) splenectomy, if necessary
  - ◘ Figure 9.10

9.4.4 Solid Pseudopapillary Neoplasia (SPN)

Definition
- Solid, only secondary pseudocystic-degenerative tumors
- <5% of cystic pancreatic tumors
- Typically solid tissue at the edge and hemorrhagically disintegrating centrally

Epidemiology (◘ Table 9.6)
- Young women (20–30 years)
- Low malignancy potential, often very large tumors
- Metastases (liver and peritoneum): In 10–15% of cases with a long time interval to resection of the primary site, then resection again
- 5-year survival = 97%

Symptoms
- Asymptomatic
- Mostly incidental finding

Diagnosis
- Multi-slice CT
- MRI
- Endosonography

Therapy

Always Operative
- Even in metastatic stage

Principles

- Distal pancreatic resection with/without splenectomy
- Pancreaticoduodenectomy (PPPD/Whipple)

Surgical Procedure

Laparoscopic Spleen-Preserving Pancreatic Left Resection

- Y-positioning (= suppine position with spread leg; = French position)
- Access by means of a total of 4 trocars in a semilunar line around the main findings
- Pneumoperitoneum
- Exploration of the abdominal cavity for pathologies not previously described (liver/peritoneum)
- Intracorporeal sonography of the liver and the peripancreatic region as well as the pancreas
- Positioning in anti-Trendelenburg position, beach-chair positioning
- Visualization of the pancreas by mobilization of the left colonic flexure as well as the transverse colon up to the right flexure
- Opening of the omental sac
- Visualization of the gastroepiploic artery and the confluens venosum of portal vein to avoid complications
- Dissection of adhesions between upper pancreatic margin and stomach and lymphadenectomy
- Pancreas mobilization starting at the lower edge, from here visualization of the splenic vein and the venous confluence
- Visualization of the celiac trunc and the splenic artery
- Completion of the oncological lymphadenectomy at the upper pancreatic margin
- Dissection + transection of the small vessels of the pancreatic body and tail in an alternating manner centrally (confluens venosum) and peripherally (splenic hilus) = e.g. Ligasure device or PDS/metal clips
- Separation of the pancreas tail with a linear stapler (GIA with coating if necessary) and salvage using a salvage bag
- Insertion of two drains dorsal and ventral to the pancreas
- Further operative possibility = method according to Warshaw:
  - Spleen supply only via left gastroepiploic artery and short gastric arteries
  - Splenic artery and vein are severed (short gastric vessels)
  - **Caution**: Higher rate of secondary splenectomies for ischemia.

9.4.5 Guidelines

Tanaka M, Chari S, Adsay V, Fernandez-del Castillo C, Falconi M, Shimizu M, Yamaguchi K, Yamao K, Matsuno S, and International Association of Pancreatology (2006) International consensus guidelines for management of intraductal papillary mucinous neoplasms and mucinous cystic neoplasms of the pancreas. Pancreatology 6:17–32.

Tanaka M, Fernandez-del Castillo C et al. (2012) International consensus guidelines 2012 for the management of IPMN and MCN of the pancreas. Pancreatology 12: 183–197.

Tanaka M, Fernández-del Castillo C, Kamisawa T, Jang JY, Levy P, Ohtsuka T, … Wolfgang CL (2017) Revisions of international consensus Fukuoka guidelines for the management of IPMN of the pancreas. Pancreatology 17(5):738–753.

9.5 Endocrine Neoplasms

Key Points

- Rare, approx. 3% of all pancreatic neoplasms
- 5-year survival of malignant neuroendocrine tumors of the pancreas approx. 30–40%
- Grouping into functional and nonfunctional neuroendocrine tumors

9.5.1 Definition

- Neuroendocrine tumors (NET) of the pancreas = rare tumors
- Initiation from endocrine cells
- Classification of NET of the pancreas:
  - Functional (hormone-active) NET (gastrinoma, insulinoma, VIPoma, somatostatinoma, PPoma): Production and release of hormones
  - Non-functional (hormone-inactive) NET

9.5.2 Epidemiology

- Incidence: 0.4–1.5 new cases per year/100,000 population
- Increasing prevalence
- Insulinoma and gastrinoma (Zollinger-Ellison syndrome) = 1:500,000 per year
- Glucagonoma (diabetes dermatitis syndrome) = very rare
- Vipoma = Verner-Morrison Syndrome
- Nonfunctional NET of the pancreas (exclude MEN-1 syndrome in case of familial clustering)

9.5.3 Symptoms

Insulinoma

- Whipple triad:
  - Hypoglycaemia (glucose <45 mg/dL) + associated neurological symptoms (= feeling of weakness, confusion, dizziness, visual disturbances, headache, loss of consciousness)
  - Autonomic symptoms (palpitations, tachycardia, sweating and sometimes aggressiveness)
  - Rapid improvement in symptoms with glucose infusion
- Weight gain (20% of patients)
- Mechanical complications possible, but rarely due to the rather small tumors
- Mostly very small tumors
- Malignant insulinomas (10%): Production of various hormones: calcitonin, melanocyte-stimulating hormone (MSH), adrenocorticotropic hormone (ACTH), etc. = variable symptomatic picture

Gastrinoma (Zollinger-Ellison Syndrome)

- Gastrin overproduction leads to:
  - Excess stomach acid = multiple ulcerations
  - Upper abdominal pain (multiple refractory gastric ulcers)
  - Reflux Disease
  - Complications of ulcers: Upper GI (gastrointestinal) bleeding + gastric or duodenal perforation

VIPom

- Massive diarrhea
- Mechanism = release of vasoactive intestinal peptide
- Resulting in:
  - Dehydration
  - Hypochloridemia
  - Hypokalemia
  - Hypomagnesemia

Glucagonom

- Severe migratory necrotizing exanthema
- Moderately elevated blood glucose levels
- Weight loss
- Anemia
- Stomatitis

Somatostatinoma

- Often clinically inapparent
- Increased fat storage: due to partial inhibition of thyroid function
- gastric distention
- Inhibition of hormones in the gastrointestinal tract results in
  - Malabsorption signs with fatty stools
  - Gallstones due to gallbladder motility disorders

Pancreatic Carcinoid Syndrome

- Paroxysmal flush
- Intestinal complaints
- Diarrhea
- Signs of right heart failure

Non-Functional NET (95%)

- Generally late diagnosis, often incidental findings
- Abdominal discomfort
- Weight loss
- Prognosis and grading according to grading (G1-G3) and proliferation rate (Ki-67 index <2%, 2–20%, >20%)

9.5.4 Diagnosis

Laboratory Diagnosis

- Determination in serum
- Detection of all hormones in serum with associated NET

Chromogranin A

9

- General marker for NET
- Also good follow-up parameter for diagnosis of recurrence

Caution
False-positive chromogranin A levels with proton pump inhibitor (PPI) therapy (discontinue at least 1 week before testing).

Gastrin

- In Zollinger-Ellison syndrome:
  - Fasting gastrin level >1000 pg/mL and gastric pH of <2
  - Secretion test >200 pg/mL above basal level
  - Also discontinue PPI inhibition (false positive levels of gastrin)

Fast Test

- For insulinoma: until hypoglycemia is reached

Insulin, Plasma Glucose

- Insulin (μU/mL)/plasma glucose (mg/dL) ratio >0.33
- C-peptide >0.7 mg/L (differential diagnosis hypoglycaemia facitata due to insulin injection)

5-Hydroxyindoleacetic Acid

- Degradation product of serotonin
- In the acidified 24-h collected urine
- Increased in carcinoid syndrome and small bowel NET

Imaging Techniques

Contrast Enhanced Ultrasound

- Echo-negative structure, more often hypervascular perfusion
- Not sufficient to confirm the diagnosis

Endosonography

- Very good representation of the positional relationship to surrounding organs
- Superior to other methods in localization diagnosis
- Good method for long-term follow-up of MEN-1 syndrome

Multidetector CT

- Hyperintense visualization of the NET in the early contrast phase (hypervascularized)

9.5.5 Therapy

Benign Solitary NET with Local Resection Option (>2 cm)

- Enucleation

Caution
High pancreatic fistula rate after enucleation up to 80%!

NET Without Local Resection Option

- Operation by location:
  - Pancreatic head resection
  - Central pancreatic resection
  - (Spleen-preserving) pancreatic left resection
  - Systematic lymphadenectomy in case of Ki-67 index >2%, CT suspicious LN metastases or tumor size >4 cm

Local Recurrences or Metastases of NET

- Surgical therapy

Diffuse Metastasized NET

- Treatment with somatostatin alone
- Treatment with somatostatin + α-interferon

Surgical Procedure

Central Pancreatectomy with Pancreatogastrostomy

- Supine positioning
- Transverse laparotomy of the upper abdomen or median laparotomy
- Exploration of the abdominal cavity for pathologies not previously described
- Opening of the omental sac
- Mobilization of the lower edge of the pancreatic neck and body
- Visualization of the superior mesenteric vein, at the inferior border of the pancreas
- Mobilization of the upper edge of the pancreas (lymphadenectomy in the area of the hepatica artery)
- Dissection of the pancreas from the portal vein
- Ventral luxation of the pancreas with loops around the pancreatic body/neck
- Identification of the splenic vein and transsection of the pancreas
- The splenic artery is usually located separately from the neck and proximal pancreatic body
- After complete exposure of the pancreatic body = transection with stapler (endo-GIA) on the mesentericoportal axis
- Stapling of the proximal pancreatic remnant or two-row suturing (PDS 4-0 MH, V-shape closure)
- Pancreatogastrostomy (or pancreato-pancreaticojejunostomy) between the distal pancreatic remnant and the posterior wall of the stomach or intestine (jejunum), after removal of the row of staples in the area of the pancreatic duct (creation as described above)
- Insertion of 2 drains at the distal and proximal pancreatic remnant

9.5.6 Guidelines

Falconi M, Bartsch DK, Eriksson B, Kloppel G, Lopes JM, O'Connor JM, Salazar R, Taal BG, Vullierme MP, O'Toole D, Barcelona Consensus Conference (2012) ENETS Consensus Guidelines for the management of patients with digestive neuroendocrine neoplasms of the digestive system: well-differentiated pancreatic non-functioning tumors. Neuroendocrinology 95:120–134.

References

Cano DA, Hebrok M, Zenker M (2007) Pancreatic development and disease. Gastroenterology 132(2):745–762

Schumpelick V (ed) (2011) Gastroenterologische Chirurgie, 3rd edn. Springer, Berlin, p 805

Strobel O, Büchler MW, Werner J (2009) Duodenumerhaltende Pankreaskopfresektion. Chirurg 80:22–27. https://doi.org/10.1007/s00104-008-1577-8

Künzli BM, Friess H, Kleeff J, Yekebas E, Mann O, Izbicki JR, Büchler MW (2004) Kurativ-operative Therapie des Pankreaskarzinoms. Onkologe 10:1285–1300

Oken MM, Creech RH, Tormey DC, Horton J, Davis TE, McFadden ET, Carbone PP (1982) Toxicity and response of the Eastern Cooperative Oncology Group. Am J Clin Oncol 5(6):649–655

Grützmann R, Post S, Saeger HD, Niedergethmann M (2011) Intraduktale papillär-muzinöse Neoplasie des Pankreas. Dtsch Arztebl Int 108(46):788–794

Kidney Transplantation

Bernd Jänigen, Franck Billmann, and Przemyslaw Pisarski

Contents

F. Billmann, T. Keck (eds.), *Essentials of Visceral Surgery*,
https://doi.org/10.1007/978-3-662-66735-4_10

10.1 Introduction

- First successful kidney transplantation (KTx) in 1954 in identical twins in Boston, USA
- Safe standard procedure with very good success:
  - 2018 in Germany: 2191 NTx, thereof 638 living donations
- Problem: Serious organ shortage. Reasons = complex, additional decrease since scandal with organ transplantation
- Alternative: Therapy of terminal renal failure by replacement procedures:
  - Hemodialysis (HDi)
  - Peritoneal dialysis (CAPD)

10.1.1 Legal Framework

- German Transplantation Act (GTA/TPG) implemented in 1997, last amendment 2012
- Goal: Promote willingness to donate organs
- Content German Transplant Act (GTA):
  - Public education
  - Organ donation (post-mortem and living)
  - Organ allocation
  - Organ Transplantation

- Since the introduction of the GTA: Irreversible loss of brain function (formerly: brain death) = recognition as criterion of death
- Transplantation according to urgency, likelihood of success and equality of chances

10.1.2 Structure in Germany

- Organization of organ donation: German Foundation for Organ Transplantation (DSO)
- Organ allocation: Eurotransplant (ET)
- Organ transplantation: Transplant Centres

Organ donation, allocation and transplantation by **independent** institutions.

German Foundation for Organ Transplantation

- Structure—7 regions
- Coordination and implementation of organ donation

Eurotransplant

- Non-profit organisation based in Leiden (The Netherlands)
- Organ Allocation for:
  - Austria, Belgium, Croatia, Germany, Hungary, Luxembourg, Netherlands, Slovenia
- For Germany: Allocation according to allocation guidelines of the German Medical Association (Bundesärztekammer)

Transplant Centers

- Preparation of the potential recipients
- Carrying out organ transplantation
- Follow-up of the recipients after transplantation

10.2 Indication for Transplantation and Preparation of the Recipient

- Indication for kidney transplantation: Basically in all patients with end-stage renal diseases (ESRD)
- Prior to registration in the waiting list: Obligatory medical evaluation of the recipient concerning indication of KTx and operability

10.2.1 Indication for Transplantation

Indication = ESRD [End-Stage Renal Disease]

- Liberal indication due to high comorbidity and loss of quality of life due to alternative procedures

- Waiting time for a post-mortem organ: currently approx. 8–10 years
- Alternative: Living donation: Also possible preemptively (before the onset of dialysis requirement): sensible starting at approximate glomerular filtration rate (GFR) <15 mL/min

Contraindications

- Severe acute or chronic infections
- Malignant disease (waiting period between 1 and 5 years)
- Severe cardiovascular diseases
- Severe pulmonary diseases
- Severe psychiatric illnesses
- Severe extrarenal diseases
- Alcohol or drug abuse
- Non-adherence: due to the need for immunosuppression

Causes of End-Stage Renal Disease

- Glomerulonephritis
- Interstitial nephritis
- Congenital malformations
- Bilateral nephrectomy for tumor or trauma
- Metabolic diseases (e.g. diabetes, oxaluria, etc.)
- Drug toxicity
- Hereditary diseases
- Obstructive diseases
- Reflux nephropathies
- Systemic diseases
- Haemolytic-Uraemic Syndrome (HUS)
- Irreversible acute renal failure
- Vasculopathies

Most Common Underlying Condition for New Waiting List Enrollment in 2018 (*n* = 2348) (Eurotransplant Statistics)

- Cystic kidney disease: 421
- Chronic nephritic syndrome: 333
- Chronic kidney disease: 372
- Type 1 diabetes: 220
- Hypertensive kidney disease:206
- Nephrotic syndrome: 127
- Chronic tubulointerstitial nephritis: 40
- Rapid progressive nephritic syndrome: 40
- Other diagnoses: 589

10.2.2 Recipient Preparation

Detailed Information—Medical Aspects

- Before evaluation of transplantability and qualification for the waiting list
- About all aspects of kidney transplantation:
  - Registration in the waiting-list
  - Waiting time
  - Transplantation
  - Need for immunosuppression
  - Risks and complications
  - Results

Medical Evaluation

- For each organ recipient
- Objectives/content:
  - Determination of general operability
  - Exclusion of contraindications
  - Compliance review

Caution

Due to the permanent immunosuppression required postoperatively, one focus of preoperative diagnosis is the exclusion of possible sources of infection.

Diagnostic Procedure

- Preparation of the recipient = ideally at an early stage before the onset of the dialysis requirement (since a preemptive transplantation can take place in the case of a living donation)
- Recipient diagnosis in close cooperation with the responsible dialysis center

Detailed Anamnesis and Clinical Examination

- Underlying renal disease
- Dialysis initiation and procedures
- Tumor disease
- Cardiovascular risk factors and pre-existing conditions
- Pre-existing pulmonary disease
- Previous operations
- Infection status
- Addictive disorders
- Family medical history

- Current medication
- Clinical examination
- Vascular status

Laboratory Tests

- Blood count, kidney function, electrolytes, liver function, coagulation, inflammatory signs, endocrine diagnosis (Hb_{A1c}, parathormone, thyroid levels), PSA (prostate specific antigen, men >45 years)
- Virology/Bacteriology: Hepatitis B (HBV) and C (HCV); human immunodeficiency virus (HIV), Epstein-Barr virus (EBV), cytomegalovirus (CMV), herpes simplex virus (HSV), varicella-zoster virus (VZV), syphilis (TPHA)
- Determination of the blood group
- HLA ("human leucocyte antigen") typing
- Donor-specific antibodies
- Urinalysis
- Cross-match (living donation)

Apparative Examination

- ECG
- Chest X-ray
- Lung function
- Cardiac echocardiography
- Exercise ECG, myocardial scintigraphy, coronary angiography if necessary
- Abdominal sonography
- Vascular status—if necessary pelvic CT native/angiography
- CCDS (color-coded Doppler sonography) carotid, if necessary,
- Urologic evaluation—including cystoscopy

Screening

- Urological screening (men >45 years)
- Gynaecological screening (women)
- Colonoscopy (>50 years)

Evaluation by Specialist

- ENT
- Dentist
- Dermatologist
- Urologist
- Psychological examination, if necessary

Vaccinations

- Influenza
- Tuberculosis
- COVID
- Hepatitis A and B
- Tetanus
- Diphtheria
- Polio
- Pneumococcus
- Meningococcus
- Live vaccines: varicella, measles/mumps/rubella (these are contraindicated under immunosuppression)

Caution

If other diseases are diagnosed, therapy must have been started or completed before registration in the waiting list (e.g. focal treatment for ENT/dental infections, interventional and surgical therapy for CHD, cholecystectomy for symptomatic cholecystolithiasis).

10.2.3 Registration in the Waiting List

Indication/Registration

- Indication is made individually by an interdisciplinary conference (6-eyes-principle)
- Registration with Eurotransplant as soon as
  - the treating transplant centre has determined indication and
  - all necessary examinations are available

Waiting time = time from the first day of dialysis. The time of registration in the waiting list and the registration status have no influence on this.

- Currently more than 7500 patients in Germany are on the kidney waiting list

Urgency Status

- Distribution (allocation) of organs:
  - Through Eurotransplant
  - According to the urgency status (Table 10.1)
- Causes for immunisation:
  - Previous transplants
  - Blood transfusions
  - Pregnancies

Table 10.1 Urgency levels according to Eurotransplant (► http://www.eurotransplant.org)

Notification status (MUC)	Description transplantability	Urgency	Allosensitisation (PRA)
HU	"High urgency"	Urgent	–
T	"Transplantable"	Normal	None; PRA <6%
I	"Immunized"	Normal	Present; 6 <PRA <85%
HI	"Highly immunised"	Normal	Present; PRA >85%
NT	"Not transplantable"	None	–

MUC Medical Urgency Codes, *PRA* panel reactive antibodies: Indicates the percentage of the recipient's antibodies against HLA versus the cross-section of the population

- High-urgency status = extremely rare. Prerequisites:
  - Lack of dialysis access option (vascular surgery report required)
  - Life-threatening situation that can only be resolved by a kidney transplant
  - Severe bladder problems (recurrent cystitis, haematuria) after simultaneous pancreas-kidney transplantation with bladder drainage of exocrine pancreatic secretions. These may occur with loss of graft kidney function and functioning pancreas graft

Overview: HU ("high urgency") status:
- Application to Eurotransplant
- Review by expert panel

10.3 Deceased Organ Donation

Key Points

- In case of consent to organ donation + presence of irreversible loss of brain function: coordination of organ donation by the German Foundation for Organ Transplantation (DSO)
- Procedure: Exclusion of contraindications, donor notification to Eurotransplant (ET), allocation of the organ, followed by donor surgery

10.3.1 Organ Donation and Donor Selection

Organ Donation

- Notification of a potential organ donor by the organ retrieval hospital to the DSO
- Consent to Organ Donation:
  - Existence of written will (e.g. donor card)
  - Oral will (relatives)
  - Presumed will of the patient (relatives)
  - Decision according to the relatives' own values if the patient's presumed will is unknown
- Irreversible loss of brain function:
  - Clinical diagnosis by two specialists experienced in the care of severely neurologically ill patients (one of whom is a specialist in neurology/neurosurgery)
  - Apparative diagnosis: e.g. detection of cerebral perfusion arrest, EEG with zero-line

Caution

- Notification to Eurotransplant + further diagnosis: Only permitted after irreversible loss of brain function and if consent to organ donation has been given.
- Donation in case of cardiocirculatory death: not allowed in Germany
- Eurotransplant: Deadline of 6 h for the allocation of organs

Donor Selection

- Exclusion of a contraindication to organ donation:
  - Generalized, chronic infection [HIV, HBV, HCV]
  - Malignant disease (waiting period usually = 5 years)
  - Exceptions = non-metastatic brain tumours, skin tumours (excluding malignant melanoma), early-stage prostate tumours
  - Kidney disease
- Carrying out the donation operation in the donor hospital
- Exact timing depends on the schedule of transplant centers that accept organs with short ischemia time (especially heart, lung)

Ischemia Times of Organs

- Heart: <6 h
- Lungs: 8 h
- Liver: 12 h
- Pancreas: 12 h
- Kidney: 30 h

10.3.2 Organ Allocation

- Organ allocation by Eurotransplant

Allocation Programs

- AM (Acceptable Mismatch) Program:
  - All highly immunized patients (PRA >85%)
  - Based on the available HLA typing, organs are selected that are most likely to result in a negative cross-match
  - Patients in the AM program have priority and are allocated before all other patients
- ETKAS program (Eurotransplant Kidney Allocation System, donors <65 years)
  - Allocation within the blood groups
  - Organ allocation (◘ Table 10.2)
- ESP program (Eurotransplant Senior Program, donors ≥65 years)
  - Recipient ≥65 years
  - Regional allocation: short ischemia time
  - Allocation only based on waiting time
  - Waiting time shorter compared to ETKAS
  - No HLA match: immunological risk difficult to assess and usually higher

◘ Table 10.2 ETKAS scoring system (Eurotransplant Kidney Allocation System: ► http://www.eurotransplant.org)

Scoring based on the following seven factors	
1. HLA typing (HLA-A, -B and -DR loci)	Per fitting HLA match (max. 6) 66.6 points, max. 400 points HLA bonus for paediatric recipients (double points)
2. Mismatch probability (MMP)	Calculation of the probability to get a 0- or 1-mismatch kidney depending on the results of AB0- and PRA-screening
3. Waiting time	33.3 points per waiting year
4. Paediatric bonus:	100 extra points. Definition of paediatric recipient: Dialysis started before the age of 18 years Listing possible from GFR <20 mL/min
5. Distance between collection centre and recipient centre (max. 300 points)	For Germany: Organ from D: +100 points, organ from federal state of recipient centre: +200 points
6. High urgency (HU) status	HU recipient = 500 extra points
7. Kidney after other organ transplantation (except pancreas)	If kidney transplant required 90–360 days after other organ transplant and dialysis requirement existed prior to other transplant = 500 extra points

HLA human leucocyte antigen, *PRA* panel reactive antibodies

10.3.3 Organ Retrieval

Principle

- All kidneys from donors <2 years of age must be *retrieved* en bloc
- Kidneys from donors between 2 and 5 years of age should be *retrieved* en bloc, but may be divided depending on the recipient profile
- Kidneys from donors >5 years of age are *retrieved* as single kidneys as described below

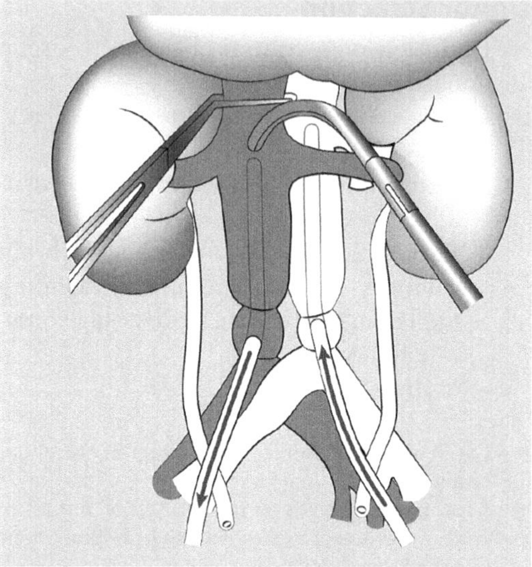

■ **Fig. 10.1** Situs during perfusion

Surgical Procedure

Visceral Organ Perfusion (■ Fig. 10.1)

- Insertion of a perfusion cannula in the aortic bifurcation or the common iliac vessel
- Free preparation of the subdiaphragmatic aorta (above the truncus coeliacus)
- Ligation of both iliac arteries distal to the catheter as well as the distal vena cava
- Full heparinisation before the cross clamp
- Ligation/clamping of the aorta subdiaphragm—cross clamp
- Immediate start of perfusion, usually with cooled (4 °C) histidine tryptophanetoglutarate (HTK) solution (approx. 8 L)
- Incision of the distal inferior vena cava as well as the thoracic inferior vena cava, if necessary insertion of a drainage catheter
- Cooling of the situs with slush ice/Ringer solution

Surgical Procedure

Kidney Retrieval

- Exposure of the orifice of the left renal vein and dissected at the level of the orifice into the vena cava
- Transverse transection of the inferior vena cava directly at the upper edge of the confluence of the right renal vein
- Longitudinal opening of the aorta starting at the aortic bifurcation and extending to the renal arteries
- Separation of the aorta just above the renal arteries, cutting of the aortic posterior wall, the aorta is left as a patch
- Transverse transection of the vena cava in the area of the incision
- After removal of the liver and, if necessary, the pancreas, the kidneys are detached from the retroperitoneum laterocranial.

- The ureter should be removed as long as possible (clearly beyond the pelvic axis) with surrounding fatty tissue to protect the accompanying vessels

Kidney packing

Caution
Wide variation in renal arterial supply:
- Often additional superior and/or inferior pole vessels (sometimes several centimeters distant from the main artery)
- Atypical course of the vessels (e.g. right inferior pole artery often ventral to the vena cava)
- Ideally, polar arteries should be harvested together with the main artery on a patch

10.4 Living Kidney Donation

Key Points

- Living donation = alternative to postmortem kidney transplantation
- Precise regulation in the GTA (e.g. who is eligible as a donor)
- Legal guidelines: Very strict in Germany compared to other countries
- For any living donation: Presentation to an Ethics Committee after extensive medical evaluation; then scheduling of organ donation
- Organ donation (open or laparoscopic): immediately before transplantation

10.4.1 Prerequisites

- Adults at least 18 years of age
- First and second degree relatives
- Spouse, partner
- Persons who have a special personal relationship with the donor

10.4.2 Legal Limits in Germany

- Altruistic donation
- Cross-over: Two pairs crossed over in case of AB0 incompatibility, positive cross-match or immunisation
- Chain transplants: Many pairs crossed over in AB0 incompatibility, positive cross-match or immunisation

10.4.3 Advantages of Living Kidney Donation

- Short waiting time or preemptive transplantation
- Better survival of the transplanted kidney
- Better overall survival of the recipient
- Mostly direct organ function due to short ischemia time

Absolute priority for living kidney donation = safety of the donor (kidney donor = healthy person with no medical indication for surgery).

10.4.4 Donor Evaluation [Preparation and Diagnosis]

Initial Interview with the Potential Donor

- Verification of the conditions
- Information about risks for the donor and opportunities for the recipient
- Exclusion of obvious contraindications by anamnesis
- Blood group, HLA typing and cross-matching

Detailed Medical Examination (Often Inpatient)

- Anamnesis
- Medication
- Clinical examination
- Lab test
- Extended virologic examination including e.g. HBV, HCV, HIV, CMV, EBV, etc.
- 24 h collection urine

- Urine status/sediment
- Lung function
- ECG
- Stress ECG
- Heart Echography
- If necessary, long-term blood pressure measurement
- OGTT (oral glucose tolerance test)
- Chest X-ray
- Kidney duplex sonography
- Abdominal Sonography
- Psychiatric evaluation if necessary
- Angio-CT/MRI
- Renal scintigraphy
- Screening depending on the age of the donor

Presentation to an Ethics Committee

- Directly in advance detailed explanation by doctor and informed consent
- Verification of voluntariness
- Exclusion of organ trafficking
- Verification of the conditions

10.4.5 Donor Operation

OP Procedure

- Open surgery
- Laparoscopic
- Retroperitoneoscopic

Open Surgery

- Advantages:
  - Good overview
  - Good control of the situs
- Disadvantages:
  - Cosmetic (pararectal or lumbar scar)
  - Risk of incisional hernia
  - Risk of abdominal wall relaxation
  - More postoperative pain
  - Longer convalescence

Surgical Procedure

Open Nephrectomy (Minimal Incision; ◘ Fig. 10.2)

- Positioning: Supine

- Pararectal section starting from the costal arch (8–10 cm)
- Severing the lateral abdominal wall
- Medialisation of the peritoneal sac
- Exposing the lower pole of the kidney
- Mobilisation of the entire kidney from laterocaudal
- Exposure and preparation of the ureter to just below the iliac axis
- Transection of the ureter (ligation distally, proximally the ureter is not closed)
- Preparation of the renal vessels from the renal hilus toward central
- Heparin administration before clamping optional
- Clamping of the renal vessels centrally and dissection of the vessels
- Transfer of the kidney for perfusion, cooling and preparation
- Supply of the vessel stumps with non-absorbable suture material
- Drainage, wound closure

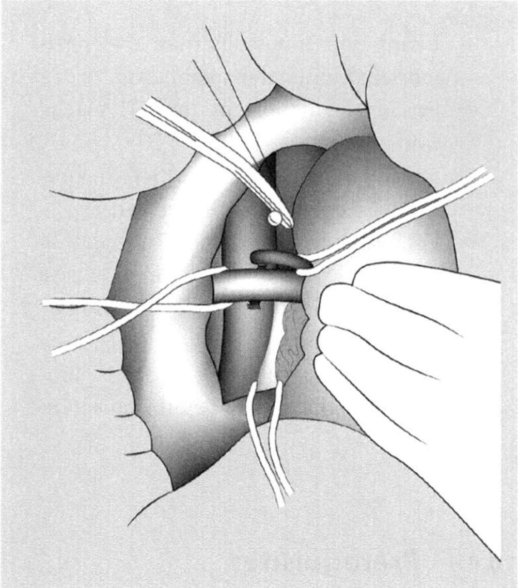

◘ **Fig. 10.2** Open living kidney donation on the left. The V. ovarica/testicularis and V. suprarenalis are already detached and ligated. The renal vein and artery are centrally connected. Caudally the ureter is visible

Laparoscopic/Retroperitoneoscopic

- Advantages:
  - Good overview
  - Cosmetics (Pfannenstiel incision)
  - Less pain
  - Shorter convalescence
  - Lower risk of hernia
  - No relaxation of the abdominal wall
- Disadvantages:
  - Loss of 0.5–1 cm vessel length (can be optimized with narrower staple suture devices)
  - In case of conversion, loss of time due to emergency laparotomy

Surgical Procedure

Laparoscopic (Hand-)Assisted Nephrectomy (◘ Fig. 10.3)

- Positioning: back with slightly raised operating side, on vacuum mattress with pelvic support on opposite side
- Five trocars (3 × 12 mm, 2 × 5 mm). Placement: 12-mm trocars in the latter Pfannenstiels incision, subumbilical and in the upper abdomen medioclavicular on the contralateral side. 5-mm trocars in the axillary line on the explantation side and epigastric.
- Entering the retroperitoneum with mobilization of the colon (+duodenum on the right, +pancreas tail and spleen on the left)
- Right transection of the ovarian vein (technically easier)
- Exposure and transection of the ureter just below the pelvic axis, the stump is clipped distally
- Preparation of the ureter up to the hilus
- Mobilisation of the kidney from laterocaudal and cranial in rendezvous
- Exposure of the vessels from the hilus to central
- On the left side, pay attention to the ovaric vein, suprarenal vein and lumbar branches. These must be carefully dissected out and severed between PDS (polydioxanone) clips.
- Pfannenstiel incision (6–8 cm) and insertion of the port
- Completing the preparation on the upper pole and vessels
- Central renal artery and vein disconnection with endo-GIA (vascular)
- Recovery of the kidney and transfer for perfusion, cooling and dissection
- Drainage, wound closure

Surgical Procedure

Perfusion Living Donation

- Start cooling in 4 °C cold solution (HTK solution, etc.)
- Irrigation of the kidney with 100 mL heparin solution (50 IU/mL) via the renal artery (in the case of minimally invasive removal, removal of the staple suture line)
- Flush the kidney with approx. 500 mL perfusion solution until clear reflux via renal vein.
- Preparation analogous to back-table preparation for postmortem organs
- Store at 4 °C until transplantation

10.4.6 Risks and Complications

Mortality

- Total mortality = 0.03%

After kidney removal, creatinine levels may be elevated.

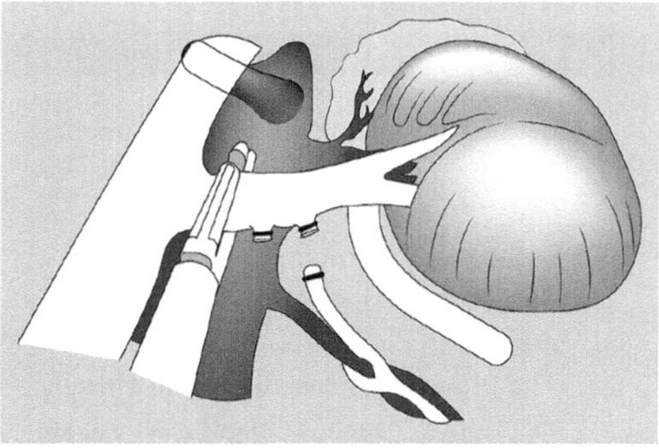

◘ **Fig. 10.3** The renal vessels are placed as centrally as possible with an endo-stapler. This results in a loss of approx. 0.5–1 cm of vessel length (width of the stapler)

Morbidity

- Morbidity: low
  - Bleeding
  - Nausea/vomiting
  - Wound infections
  - Chronic pain
  - Thrombosis
  - Embolism
  - Pneumonia

Long-Term Risks

- Proteinuria
- Arterial hypertension: in about one-third of the cases
- Risk of needing dialysis: approx. 0.2% (donor) vs. 0.02% (comparable non-donor)
- Surgical complications

The living kidney donor carries a small residual risk. Therefore, a detailed explanation in the transplant centre (surgeon and nephrologist) is essential before living kidney donation. Perioperative graft loss is particularly stressful.

10.4.7 Donor Aftercare

- By family doctor or nephrologist
- 3–5 controls during the first year
- After the first year once a year
- Recommendation: kidney function, protein excretion and blood pressure control

10.5 Kidney Transplantation

Key Points

- Before the start of the recipient operation: preparation of the organ "back-table".
- Subsequent retroperitoneal implantation of the kidney (standardized technique)
- The presence of vascular anomalies in the donor organ/recipient can make kidney transplantation very difficult or, extremely rarely, even impossible

10.5.1 Back-Table Preparation of the Kidney

- Living kidney donation: Back-table preparation immediately following removal and perfusion
- Post-mortem kidney removal: back-table preparation is the responsibility of the recipient centre

Surgical Procedure

Back-Table Preparation

- Tracing of the vessels to the hilus, excess fatty tissue is removed with clamps and ligatures
- Lateral branches, such as branches to the adrenal gland, are ligated
- If necessary, vessel reconstruction in case of vessel variations, e.g. polar arteries, accessory vessel supply
- Exposure of the ureter: The accompanying vessels must be spared at all costs to minimize the risk of ureteral necrosis
- **Caution**: Ureter fissus as a norm variant

Checking the seal of the vessels

10.5.2 Surgical Technique of Transplantation

Implantation Site

- Iliac fossa (mostly right), simpler venous vascular access
  - Extraperitoneal position
  - Easy vascular and bladder access
  - Short distance to the bladder
  - Good accessibility for biopsy, ultrasound

Surgical Procedure

Kidney Transplantation (◘ Fig. 10.4)

- Positioning: Supine

- Preparation: Central venous catheter, sterile insertion of a bladder irrigation catheter, filling of the bladder
- Hockey stick-shaped cut in the lower abdomen
- Opening of the lateral abdominal wall: M. obliquus externus, M. obliquus internus and M. transversus
- Medialization of the peritoneal sac
- Sparing preparation of the iliac axis in order to ligate as few lymphatic vessels as possible
- If necessary, shortening of the transplant kidney vein and end-to-side anastomosis to the distal inferior vena cava, common iliac vein or external vena cava, continuous suture with non-absorbable suture material
- Implantation of the artery mostly on the A. iliaca communis (aorta or A. iliaca externa also possible), continuous suture with non-absorbable suture material
- The vessels should come to rest without kinking or torsion
- Reperfusion, if necessary haemostasis in the area of the anastomoses, the hilus and the renal capsule
- Opening the bladder roof
- Ureterocystoneostomy and antirefluxplasty according to Lich-Gregoir
- Ureter must lie free of torsion and tension
- Implantation of a DJ (double J) catheter optional
- Drainage, wound closure

Immunosuppression

- Started shortly before reperfusion by steroid bolus
- 250 mg methylprednisolone i.v.

Application of 20% mannitol and Lasix before anastomotic opening = optional and not evidence-based.

- pAVK in the recipient can significantly complicate implantation; central = create anastomosis proximal to a stenosis; if possible: thrombendarterectomy with vessel reconstruction before actual transplantation
- In paediatric recipients: anastomosis mostly to aorta and v. cava = compensation of a discrepancy of recipient and donor vessels + possibility of transplantation of kidneys from adult donors to small recipients

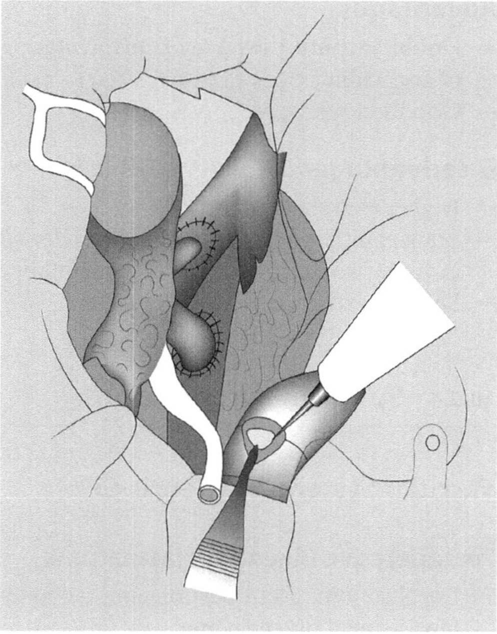

Fig. 10.4 Situs after kidney transplantation. The vessels lie stretched. The ureter is then anastomosed with the bladder

Caution
A living donor transplant is technically more challenging due to the lack of an arterial patch.

10.5.3 En Bloc Renal Transplantation

Principle

- Organs from donors <5 years and <10 kg weight
- Aorta and v. cava of the donor serve as vascular elongation for connection to recipient vessels

Advantages

- Double nephron mass by transplantation of two kidneys
- Good long-term prognosis

Disadvantages

- Higher complication rate
- Transplantation must be critically reviewed in young women due to possible pregnancy
- Difficult biopsy in case of rejection

10.5.4 Surgical Complications

Vascular System (Incidence <5%)

Postoperative Bleeding/Haematoma

- Localisation: Retroperitoneum, anastomoses, renal parenchyma
- Occurrence: Immediately postoperative
- Cause: coagulation disorder, medication (ASS) and infections
- Therapy: Depending on dynamics and clinical presentation, reoperation if necessary

Arterial Thrombosis

- Symptom: Sudden stop of diuresis
- Occurrence: Early postoperative
- Diagnosis: Color-coded duplex sonography
- Therapy: Immediate reoperation and attempt at revascularization

Graft Vein Thrombosis

- Symptoms: Sudden stop of diuresis
- Occurrence: Early postoperative
- Diagnosis: Color-coded duplex sonography
- Therapy: Immediate reoperation and attempt at thrombectomy

Renal Artery Stenosis

- Symptoms: creatinine increase, arterial hypertension
- Occurrence: Medium/long term after transplantation
- Diagnosis: Color-coded duplex sonography
- Therapy: If possible, interventional therapy with stent, reoperation is likely to cause complications

Urological Complications (Incidence 2–10%)

Urinary Leakage

- Localization: Laterocranial to the bladder
- Symptoms: pain, creatinine increase, signs of infection
- Diagnosis: Sonography, puncture, Mibi (microbiology)/creatinine in the punctate, localization by retrograde pyelography
- Cause: Frequently high bladder pressure in contracted bladder, ureteral necrosis, injury to urinary drainage system during transplantation
- Therapy: Depending on location, low-pressure drainage with indwelling bladder catheter (BDK), Splint if necessary, ureteral reimplantation if necessary

Ureteral Stenosis

- Localization: Mostly prevesical
- Symptoms: Urinary retention, pain, creatinine increase, late signs of infection
- Diagnosis: Sonography, retrograde pyelography
- Cause: Often swelling in the anastomosis area, scarred stricture of the anastomosis, ureteral necrosis
- Therapy: Splint, in case of persistence ureteral reimplantation

Ureteral Necrosis

- Localization: Prevesical
- Symptomatology: Clinical presentation of ureteral leakage or ureteral stenosis
- Diagnosis: Depending on the symptoms
- Therapy: Reimplantation of the ureter with resection of the necrotic portion

Lymphatic Complications (Incidence 2–18%)

Lymphocele

- Localization: Mostly mediocaudal to the kidney

- Symptoms: Urinary retention, pain, increase in retention levels
- Diagnosis: Sonography, puncture
- Therapy: Laparoscopic or open fenestration after intraperitoneal

10.6 Postoperative Treatment

Key Points

- After kidney transplantation: monitoring of the patient, if possible intermediate care unit
- After approx. 5 days: start of intensive training of the patients (focus = regular intake of medication)

10.6.1 Inpatient Stay

- Length of stay: approx. 14–21 days

Content

- Monitoring of urine production
- Balanced electrolyte and water balance
- Early mobilisation
- Adjusting immunosuppression
- Prophylaxis: Ulcer (pantoprazole), Candida infections (fluconazole), Pneumocystis jirovecii (cotrimoxazole), CMV (valganciclovir; ◘ Table 10.3)

Delayed Graft Function (DGF)/Acute Tubular Necrosis (ATN)

- Ischemia reperfusion injury
- Incidence: Up to 30% in postmortem renal transplantation, incidence increases with increase of cold ischemia time
- No therapy possible, ensure sufficient fluid intake, adequate immunosuppression
- Problem: Differential diagnosis of other causes of graft failure:
  - Acute rejection: biopsy
  - Circulatory disorder: Color-coded duplex examination

◘ **Table 10.3** Valganciclovir prophylaxis

Risk constellation	Duration of therapy
High risk: Donor +/ Recipient –	6 months
Medium risk: Donor +/ Recipient +	3 months or biweekly CMV PCR
Moderate risk: Donor –/Recipient +	3 months or biweekly CMV PCR
Low risk: Donor –/ Recipient –	No prophylaxis
For induction therapy:	
Antithymocyte globulin	6 months
AB0-incompatible transplantation	3 months
Basiliximab	3 months

Caution
A clinical assessment is not possible in DGF/ATN due to lack of excretion. Therefore, in this situation, a kidney biopsy is always indicated after 7 days.

10.6.2 Immunosuppression

Key Points

- Highest immunological risk = at the time of transplantation
- Risk decreases exponentially over time

Immunosuppressive Therapy

- Induction phase (transplantation and early postoperative phase)
  - Triple therapy (see below) in higher dosage
  - If necessary, (in case of high immunological risk) additional induction therapy with: Monoclonal (non-depleting) antibodies (e.g. basiliximab) or polyclonal (depleting) antibodies (e.g. antithymocyte globulin)

- Maintenance phase (starting approx. 6 months after transplantation)
  - Triple therapy in low dosage

Standard Triple Therapy

- Calcineurin inhibitor (Tacrolimus)
- Antimetabolite (mycophenolate mofetil, azathioprine)
- Glucocorticoids (prednisolone)

Immunological Risk Factors

- Long cold ischemia time
- Low histocompatibility (≥3 HLA mismatches)
- Donor organ (donor >40 years)
- Recipients (<50 years)
- Retransplant
- Immunized recipient (PRA level elevated)

Immunosuppressive Agents

- Mechanism of action, side effects and application ◘ Table 10.4
- Dosing according to phase ◘ Table 10.5

◘ **Table 10.4** Functionality, side effects and use of immunosuppressants

Active ingredient group	Active substance	Mechanism of action	Side effects	Application
Glucocorticoids	Prednisolone	Inhibition of the entire immune response (non-specific)	Cushing's habitus, hypertension, hyperlipidemia, osteoporosis, leukocytosis, cataract, psychosis, pancreatitis, gastrointestinal bleeding, gastric/duodenal ulcers, skin atrophy, diabetes, impaired wound healing	Maintenance therapy, rejection therapy
Calcineurin inhibitors	Ciclosporin A	Inhibits calcineurin by binding to immunophilin	Hypertension, nephrotoxicity, hirsutism, gingival hyperplasia, CNS toxicity	Maintenance therapy
	Tacrolimus	Inhibits calcineurin by binding FK-binding protein	Nephrotoxicity, CNS toxicity, diabetes, hypertension	
Antimetabolite	Mycophenolic acid	Blocks ionosine mono-phosphate dehydrogenase	Gastrointestinal side effects, leukopenia, anaemia, wound healing disorders	Maintenance therapy
	Azathioprine	Interferes with lymphocyte proliferation	Pancytopenia, alopecia, cholestatic hepatosis, pancreatitis	
m-TOR inhibitors	Sirolimus, Everolimus	Blocks T-cell activation	Hyperlipidemia, thrombocytopenia, pneumonia, rash, wound healing disorder	Maintenance therapy

Table 10.4 (continued)

Active ingredient group	Active substance	Mechanism of action	Side effects	Application
Monoclonal antibodies	Basiliximab, Dacli	IL-2 receptor blockade	Nausea, drowsiness	Induction Therapy
	Rituximab	CD-20 receptor blockade	Nausea, edema, skin rash, leukopenia, thrombocytopenia	AB0-incompatible transplantation
Polyclonal antibodies	Antithymocyte globulin	Lymphocyte depletion (unspecified)	Allergic reaction, leukopenia, anaemia, opportunistic infections, increased risk of malignancy	Induction therapy, rejection therapy

Table 10.5 Phase-appropriate dosage of immunosuppressants

Active ingredient group	Dose	Target mirror
Glucocorticoids	– Initially 3 mg/kg BW/intraoperatively then tapered to 0.1 mg/kg BW/day (approx. 3–6 months) – Rejection therapy: 500 mg Boli for 3 days	
Tacrolimus	0.1–0.2 mg/kg BW/day	8–12 ng/mL (6–8 weeks) 6–8 ng/mL (after 6–8 weeks) 4–6 ng/mL (after 3 months)
Ciclosporin A	3–6 mg/kg BW/day	150–250 ng/mL (6–8 weeks) 100–150 ng/mL (after 6–8 weeks) 50–100 ng/mL (after 3 months)
Mycophenolate mofetil	2 × 1 g daily 2 × 750 mg daily after 3 months 2 × 500 mg after 6 months	
Azathioprine	Initial 2–3 mg/kg BW/day Long-term 1–2 mg/kg BW/day	
Basiliximab	2 × 20 mg (preoperative and day 4)	
Rituximab	AB0i: 375 mg/m^2 BSA 4 weeks before planned transplantation	
Antithymocyte globulin	1.5 mg/kg BW/day Cumulative dose max. 6–10 mg/kg BW	

BW body weight, *BSA* body surface

Caution

In all immunosuppressed patients:
- Significantly increased risk of infection
- Therefore, early anti-infective therapy is obligatory.
- Opportunistic infections must be included in the differential diagnosis

Individual immunosuppression of each patient weighing the immunological risk versus the risk of infection.

ABO-Incompatible Transplantation (Living Donation)

- Special preparation of the recipient
- In Europe: 375 mg/m^2 BSA (body surface area) rituximab (Mabthera®) 4 weeks before planned transplantation
- 1 week before transplantation start immunoadsorption/plasmapheresis: removal of circulating blood group antibodies against donor blood group
- IgG titre in target range (IgG <4), then transplantation
- Triple therapy: Start 1 week preoperative
  - Induction with basiliximab
  - 1 week postoperative daily: Titre control and immunadsorption in case of rising titres (in our lab IgG >8)
  - 2 weeks postoperative every 2 days: Titre control and immunadsorption in case of rising titres (in our lab IgG >16)
  - Accommodation (exact mechanism unclear): From >2 weeks postoperative: No more titre controls
- Results regarding long-term function of the grafts identical to AB0-compatible living donation
- Higher risk of developing lymphoceles: Preoperative mycophenolate mofetil administration or immunoadsorption as a cause are discussed

AB0-incompatible living kidney donation for blood group incompatibility = safe standard therapy.

10

10.6.3 Organ Rejection

Hyperacute Rejection

- Extremely rare since the introduction of the cross-match
- Aetiology: Circulating antibodies against the donor organ
- Minutes after reperfusion of the graft
- Cross-match: Compatibility testing of recipient serum with donor blood, spleen or lymph node cells

Acute Rejection

- Rejection within days to months after transplantation: In approx. 10% of all kidney transplants
- Clinical presentation: creatinine increase >20%, decrease in excretion, painful, swollen graft
- Color-coded duplex sonography: increase in intrarenal resistance index
- Gold standard: kidney biopsy (Banff classification; ◘ Table 10.6)
- Therapy:
  - T-cell mediated rejection: steroid boli
  - Vascular rejection: antithymocyte globulin
  - Humoral rejection: antithymocyte globulin, plasmapheresis
  - For all forms, increase the dose of maintenance immunosuppression

Chronic Rejection

- Rejection within months to years after transplantation
- Pathomechanism:
  - Formation of donor-specific antibodies (de novo DSA), connection with poor adherence (immunosuppressants) is currently being discussed
  - Recurrent subclinical rejections
  - Presence of memory cells (B lymphocytes) for the formation of donor-specific antibodies, not detected by

Table 10.6 Banff classification of acute and chronic renal rejection

Grade	Definition
Acute kidney rejection	
Borderline damage	Focal mild tubulitis (1–2 mononuclear cells per cross-section) without intimal arteritis
IA	Significant interstitial infiltration (>25% of parenchyma affected) and focal, moderate tubulitis (>4 mononuclear cells per tubular cross-section or 10 tubular cells)
IB	Significant interstitial infiltration (>25% of parenchyma affected) and focal, severe tubulitis (>10 mononuclear cells per tubular cross-section)
IIA	Significant interstitial infiltration with mild to moderate intimal arteritis
IIB	Significant interstitial infiltration with moderate intimal arteritis (>25% of vessel lumen)
III	Transmural arteritis or fibrinoid changes and necrosis of the smooth muscle cells of the media
Chronic kidney rejection	
I	Signs of minor chronic ischemia with mild graft glomerulopathy, minor interstitial fibrosis, and tubular atrophy (<25% of cortical surface area)
II	Signs of moderate chronic ischemia with moderate graft glomerulopathy, moderate interstitial fibrosis and tubular atrophy (26–50% of cortical surface area)
III	Signs of severe chronic ischemia with severe graft glomerulopathy, extensive interstitial fibrosis, and tubular atrophy (>50% of cortical surface area)

cross-match and HLA typing (e.g. in the case of living donation from child's father to mother)
- Clinical presentation: Slow, continuous deterioration of renal function.
- Therapy:
  - Increasing immunosuppression
  - For donor-specific antibodies mostly frustrating

10.6.4 Infections

- Increased risk due to immunosuppression

Bacterial Infections

- Mostly urinary tract infections or pulmonary infections
- Atypical germs must be included in differential diagnosis
- Early resistance-appropriate antibiotic therapy

Opportunistic Infections

- Mostly in the first year after transplantation (higher immunosuppression)
- Mostly viral infections (CMV, BKV)
- Common pathogens:
  - CMV
  - Aspergillosis
  - Candida
  - Clostridium difficile

10.6.5 Aftercare

- After discharge from hospital:
  - Initially 2–3 times weekly in cooperation with a nephrologic centre
  - In the course increase of the interval
- One visit per year to the transplant centre
- Main focus: creatinine progression, immunosuppression

10.7 Results

- Survival rates ◘ Table 10.7

◘ **Table 10.7** 1- and 5-year survival rates of the transplant and the recipient comparing post-mortem organ donation vs. living donation

	Graft		**Recipient**	
	1 year	**5 years**	**1 year**	**5 years**
Post-mortem donation	91%	69%	96%	84%
Living donation	95%	80%	98%	91%

Spleen

Therezia Bokor-Billmann and Franck Billmann

Contents

F. Billmann, T. Keck (eds.), *Essentials of Visceral Surgery*,
https://doi.org/10.1007/978-3-662-66735-4_11

11.1 Spleen: Generalities

Key Points

- Coffee bean shaped organ; volume = 160 mL
- Intraperitoneal position, left hypochondriacal region
- Vascularization through splenic artery and vein (variations)
- Organ of filtering/degradation of erythrocytes and thrombocytes + Organ of lymphatic defence

11.1.1 Embryology and Developmental Disorders

Embryology

- Development in the dorsal mesogastrium
- Colonization of the spleen by vascular plexus
- Colonization by reticulum cells + lymphocytes (formation of splenic pulp)

Developmental Disabilities

- Aplasia (= agenesis = asplenia)
  - Complete absence of the spleen
  - Cause = Absence of the vasa splenica (developmental disorder 2nd–5th embryonic week)
  - Often associated with cardiac malformation/situs inversus
- Congenital hypoplasia
  - Primary growth inhibition of the spleen
  - Very rarely cardiac malformation/situs inversus

Splenic hypoplasia: Usually = secondary (atrophy)

11.1.2 Anatomy

Structure

Definition (◘ Fig. 11.1)

- Upper splenic pole = Extremitas superior
- Lower splenic pole = Extremitas inferior
- Posterior margin = Margo posterior
- Anterior margin = Margo anterior
- Surfaces:

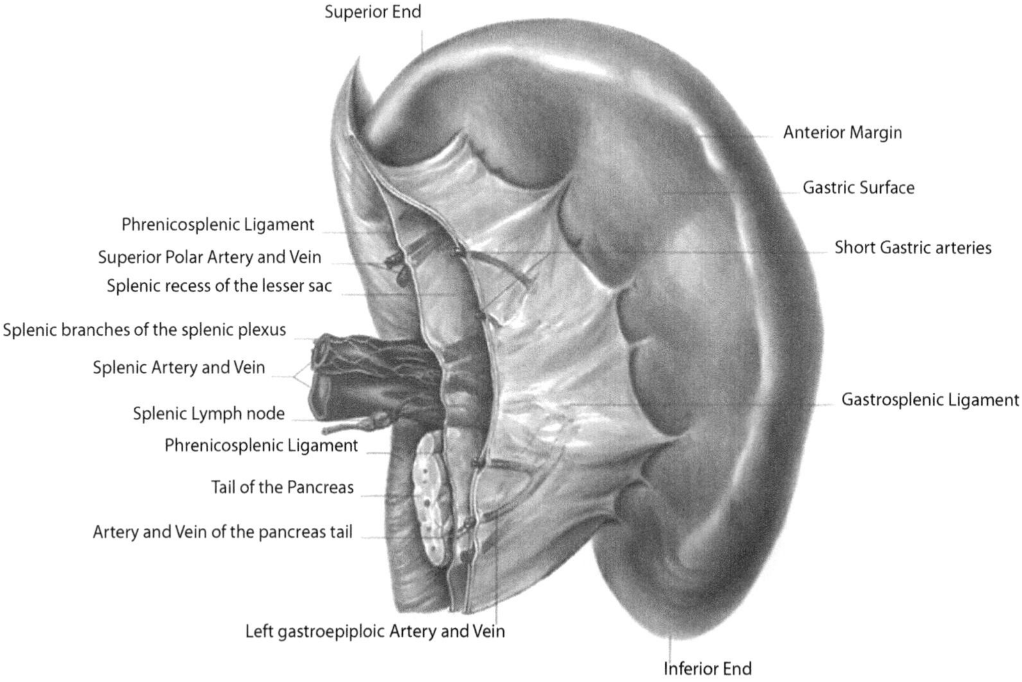

◘ **Fig. 11.1** View of the spleen from ventromedial. (From von Lanz and Wachsmuth 2004)

- Diaphragmatic surface (Facies diaphragmatica): relationship to the diaphragm
- Visceral surface (Facies visceralis): divided into two facets: Facies gastrica (for the stomach) + Facies renalis (for the left kidney); between the two: splenic hilus.

Form

- Similar to a coffee bean
- Variations: possible
- Parenchymal depression: at the anterior border of the spleen

Variations

- Double spleen: two separate, equally sized and adjacent partial spleens (rare)
- Multiple spleens: up to 10 spleens of unequal size; supplied by splenic artery
- Adjacent spleen: common (6–10% of population); very small roundish spleen adjacent to a regular spleen: CT hypervascular; DD: primitive neuroectodermal tumor

Measurements

- Depending on the blood supply of the organ/eventual pathology
- Expansion capacity of the spleen = 2–3 times the basal volume
- Decrease in height/weight from age 40 onwards

Measurements for Adults

- Length = 12.2 cm
- Width = 7.8 cm
- Thickness = 2.9 cm
- Weight (median):
  - Men = 162 g
  - Women = 155 g
- Volume (median) = 160 cm^3

Location

- Intraperitoneal, left hypochondriacal region
- Spleen longitudinal axis = course of 10th rib
- Position dependent on movements of the diaphragm (breathing)
  - Between lower margin 8th rib and upper margin 12th rib
  - Held in position by peritoneal ligaments = phrenicosplenic ligament + splenorenal ligament + gastrosplenic ligament

Vessels and Innervation

Vessels

- Splenic artery (A. splenica) = main vessel; one of the 3 branch vessels of the truncus coeliacus
- Polar arteries = variations:
  - In number: 1–5 splenic polar arteries
  - In origin: mostly from splenic artery; from left gastroepiploic (A. gastroomentalis sinistra), aorta, left gastric artery (A. gastrica sinistra), inferior pancreatic artery (A. pancreatica inferior), superior mesenteric artery (A. mesenterica superior)
- Splenic vein (V. splenica) to portal vein (V. portae hepatis)
- Blood circulation = 100–300 mL/min

Innervation

- Almost exclusively sympathetic postganglionic rr. splenici
- Few parasympathetic cholinergic fibers
- Spleen pain: Visceral pain, radiating from the front into the back

11.1.3 Physiology

Filter Function

Filter/Degradation Organ of the Altered Erythrocytes

- Filtering of pathologically altered red blood cells
- Storage of hemoglobin (destruction of the altered erythrocytes)

Storage/Degradation Organ of Platelets (and Clotting Products)

- Storage: up to 30% of circulating platelets
- Filtering of coagulation products in serum (parallel)

Lymphatic Defense Organ

- Formation of new B-lymphocytes
- Presentation of antigens to lymphocytes
- Spleen = most important organ of lymphocyte recirculation

11.2 Spleen Diseases

Key Points

- Benign diseases: Especially of hematological origin
- Malignancies: Lymphomas vs. leukemias vs. metastases
- Splenic trauma: Mostly blunt abdominal trauma; conservative vs. surgical approach.
- Post-splenectomy morbidity: vaccination (possible pre- or postoperatively)

11.2.1 Benign Haematological Diseases

Idiopathic Thrombocytopenic Purpura (ITP)

Definition

- Thrombocytopenia: platelet count $<150{,}000/mm^3$
- Normal bone marrow function
- Exclusion of another cause of thrombocytopenia

Mechanism

- Increased platelet destruction
- By autoantibodies against platelet membrane antigens
- Phagocytosis of platelets in the reticuloendothelial system (spleen)

Epidemiology

- Young women > Men
- 72% patients >10 years old
- 70% young women >40 years old

Clinical Examination

- Purpura
- Epistaxis
- Bleeding gums
- Less common: GI (gastrointestinal) bleeding, hematuria, cerebral hemorrhage.

Diagnosis

- Laboratory diagnosis: thrombocytopenia
- Exclusion of other causes of thrombocytopenia (◘ Table 11.1)
- Diagnosis follows this exclusion strategy

Table 11.1 Differential diagnoses of immune thrombocytopenic purpura

False-low platelets	– EDTA-induced in vitro platelet clumping or cold agglutinins – Giant platelets
Common causes of thrombocytopenia	– Pregnancy (pregnancy thrombocytopenia, preeclampsia) – Drug/drug-induced thrombocytopenia (heparin, quinidine, quinine, sulfonamides) – Viral infections (HIV, infectious mononucleosis, etc.) – Hypersplenism (chronic liver failure)
Other causes of thrombocytopenia	– Myelodysplasia – Congenital thrombocytopenias – Thrombotic thrombocytopenic—purpura/hemolytic uremic syndrome – Chronic disseminated intravascular coagulation
Secondary thrombocytopenias	– Autoimmune diseases (e.g. lupus) – Lymphoproliferative diseases (CLL, non-Hodgkin lymphoma)

EDTA ethylenediaminetetraacetic acid, *HIV* human immunodeficiency virus, *CLL* chronic lymphocytic leukemia

Therapy

- Depending on the severity of thrombocytopenia

Strategy

- Platelets >50,000/mm^3 + asymptomatic: monitoring
- 30,000 > Platelets >50,000/mm^3 + asymptomatic
  - Monitoring without therapy
  - Glucocorticoids: prednisone (1 mg/kg BW/day)
- Platelets >20,000/mm^3 + few symptoms: Glucocorticoids (see above)
- Platelets <20,000/mm^3 + bleeding: Inpatient treatment
  - Platelet transfusion only if there is serious bleeding.
  - I. v. immunoglobulins in case of bleeding and preoperatively (1 g/kg BW/day for 2 days)

Splenectomy

- Indications:
  - Refractory severe ITP
  - Patients requiring very high or toxic doses of glucocorticoids
  - Thrombocytopenia recurrence
  - Incomplete response after drug therapy
  - Pregnant women after drug therapy with a risk of bleeding
- Modality:
  - Open splenectomy
  - Laparoscopic splenectomy (see below)
- Result: Immediate response (within 10 days postoperatively) = 71–95%

Surgical Procedure

Laparoscopic Splenectomy

- Preoperative skin marking, pressure-free right lateral positioning, slight angulation of the operation table to increase the distance between the costal arch and the spina iliaca
- Inferior dissection of the spleen, possible partial mobilization of the left colonic flexure
- Transection of the splenogastric ligament and the gastricae-breves vessels (ligasure)
- Visualization of the splenic hilus and vessels
- Minimal skeletonization of the splenic artery and clipping by means of laparoscopic clips/vascular clips + transection
- Initial clipping of the artery: reduction of the spleen volume
- Dissection of the lateral and retroperitoneal splenic ligaments
- Identification of the pancreas tail and mobilization of the pancreas without injury

- Visualization of the splenic vein, skeletonization, clipping by means of laparoscopic clips/vascular clips and transection
- Transection the splenodiaphragmatic ligament
- Extraction of the spleen using of a laparoscopic extraction bag
- Irrigation and closure, drainage if necessary

Hereditary Spherocytosis

Definition

- Hereditary autosomal dominant disease
- Genetic defect: Alteration of the proteins of the ankyrin complex (= erythrocyte cytoskeleton protein) (e.g. ankyrin, α- and β-spectrin protein)

Mechanism

- Ankyrin/spectrin alteration/deficit = erythrocyte cell membrane deficit = erythrocytes smaller, rounder, non-deformable
- Consequence = increased osmotic fragility
- In the spleen: spherocytes increasingly trapped = erythrocytopenia (= haemolysis)

Clinical Examination

- Variable: asymptomatic carrier to severe hemolysis
- Anemia
- Possibly jaundice
- Splenomegaly

Diagnosis

- Spherocytes
- Increased reticulocyte count
- Increased osmotic fragility of erythrocytes
- Negative Coombs test

Therapy

- Splenectomy
- Mechanism: Reduction of hemolysis by abolishing destruction in the spleen; no influence on spherocytosis

Hemolytic Anemia Due to Erythrocyte Enzyme Defect

Definition

- Two enzymatic defects:
  - Glucose-6-phosphate dehydrogenase (G6PD): X-linked inheritance
  - Pyruvate kinase: autosomal inheritance
- Mechanism: defect = abnormal glucose metabolism = abnormal erythrocyte deformability = hemolysis in the spleen

Clinical Examination

- Glucose-6-phosphate dehydrogenase deficit: anemia following drug, medication, or chemical exposure
- Pyruvate kinase deficit: anemia + splenomegaly

Therapy

- Glucose-6-phosphate dehydrogenase deficit: splenectomy rarely indicated
- Pyruvate kinase deficit: splenectomy

Haemoglobinopathies

Definition

- Two entities:
  - Sickle cell anemia: Autosomal recessive disease
  - Thalassemia: Autosomal dominant disease
- Mechanism:
  - Sickle cell anaemia: deformation of erythrocytes in haemoglobin S homozygous patients = destruction of erythrocytes in spleen = anaemia; in

heterozygous patients deformation in certain reduced P_aO_2-situations
  - Thalassemia: defect in hemoglobin synthesis = hemolytic anemia

Clinical Examination

- Sickle cell anaemia: haemolytic anaemia + thrombosis = microinfarctions (especially in the spleen) + hypersplenism
- Thalassemia: Hemolytic anemia + splenomegaly + splenomegaly + hypersplenism

Hypersplenism + splenic sequestration
- For sickle cell disease and thalassaemia
- Consequence: Acute splenomegaly = severe pain + need for transfusion

Therapy

- Medical/conservative therapy: transfusions, painkillers, etc.
- Splenectomy:
  - Indication: recurrent acute sequestration crises; recurrent blood transfusions; massive splenomegaly; splenic abscesses
  - Open vs. laparoscopic splenectomy

11.2.2 Other Benign Diseases

Splenic Cysts

Classification

- True cysts (parasitic/non-parasitic)
- Pseudocysts: Mostly secondary after trauma
- Cystic-impressing tumors: cystic lymphangiomas, cavernous hemangiomas

Clinical Examination

- Mostly asymptomatic
- Symptoms: vague pain in the left upper abdomen, left back or shoulder pain, pleuritic chest pain, shortness of breath
- Acute symptoms due to hemorrhage of the cyst; usually due to increase in size of the cyst

Epidemiology

- True cysts: mostly parasitic (Ecchinococcus species)
- Non-parasitic cysts: 70–80% = pseudocysts

Therapy

- Suspicion of parasitic cysts: Preoperative serological confirmation
- Parasitic cysts/pseudocysts: splenectomy
- Non-parasitic cysts: partial splenectomy
- Pseudocysts: If <4 cm: Monitoring

Splenic Abscess

- Rare, potentially life-threatening disease
- Incidence = 0.7%
- Mortality:
  - 15–20% in previously healthy patients
  - Up to 80% in immunocompromised patients

Risk Factors

- Malignant diseases
- polycythemia vera
- Endocarditis
- Haemoglobinopathies
- I. v. drug abuse
- AIDS ("acquired immunodeficiency syndrome")
- Urinary tract infections

Clinical Examination

- Often non-specific:
  - Abdominal pain in the left upper quadrant
  - Fever
  - Peritonitis signs
  - Pleuritic chest pain

Diagnosis
- CT abdomen with contrast medium

Therapy
- Unilocular abscesses: CT-guided drainage (success rate = 75–90%) + antibiotics.
- Multilocular abscesses: Splenectomy + peritoneal drainage + antibiotics

11.2.3 Malignant Diseases

Lymphomas
- Hodgkin lymphoma: surgical therapy = staging laparoscopy
- Non-Hodgkin lymphoma: splenectomy in patients with isolated splenic involvement

Leukemia
- Hairy-cell leukemia: splenectomy in patients with splenomegaly.
- Chronic lymphocytic leukemia: splenectomy = palliative measure for symptomatic splenomegaly
- Chronic myelocytic leukemia: splenectomy = palliative measure in symptomatic splenomegaly or hypersplenism

Non-hematological Malignant Tumors
- Metastases:
  - Mostly from cancers of the breast, lung or melanoma
  - Mostly asymptomatic
  - Symptoms if: Splenomegaly/spleen rupture
  - Splenectomy = effective palliative treatment
- Vascular tumors:
  - Benign: Hemangiomas
  - Malignant: angiosarcomas, hemangiosarcomas; highly aggressive tumors = splenectomy (diagnostic, therapeutic, palliative)

11.2.4 Spleen Trauma

- See polytrauma; blunt abdominal trauma

Epidemiology
- Spleen trauma = most frequent indication for laparotomy after blunt abdominal trauma
- Mechanisms:
  - Car/truck accident most frequent
  - Other: Falls; pedestrian vs. car/motorcycle; bicycle accident; sports accidents.

Pathophysiology
- Injury by:
  - Rapid deceleration (with avulsion of the splenic ligaments) = capsular avulsion
  - Compression
  - Energy transfer through the posterolateral thoracic wall
  - Impaling through a (fractured) rib
- Spleen perfusion = 5% of cardiac output = minimal splenic trauma = severe bleeding

Diagnosis

Anamnesis
- Mostly orienting/typical
- Important = accident mechanism

Clinical Examination
- Peritoneal irritation (pain, defense)
- External signs of direct force (deformity, haematoma, etc.)
- Hemodynamic status (hypotension, tachycardia)

Ultrasound Examination

- FAST (Focussed Assessment with Sonography in Trauma)
- Non-invasive, quickly available, cost-effective
- Quickly leads to the diagnosis and treatment strategy

Diagnostic peritoneal lavage
- Obsolete
- Has been replaced by FAST and CT

- CT abdomen:
  - If patient is hemodynamically stable
  - Excellent morphological representation of the injury
  - Classification according to American Association for the Surgery of Trauma Splenic Injury Scale (◘ Table 11.2)

Therapy

- Medical/conservative vs. surgical therapy
- Surgical therapy: spleen-preserving surgery vs. splenectomy
- Indication for surgical exploration:
  - Hemodynamic instability
  - Progressive intra-abdominal blood loss (in ultrasound, CT)
  - Large hemoperitoneum
  - Relative: Pseudoaneurysm in traumatized splenic area

11.2.5 Post-splenectomy Morbidity

Asplenia: Pathophysiology

- Thromboembolic consequences:
  - Due to thrombocytosis (= increase in platelet concentration in the blood)
  - Increased risk of deep vein thrombosis + pulmonary embolism
  - Lifetime pulmonary embolism risk = 35.6% vs. 9.7% (in control group)
- Immunological consequences:
  - Due to the absence of splenic function
  - OPSI (Overwhelming Post-Splenectomy Infection)
    - Rare, but high mortality = 50–70%
    - Often prodromes (malaise, myalgias, vomiting)
    - Pneumonia
    - Rapid progression of the disease
    - Multi-organ failure: hypotension → disseminated intravascular coagulation → respiratory failure → coma → death within hours of onset.
    - Pathogen: Mostly S. pneumoniae; other pathogens: Haemophilus influenzae, Neisseria meningitis, Salmonella species

Prophylactic Therapy in Asplenia Patients

- Vaccination (◘ Table 11.3):
  - Three to four weeks preoperatively before elective splenectomy
  - Three weeks postoperatively after non-elective splenectomy
  - Pneumococcal, Haemophilus influenzae type b, meningococcal and influenza vaccinations
  - Connection to asplenia outpatient clinic
- Antibiotics: Currently no data on antibiotic prophylaxis in splenectomized patients; however, recommended in children <5, 2 years after splenectomy in children of all ages, and adults after postsplenectomy sepsis.
- From 1 million platelets/mm^3: prophylactic ASS (acetylsalicylic acid) administration (thrombosis prophylaxis)

Table 11.2 American Association for the Surgery of Trauma Spleen Injury Scale (2018 revision)

Grade[a]	AIS[b] severity	Imaging criteria (CT)	Surgical criteria	Pathological criteria
I	2	Subcapsular hematoma <10% of the surface	Subcapsular hematoma <10% of the surface	Subcapsular hematoma <10% of surface
		Parenchyma lazeration <1 cm depth	Parenchyma lazeration <1 cm depth	Parenchyma lazeration <1 cm depth
		Capsule injury	Capsule injury	Capsule injury
II	2	Subcapsular hematoma 10–50% of the surface; intraparenchymal hematoma <5 cm	Subcapsular hematoma 10–50% of the surface; intraparenchymal hematoma <5 cm	Subcapsular hematoma 10–50% of the surface; intraparenchymal hematoma <5 cm
		Parenchymal laceration 1–3 cm	Parenchyma laceration 1–3 cm	Parenchymal laceration 1–3 cm
III	3	Subcapsular hematoma >50% of the surface; ruptured subcapsular or intraparenchymal hematoma ≥5 cm	Subcapsular hematoma >50% of the surface or progressive in size; ruptured subcapsular or intraparenchymal hematoma ≥5 cm	Subcapsular hematoma >50% of the surface; ruptured subcapsular or intraparenchymal hematoma ≥5 cm
		Parenchymal laceration >3 cm in depth	Parenchymal laceration >3 cm in depth	Parenchymal laceration >3 cm in depth
IV	4	Any injury with lesion of the splenic vessels or active intracapsular splenic hemorrhage	Parenchymal laceration with involvement of segmental or hilar splenic vessels with >25% devascularization	Parenchymal laceration with involvement of segmental or hilar splenic vessels with >25% devascularization
		Parenchymal laceration with involvement of segmental or hilar splenic vessels with >25% devascularization		
V	5	Any injury with lesion of the splenic vessels and active bleeding into the peritoneal space; injury of spleen-adjacent structures	Hilar vascular injury with splenic devascularization	Hilar vascular injury with splenic devascular-ization
		Destroyed spleen	Destroyed spleen	Destroyed spleen

Vascular injury defined by pseudoaneurysm or arteriovenous fistula; presents as focal collection of contrast from a vessel with decrease in intensity on delayed imaging. Active bleeding from a vascular lesion defined as contrast leakage from a vessel, focal or diffuse, with increase in size or decrease in intensity on delayed imaging. Vascular thrombosis can lead to infarction of the organ

[a] Grade classification based on highest classification by imaging, surgery or pathology. For multiple injury: Grade + 1 to Grade III

[b] *AIS* abbreviated injury scale

Table 11.3 Recommended vaccinations for asplenia patients

Vaccination[a]	Before elective splenectomy[b]	After splenectomy[c]
Pneumococcal vaccination	– Sequential vaccination with conjugate vaccine (PCV13 Prevenar 13®) followed by PPSV23 (Pneumovax 23®) 8 weeks later (children <24 months should be vaccinated with PCV13 only) – Repeat vaccination (PPSV23) and booster every 6 years	– If vaccination has not yet taken place, sequential PCV13 and PPSV23 8 weeks later – If vaccination with PCV13 has already taken place, then only PPSV23 at the earliest 2 weeks after splenectomy (if follow-up uncertain PPSV23 before discharge) – Repeat vaccination (PPSV23) and booster every 6 years
Haemophilus influenzae type b vaccination	– Single vaccination with single vaccine Act-Hib® or Hiberix® – No repetition/refresher	Id. as before elective splenectomy
Meningococcal vaccinations	– Vaccination against meningococci of serogroups ACWY – Children >2 months and adults: single dose of a 4-valent conjugate vaccine MenACWY (Menveo®, Nimenrix®) – Currently no refresher recommended	Two doses of MenACWY with an interval of 8–12 weeks between doses
	– Vaccination against meningococci of serogroup B – Since 2015 STIKO recommendation for vaccination using Bexsero® or Trumenba® (risk assessment by the treating physician) – Currently no refresher recommended	Id. as before elective splenectomy
Influenza vaccination	– Annual influenza vaccination in autumn – Children and adolescents up to 17 years of age may be vaccinated with inactivated vaccine or live nasal attenuated vaccine (LAIV)	Id. as before elective splenectomy

[a] Recommendations of the Robert Koch Institute "Vaccinations in Asplenia"
[b] If possible, the vaccinations should have taken place at least 2 weeks before the operation
[c] After splenectomy, vaccination can be given as soon as the patient is in a stable general condition

References

von Lanz T, Wachsmuth W (2004) Praktische anatomie. Hals. Springer, Berlin

Further Reading

Beauchamp RD, Holzman MD, Fabian TC, Weinberg JA (2008) The spleen. In: Townsend CM Jr, Beauchamp RD, Evers BM, Mattox KL (eds) Sabiston textbook of surgery. The biological basis of modern surgical practice, 18th edn. Saunders, Elsevier, Philadelphia

Bhangu A, Nepogodiev D, Lal N, Bowley DM (2012) Meta-analysis of predictive factors and outcomes for failure of non-operative management of blunt splenic trauma. Injury 43:1337–1346

Cooper N, Ghanima W (2019) Immune thrombocytopenia. N Engl J Med 381:945–955

Feig BW, Ching CD (2019) The MD Anderson surgical oncology handbook, 6th edn. Wolters Kluwer, Philadelphia

Germer CT, Keck T, Grundmann RT (2017) Evidenzbasierte Viszeralchirurgie benigner Erkrankungen. Springer, Berlin

Iolascon A, Andolfo I, Russo R (2019) Advances in understanding the pathogenesis of red cell membrane disorders. Br J Haematol 187:13–24

Keck T, Germer CT (2017) Minimal invasive Viszeralchirurgie. Springer, Berlin

Leonhardt H, Tillmann B, Töndury G, Zilles K (2003) Lehrbuch und Atlas der Anatomie des Menschen, Innere Organe, vol 2, 3rd edn. Thieme, Stuttgart

Piel FB, Steinberg MH, Rees DC (2017) Sickle cell disease. N Engl J Med 376:1561–1573

Piel FB, Weatherall DJ (2014) The α-thalassemias. N Engl J Med 371:1908–1916

Rauber A, Kopsch F (1948) Lehrbuch und Atlas der Anatomie des Menschen, Eingeweide, vol 2, 17th edn. Thieme, Leipzig

Robert Koch Institut (2019) Impfungen bei Asplenie. https://www.rki.de/sharedDocs/FAQ/Impfen/AllgFr_Grunderkrankungen/FAQ01.html. Accessed on 7.6.2021

Rubin LG, Schaffner W (2014) Clinical practice. Care of the apslenic patient. N Engl J Med 371:349–356

Standring S (2009) Gray's anatomy. the anatomical basis of clinical practice, 40th edn. Churchill Livingstone, Elsevier, London

The American Association for Surgery of Trauma (2018) Injury scoring scale. A resource for trauma care professionals. http://www.aast.org/library/traumatools/injuryscoringscales.aspx#spleen. Accessed on 7.6.2021

Theilacker C, Ludewig K, Serr A, Schimpf J, Held J, Bögelein M, Bahr V, Rusch S, Pohl A, Kogelmann K, Frieseke S, Bogdanski R, Brunkhorst FM, Kern WV (2016) Overwhelming postsplenectomy infection: a prospective multicenter cohort study. Clin Infect Dis 62:871–878

von Lanz T, Wachsmuth W (2004) Praktische Anatomie. Bauch. Springer, Berlin

Zilles K, Tillmann B (2010) Anatomie. Springer, Berlin

Peritoneum

Jörg Pelz

Contents

F. Billmann, T. Keck (eds.), *Essentials of Visceral Surgery*,
https://doi.org/10.1007/978-3-662-66735-4_12

12.1 Anatomy and Physiology of the Peritoneum

12.1.1 General Anatomy

Definition

- Peritoneum = serous membrane
- One of the largest organ in terms of area
- Mesothelial covering of the abdominal cavity and the organs therein (peritoneum viscerale) (excluded: retroperitoneal and extraperitoneal organs)
- Total area: 1.6 and 2.0 m^2
- Blood flow: approx. 100–200 mL/min
- Lymphatic absorption rate
  - Approx. 1–2 mL/min
  - Drainage via the lymphatic channels to the thoracic duct

Structure (Histology)

- Mesothelium (Tunica serosa) = serous membrane
- Extracellular matrix (lamina propia)
- Connective tissue layer (Tela subserosa)
- Thickness = 90–130 µm

Division

- Visceral peritoneum (Peritoneum viscerale) (80%)
  - Covering of the abdominal viscera and organs
  - Innervated = pain (visceral pain)
- Parietal peritoneum (Peritoneum parietale) (20%)
  - Covering of the inner side of the abdominal wall (somatic pain)
- Peritoneal fluid (physiologically production 50–70 mL/day)

12.1.2 Physiology (Tasks) of the Peritoneum

Organ Mobility

- Mobility (sliding) of the abdominal organs
- Through liquid film on the serosal epithelium

Resorption

- Within minutes; in cranial direction transdiaphragmatic
- Metabolically highly active membrane (semi-permeable)
- Used for peritoneal dialysis or intraperitoneal chemoperfusion/therapy

Immunological Tasks (= Defence)

- Especially for infections of the abdominal cavity
- Inflammatory process (vasodilation, phagocytic clearance)
- Involved in macrophage activation
- Humoral immunity by complement system
- Clearance limitation: Critical limit at >105 germs/mL
- High regeneration capacity

12.2 Benign Diseases of the Peritoneum

Key Points

- Peritonitis (inflammation of the peritoneum)
  - Manifestation up to a severe septic course
  - Medical/conservative vs. surgical treatment
- Peritoneal adhesions = most frequent cause of small bowel obstruction (ileus)
  - Surgical therapy for ileus

12.2.1 Peritonitis

Definition

- Inflammation of the peritoneum
- Evolution: Up to a severe septic course

Etiology

Primary Peritonitis (Without Previous Abdominal Disease)

- About 1% of peritonitis

- By hematogenous seeding of bacteria
- Frequent association with liver cirrhosis

Secondary Peritonitis
- Inflammations (cholecystitis, appendicitis, etc.)
- Perforation of an abdominal organ (gastric ulcer, anastomotic insufficiency, etc.)
- Perforation of the abdomen (e.g. stab wounds)

Spontaneous Bacterial Peritonitis (e.g. in Ascites, Liver Cirrhosis)

Special Form: Peritonitis After CAPD Catheter Insertion
- Frequently!
- CAPD: "continuous ambulatory peritoneal dialysis".

Classification
- According to aetiology (see above)
- According to localization
  - Local peritonitis
  - Diffuse (generalized) peritonitis
- According to clinical course
  - Acute peritonitis
  - Chronic peritonitis
  - Localized peritonitis
  - Generalized peritonitis

Symptoms
- Abdominal tension
- Fever
- Increase in inflammatory signs (leukocytosis, CRP, erythrocyte sedimentation rate ESR, procalcitonin)
- Pain (localized/generalized)
- Fluid shift

Diagnosis
- Anamnesis
- Clinical examination
  - Abdominal tenderness and guarding
  - Abdominal rigidity
  - Pain localization
- Laboratory (leukocytosis, CRP elevation)
- Ultrasound
- Computer tomography CT
  - Contrast medium image of the parietal peritoneum
  - Search of the source of peritonitis
  - Peritoneocentesis as direct pathogen detection

Therapy

Surgical Therapy
- Eradication of the source of infectious (if present)
- Closed peritoneal lavage
  - Irrigation of the peritoneal space (through drains placed during the operation) after appropriate operations
  - For accelerated removal of inflammatory secretion/pus as a consequence of various surgical diseases of the abdominal cavity
  - **Caution**: Often irrigation limited to area directly adjacent to drains (not entire peritoneal cavity)
- Staged lavage (= programmed lavage)
  - For high-grade inflammatory diseases of the abdominal cavity
  - Planned relaparotomy (with irrigation) performed at set intervals evidence-based worse than on-demand lavage (according to patient's clinical condition)

> **Caution**
> In pancreatitis usually conservative approach.

Conservative Therapy
- Calculated antibiotic administration
- Adequate fluid management (volume and catecholamine controlled, hemodynamic monitoring)
- Intensive care unit monitoring for severe peritonitis

12.2.2 Peritoneal Adhesions

Epidemiology
- Mostly postoperative

- Most frequent cause of small bowel obstruction (ileus = approx. 60% of obstructions)
- More often in the lower abdomen:
  - After gynecological surgery
  - After appendectomy
  - After colorectal resection

Clinical Presentation

- Asymptomatic to full image of ileus (► Sect. 16.2)
- Usually nonspecific, occasionally crampy abdominal pain

Diagnostic Imaging

- CT: Indirect evidence of adhesions: dilated small bowel loops on the anterior abdominal wall; caliber change of the small bowel.
- MRI: MRI-sellink if necessary

Therapy

- Asymptomatic adhesions/nonspecific pain:
  - Symptomatic therapy preferred
  - Adhesiolysis: Only in individual cases, due to high incidence of recurrence.
- In case of manifest ileus: surgical therapy (► Sect. 16.2)

12.3 Pseudomyxoma Peritonei

12.3.1 Definition

- Accumulation of mucus masses in the abdominal cavity due to a mucus-forming tumour. Lymph node (<5%) or distant metastases may rarely occur.

12.3.2 Classification

- Three groups (1995 classification)
  - "Disseminated peritoneal adenomucinosis (DPAM): Rather benign appearance.
  - "peritoneal mucinous carcinomatosis" (PMCA): cause = disseminated carcinoma cells, malignant appearance
  - Intermediate category

Controversy: Benign disease vs malignant disease without infiltrative growth.

12.3.3 Aetiology

- Mucinous cystadenoma (= mucocele) of the appendix vermiformis
  - Second most common tumor of the appendix (after appendiceal carcinoid)
  - In case of accidental detection: indication for metachronous or synchronous right hemicolectomy (better outcome)
  - In 50% of cases further intra-abdominal manifestation at diagnosis
- Mucinous tumor of the ovary (= mucocele)
  - Rare
- Tumour cell spillage of malignant tumours of the abdominal cavity (e.g. appendix, ovary, colon, uterus)

12.3.4 Clinical Presentation

- Local problems due to displacing growth, subileus

12.3.5 Therapy

- ► Section 12.5: Cytoreductive surgery (CRS) + hyperthermic intraperitoneal chemotherapy (HIPEC)
- Poor/no effect of systemic chemotherapy
- Absolute indication for HIPEC therapy (highest evidence)
- Right hemicolectomy for R0-resected "low-grade tumours" = not recommended

12.3.6 Prognosis

- With CRS + HIPEC: 10-year survival rate approx. 70%
- Low-grade tumor with significantly better outcome

12.4 Malignant Diseases of the Peritoneum

Key Points

- Peritoneal carcinomatosis = most frequent secondary, malignant disease of the peritoneum
- Therapy: Paradigm shift with cytoreductive surgery (CRS) + HIPEC
- CRS + HIPEC:
  - Significant survival benefit in selected tumor entities
  - Optional treatment strategy in the current S3 guidelines for colorectal cancer
  - High morbidity between 25% and 60%
  - Mortality between 2 and 10
  - The impact of chemoperfusion is unclear!

12.4.1 Mesothelioma

Definition

- Primary malignant disease of the peritoneum

Epidemiology

- Most common primary malignant disease of the peritoneum
- Mostly limited to the abdomen
- Median survival = 4–12 months (due to advanced stage at diagnosis)
- history of asbestosis: 50–70% of patients

Clinical Presentation

- Abdominal pain
- Ascites
- Weight loss

Prognosis

- Frequent infiltration of the other intra-abdominal organs (liver, intestine, bladder, abdominal wall)
- Men with significantly worse outcome
- Median (overall) survival of 33 months
- Better survival in epithelioid subtype and after CC-0 resection

Therapy

- Difficult to treat
- Goal = complete surgical resection
- Concept of CRS + HIPEC

12.4.2 Peritoneal Carcinomatosis

Epidemiology

- Synchronous peritoneal carcinomatosis in 5–10% of all gastrointestinal tumors
- Another 5–15% = metachronous
- Mean survival time of these patients is severely limited

Clinical Presentation

- History of malignancy
- Abdominal pain
- Ascites
- Weight loss

Diagnosis

- Pretherapeutic staging = essential

Imaging Techniques

- CT, MRI or PET-CT
- Frequent understaging:
  - Sensitivity between 50 and 96
  - Specificity between 62 and 100
  - Radiologic diagnosis of carcinomatosis of the small intestine: in only 50% of cases

Staging Laparoscopy

- Small tumor nodules can be detected earlier
- Biopsy and pathological workup possible
- If necessary, limited tumor removal is possible laparoscopically
- Disadvantage: Second-look operation is usually necessary

Therapy

- Cytoreductive therapy alone not sufficient for cure
- Systemic chemotherapy = currently palliative standard treatment procedure
- Interdisciplinary treatment concept = central (tumor board)
- Development of new therapeutic strategies (CRS + HIPEC; ► Sect. 12.5)

Systemic Chemotherapy

- Always as an interdisciplinary approach
- Important factor in multimodal treatment
- Results:
  - Median survival = 9–12 months (palliative chemotherapy)
  - Median survival = up to 20 months (modern combination chemotherapeutics)
  - Median survival = up to 30 months in selected patients
- Pros:
  - Systemic effect (influence also on potential distant metastases)
  - Fewer complications when compared with surgery
- Disadvantages:
  - Still limited efficacy in peritoneal carcinomatosis

12

12.5 Cytoreductive Surgery (CRS) and HIPEC

- Definition:
  - Combination of cytoreductive surgery (CRS) followed by hyperthermic intraperitoneal chemoperfusion (HIPEC)

12.5.1 Curative CRS and HIPEC

Theoretical Approach

- Cytoreductive surgery: goal = removal of all visible tumor manifestations
- HIPEC: goal = destruction of remaining tumor cells after CRS
  - Chemotherapeutic agents can be distributed throughout the abdomen
  - Intraoperative application = dose-intensified + timely adjuvant/additive chemotherapy with cytotoxic concentration (not possible with systemic administration)
  - Schematic representation of a HIPEC perfusion: ◘ Fig. 12.1

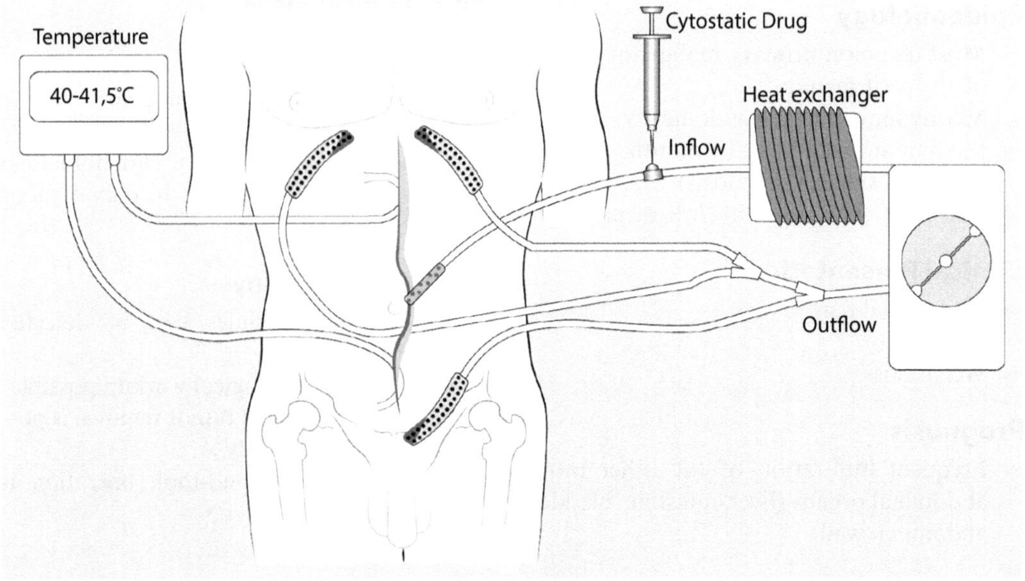

◘ **Fig. 12.1** Schematic representation of HIPEC according to Pelz

Surgical Procedure

Cytoreductive Surgery

- Median laparotomy from the xyphoid process to the symphysis pubica
- Incision of the abdominal wall without incision of the peritoneum, detachment of the closed parietal peritoneum
- Opening the peritoneum
- Staging = documentation of the Peritoneal Cancer Index (PCI) according to Sugarbaker (a total of 13 regions to be assessed) = prognostic factor and relevant for indication:
  - Abdominal cavity divided into 9 regions
  - Small intestine into further 4 regions
  - Point system depending on tumor size in each region: Absence of tumor = 0 points (LS0); up to 0.5 cm = 1 point (LS1); up to 5 cm = 2 points (LS2); > 5 cm = 3 points (LS3)
  - PCI between 0 and 39 points (◘ Fig. 12.2)
- Removal of all visible tumor manifestations (up to multivisceral resection); if a stoma is necessary: Only after HIPEC
- Postoperative classification: Completeness of Cytoreduction (CC) according to Sugarbaker (◘ Fig. 12.3) = prognostic factor
- Therapy goal = CC-0 or CC-1
- Placement of 4 26-CH silicone drains (= preparation HIPEC and drainage):
  - One inflow: At the site of greatest tumor burden
  - Three drains: Subphrenic right, subphrenic left, Douglas…
  - Two intra-abdominal temperature probes
- HIPEC:
  - Following cytoreductive surgery (◘ Fig. 12.1)
  - Inflow temperature 41–43 °C
  - Perfusion time 30–120 min
  - Open or closed perfusion
  - Chemotherapeutics
  - At present, there is no uniform recommendation on the type and dose of cytostatic drug to be used

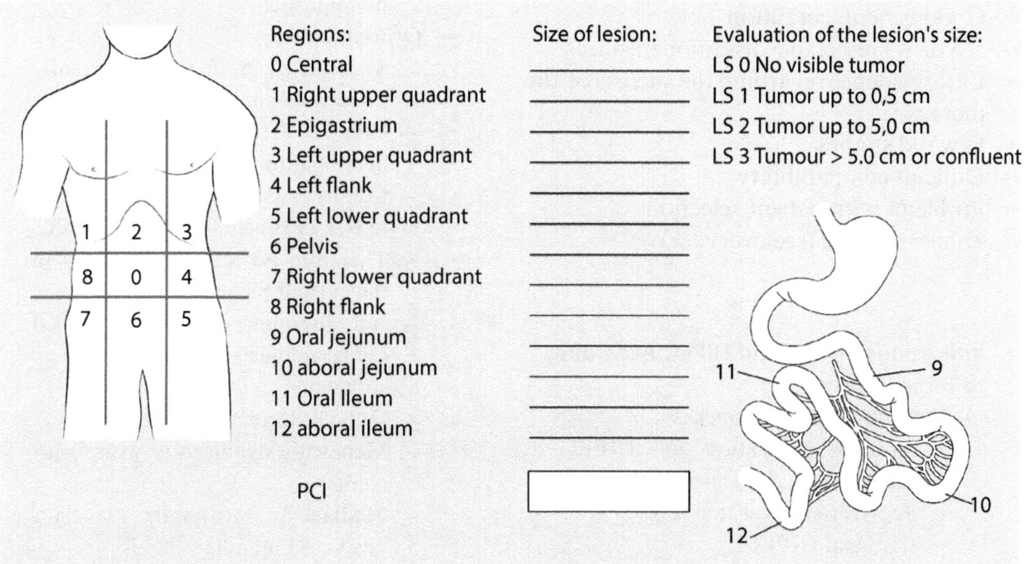

◘ **Fig. 12.2** Peritoneal carcinoid index according to Sugarbaker. (Mod. according to Jacquet and Sugarbaker 1996)

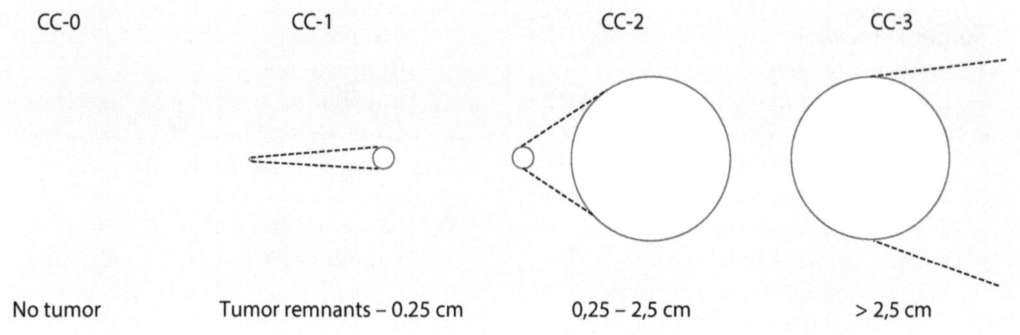

Fig. 12.3 Completeness of Cytoreduction (CC score) according to Sugarbaker. Assessment of postoperative tumor burden after cytoreductive surgery. Surgical score *CC-0* means that no tumor was left; *CC-1* tumor remnants up to 0.25 cm, *CC-2* tumor remnants of 0.25–2.5 cm, *CC-3* tumor remnants larger than 2.5 cm. (Mod. according to Jacquet and Sugarbaker 1996)

Concept and Goals

- Resection of the primary tumor
- Macroscopic complete removal of all accessible tumor metastases
- HIPEC (= hyperthermic intraperitoneal chemoperfusion) = destruction of remaining tumor cells after CRS
- The value of hyperthermic perfusion is unclear. Preliminary publications of the PRODIGE-7 study do not show any survival benefits with the use of oxaliplatin.

12

Indication

- Limited tumor extension
- Good general condition
- No or <3 resectable distant metastases
- Little evidence regarding the success of the therapy
- Few/old studies
- Difficult comparability
- Problems with patient selection
- Tumor entities: (see overview)

Indications of CRS and HIPEC According to Tumor Entities

- Pseudomyxoma peritonei:
  - Absolute indication for HIPEC therapy = Highest level of evidence
  - Ten-year survival rate of 69% after CRS and HIPEC
  - Low-grade tumor with significantly better outcome
  - Right hemicolectomy not recommended for R0-resected low-grade tumors
- Colorectal cancer:
  - Only one randomized trial (Verwaal et al. 2003) = significant survival benefit with respect to HIPEC therapy
  - Five-year survival = 54%; median survival = 62 months in highly selected patients (= benefit for patients likely linked with surgery)
  - Careful patient selection = absolute prerequisite!
- Ovarian cancer:
  - Systemic chemotherapy = currently therapy of choice
  - CRS + HIPEC currently under investigation
  - Controversial publications: tendency to lack of benefit for CRS + HIPEC
  - Therefore no recommendations in the current S3 guidelines
  - Interdisciplinary approach needed (gynaecologist + surgeon)
- Mesothelioma:
  - Difficult to treat tumor
  - Men with significantly worse outcome
  - Median (overall) survival = 33 months
  - Better survival in epithelioid subtype and after CC-0 resection

- Stomach:
  - Overall poor prognosis
  - Systemic therapy = therapy of choice
  - Median survival = 15 months
  - Perioperative lethality rate of 4.9%
  - Contraindication for PCI >10 and/or signet ring cell carcinoma
  - Rather HIPEC in synchronous peritoneal carcinomatosis (Gastripec randomized trial)
- Intra-abdominal sarcoma:
  - Very poor prognosis despite multimodal therapy
  - Median survival = 26 months
  - Systemic chemotherapy = therapy of choice
  - Only in studies
- Tumors of the hepatobiliary system:
  - Very poor prognosis
  - Systemic chemotherapy = therapy of choice
  - Only in studies

Risk-Benefit Analysis

- To be determined individually for each patient
- Interdisciplinary consideration in a tumor board
- No uniform standards for the indication of CRS + HIPEC
- Individual and interdisciplinary assessment of risks: potential benefit must be higher than risk of complications
- **Caution**: Delay of palliative systemic chemotherapy

12.5.2 Prophylactic/Adjuvant CRS and HIPEC

- Theoretical approach
  - Risk minimization of metachronous peritoneal carcinomatosis
  - Use in high-risk patients
- The Prophylochip study failed to show any benefit in these patients

Indications

- High-risk patients
- T3/4 carcinomas with tumor rupture
- Mucinous or signet-ring cell carcinoma
- Isolated omental metastases/Krukenberg tumors

Evidence

- Currently no evidence
- Some evidence for a significant improvement in tumor-free survival
- No increase in complication rate due to chemoperfusion
- Randomized trial ongoing (prophylactic HIPEC)

Learning Curve

- Significant reduction in morbidity and lethality

12.5.3 Palliative Therapeutic Concepts for Ascites

- Therapy of choice for ascites = paracentesis
- Systemic chemotherapy = conditional control of malignant ascites
- HIPEC for ascites control (short-term effect only)

12.5.4 Complications

- With the use of CRS and HIPEC complication rate increases with the extent of resection
- Complication rate depends on the type and dose of cytostatic drug used

Most Common Complications

- Anastomotic insufficiency (4.5–33%, depending on author and tumor)
- Fistula (3–6%)
- Intra-abdominal abscess (10–17%)
- Bleeding (1.5–12%)
- Ileus (2–17%)
- Wound healing disorders (2–15%)
- Toxicity (20–26%)
- Nephrotoxicity 16–19%
- Haematotoxicity 14–20%

Strategies to Minimize Complications

- Patient selection
- Learning curve
- As few gastrointestinal anastomoses as possible
- Protective stomas should be generously indicated (especially for anastomoses in the rectal region)
- Monitoring in the intensive care unit
- Close monitoring of laboratory parameters = obligatory (focus on blood count)
- Postoperative chest X-ray in extended peritonectomy of the diaphragm
- Chemoperfusion always with a certified perfusion device
- Establishment of Centers of expertise

Learning Curve/Patient Selection

- Learning curve: 100 procedures required to:
  - Reduction of complications
  - Improvement of CC-0 resection rate from 35.6% to 65.1%
  - Reduction in morbidity from 71.2% to 34.1%
  - Reduction in the average length of stay in hospital from 21 to 17 days
  - Reduction of the reoperation rate from 30% to 10%.
  - Planning and training
- Patient selection by:
  - Advanced imaging
  - Interdisciplinary discussion (tumor board)
  - Individualized decision—by means of e.g. Peritoneal Surface Disease Severity Scores (PSDSS; Pelz et al. 2009)
  - Lack of standardization of selection criteria for surgical therapy (guidelines from the 2006 consensus conference in Milan)

12.5.5 Results

- Significant survival benefit in selected tumor entities
- Optional situation in the current german S3 guidelines for colorectal cancer (▣ Fig. 12.4)
- High morbidity between 25% and 60%
- Mortality between 2% and 10%
- Quality of life:
  - Postoperative: deterioration in the first days to weeks after surgery depending on the size of the surgical intervention and the peri- and postoperative complications
  - Reaching the preoperative baseline level: After about 3–4 months
  - In a proportion of patients: Long-term improvement

12.5.6 PIPAC (Pressurized Intraperitoneal Aerosol Chemotherapy)

- The PIPAC is a palliative therapy
- Possibility of laparoscopic local therapy
- Pure chemotherapy (no cytoreduction)
- Repeatability of the therapy
- Improvement of overall survival in selected patient population
- Still little valid data

12.5.7 Guidelines

AWMF Guideline "Colorectal Carcinoma" ► https://www.awmf.org/uploads/tx_szleitlinien/021-007OLk_S3_Kolorektales-Karzinom-KRK_2019-01.pdf

AWMF Guidelines "Ovarian Cancer" ► https://www.awmf.org/uploads/tx_szleitlinien/032-035OL1_S3_Ovarialkarzinom_2020-04.pdf

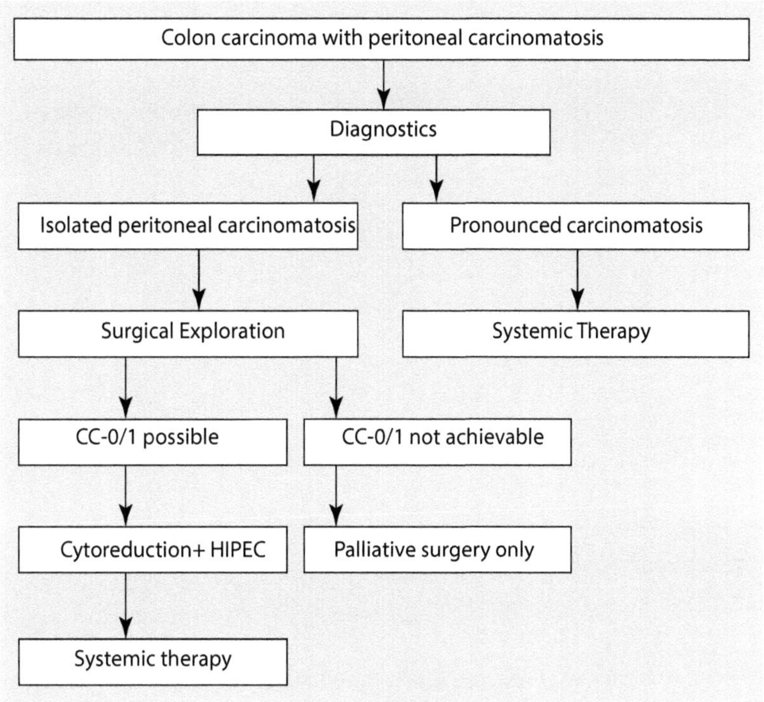

Fig. 12.4 Clinical pathway using the example of colon cancer

References

Jacquet P, Sugarbaker PH. Clinical research methodologies in diagnosis and staging of patients with peritoneal carcinomatosis. Cancer Treat Res. 1996;82:359–74. https://doi.org/10.1007/978-1-4613-1247-5_23. PMID: 8849962.

Pelz JO, Stojadinovic A, Nissan A et al (2009) Evaluation of a peritoneal surface disease severity score in patients with colon cancer with peritoneal carcinomatosis. J Surg Oncol 99:9–15

Verwaal VJ, van Ruth S, de Bree E, van Sloothen GW, van Tinteren H, Boot H, Zoetmulder FA (2003) Randomized trial of cytoreduction and hyperthermic intraperitoneal chemotherapy versus systemic chemotherapy and palliative surgery in patients with peritoneal carcinomatosis of colorectal cancer. J Clin Oncol 21:3737–3743. https://doi.org/10.1200/JCO.2003.04.187

Suggested Reading

Baratti D, Kusamura S, Azmi N, Guaglio M, Montenovo M, Deraco M (2020) Colorectal peritoneal metastases treated by perioperative systemic chemotherapy and cytoreductive surgery with or without mitomycin C-based HIPEC: a comparative study using the peritoneal surface disease severity score (PSDSS). Ann Surg Oncol 27(1):98–106

Ceelen W (2019) HIPEC with oxaliplatin for colorectal peritoneal metastasis: the end of the road? Eur J Surg Oncol 45(3):400–402. https://doi.org/10.1016/j.ejso.2018.10.542. Epub 2018 Oct 31

Hernia

Jens Otto, Thorsten Lindenau, and Karsten Junge

Contents

F. Billmann, T. Keck (eds.), *Essentials of Visceral Surgery*,
https://doi.org/10.1007/978-3-662-66735-4_13

13.1 Anatomy and Classification

13.1.1 Hernia Anatomy

- Hernia gate
  - Gap in the layers of the abdominal wall, pelvic floor, diaphragm or back muscles.
- Hernia sac
  - Lining of the hernia; protrusion of the parietal peritoneum.
- Content of hernia sac
  - All components of the abdominal cavity possible.

13.1.2 Epidemiology

Hernia Incidence

- In the normal population = 2–4%.
- In older age = up to 20.
- 10–15% of general surgery procedures.

Hernia Distribution

- Proportion of external hernias = 95.
  - Inguinal hernias (75%).
  - Scar hernias (10%).
  - Umbilical hernias, thigh hernias and rare forms of hernia (5–7% each).
- Proportion of internal hernias = 5.

13.1.3 Pathogenesis and Classification

Pathogenesis

- Preformed or secondary fascia gap.
- Development of the hernia = protrusion of the parietal peritoneum through the gap.

Hernia Classification

- According to position relative to the abdominal wall (■ Table 13.1):

■ **Table 13.1** Classification of hernias according to position in relation to the abdominal wall

External hernias	Internal hernias
Inguinal hernia (inguinal hernia) Direct Indirect	Treitz hernia
Femoral hernia (thigh hernia)	Paracoecal hernia
Umbilical hernia (umbilical hernia)	Hernia through foramen omentale (Winslowi)
Paraumbilical hernia	Hernia at the mesosigma
Epigastric hernia	Hernia at the mesentery (postoperative mesoslit), Petersen hernia
Incisional hernia (also parastomal hernia)	Pelvic floor peritoneal hernia
Spieghel hernia (linea semilunaris)	Paravesical hernia
Rare hernias Bochdalek Grynfelt Trigonum lumbale (petit)	

  - External hernias: Protrusion of the peritoneum through the abdominal wall “outwards” (e.g. inguinal hernias).
  - Internal hernia: Hernia within the abdominal cavity, no external appearance (e.g. ileocecal hernias).
- According to clinical aspects:
  - Reponible/Irreponible: hernial contents to be forced back into abdominal cavity (or not).
  - Incarcerated: Non-reducible, acutely painful protrusion (incarceration).
- By etiology:
  - Congenital hernia (e.g. open processus vaginalis peritonei in indirect inguinal hernia).
  - Acquired hernia (e.g. incisional hernia).

13.1.4 Hernia-Specific Complications

Intestinal Incarceration

- Most common complication.
- Emergency situation
- Clinical presentation:.
  - Severe pain, palpable, bulging elastic tumor, local environmental irritation, irreducibility, vomiting, ileus, intestinal perforation, peritonitis.
- **Caution:** The sun must neither rise nor set over a pinched hernia (OP within max. 12 h).

Hernia

- Danger of spontaneous perforation.
- Clinical presentation: swelling, redness, hyperthermia, painfulness.

Mains Clamping

- Clinical presentation: Pressure painful, non-responsive hernia with little impairment of the patient.

13.2 General Diagnosis and Therapy Principles

13

13.2.1 Diagnosis

Physical Examination

- Palpation of the hernial gap.
- Palpate contents of hernia sac if necessary.
- Assessment of reproducibility.
- In the case of irreducible hernias, differentiation between chronic irreducibility (e.g. in the case of adhesion or excessive extent of the hernia) vs. acutely occurring irreducibility = incarceration.

Sonography

- Most important tool for assessing fracture aperture, fracture content and size indication.

Further Investigations

- MRI or CT.
- Only in the case of corresponding symptoms, complex situation (recurrent findings) or poor assessability (e.g. obesity).

13.2.2 Therapy Principles

- In the case of acute incarceration = manual reduction of the fracture tumour only within the first few hours.

Caution

Bowel perforation/reposition of gangrenous bowel with delayed attempt at reduction.

- Successful reduction = inpatient monitoring + surgical repair of the hernial gap during the same stay.
- Unsuccessful reduction = operation as soon as possible + vitality check of the content of hernia sac.

Procedure for Surgical Therapy

- Direct fascia suture/fascia doubling: Shouldice, Bassini.
- Sublay mesh implantation.
- Combination methods.
- Laparoscopic procedures: e.g. TAPP (transabdominal preperitoneal plasty), TEP (total extraperitoneal plasty).

13.3 Incisional Hernia

13.3.1 Definition

- Post-operative fascia defects in the area of a fascia scar.
- Hernial gap/hernia sac (▶ Sect. 13.1).

Distinction: Incisional hernia – rectus diastasis – burst abdomen:

- Differentiation by hernial gap and hernia sac.
- Rectus diastasis: widening of the linea alba with divergence of the rectus muscles.
- Abdominal laceration: early postoperative abdominal wound dehiscence after laparotomy.

13.3.2 Incidence

- Most frequent postoperative complication.
- Up to 18%, depending on the investigation period.
- In Germany: 100,000 incisional hernias per 700,000 laparotomies per year; only 30% of hernias with surgical treatment.
- Longitudinal laparotomies more affected than transverse laparotomies.

13.3.3 Aetiology

- Impaired scar formation due to impaired collagen metabolism (congenital/acquired).
- Multifactorial risk profile.
- Risk factors s. Overview:

Risk Factors for Incisional Hernias
- Patient-related:
  - Age (>45 years).
  - Male gender.
  - Obesity (BMI > 25).
  - Ascites.
  - COPD (chronic obstructive pulmonary disease).
  - Consuming disease.
  - Diabetes mellitus.
  - Renal failure.
  - Anemia (Hb < 10 g/dL).
  - Nicotine abuse.
  - Chemotherapy.
  - Steroid therapy.
  - Collagen metabolism disorder.
- Surgical:
  - Recurrent surgery.
  - Emergency surgery.
  - Contaminated surgical field.
  - Experience of the surgeon.
  - Fascia suture technique Prevention through small bites – technique.
  - Thread material.
- Postoperative condition:
  - Wound infection.

- In the search for the risk profile for the development of incisional hernias, the multifactorial genesis is always emphasized.
- Aim for etiological treatment (before surgical therapy or in parallel).

13.3.4 Clinical Presentation

- Mostly asymptomatic.
- Noticeable only by increase in size.
- Advancement of peritoneal organs; risk = "loss of domain".
- Entrapment symptoms (e.g., irreducibility, pain, passenger disruption): Up to 15.
  - With intestinal strangulation: Up to 2%.

13.3.5 Diagnosis

Clinical Examination

- Examination always lying down + standing (+ pressing).
- Clinical signs ► Sect. 13.3.4.

Sonography

- Standard procedure.
- Confirmation of diagnosis + exclusion of a complication.
- Extent of the hernia gap (planning of the operation).

CT or MRI

- In case of unclear findings.
- For complex recurrence findings with implanted mesh materials.
- With pronounced obesity.

13.3.6 Surgical Therapy

Operation Indication:
- Every incisional hernia = indication for surgery.
- If incarceration is suspected = emergency.

Open Procedures

Suture Procedure

- Direct suture of the fascia gap
- Only indicated for small trocar hernias with unclear initial occlusion

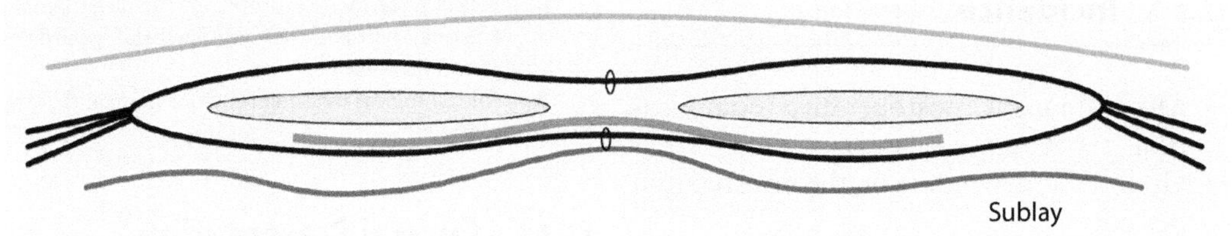

Fig. 13.1 Schematic drawing of retromuscular meshplasty (sublay position). (After Schumpelick 2011)

Sublay Technique

- Conventional standard care.
- Incisional hernia repair in the sense of abdominal wall reinforcement using a textile mesh implant in the retromuscular position (Fig. 13.1).
- Pros:
  - Extraperitoneal mesh position
  - Restoration of fascia continuity = restoration of abdominal wall function.

Abdominal Wall Replacement

- When tension-free fascial closure is impossible.
- Defect bridging by mesh.

Caution
In both the sublay technique and abdominal wall replacement, care must be taken to ensure sufficient overlap between the mesh prosthesis and the tissue of at least 5 cm in all directions.

13

Laparoscopic Procedures

- IPOM (intraperitoneal onlay mesh) = standard laparoscopic treatment.
- Advantage laparoscopic vs. open = reduced rate of wound complications.
- Basics:
  - Visualization of the entire anterior abdominal wall (= adhesiolysis).
  - Mobilisation of the content of the hernia sac, display of the complete hernia gap.
  - Cover the entire scar with an overlap of at least 5 cm on all sides (of the hernia gap and the scar; Fig. 13.2).
  - If necessary, cut through fatty tissue structures such as the ligaments falciforme and teres hepatis or open up the prevesical space in the lower abdomen.

IPOM mesh materials must achieve rapid and stable incorporation on the parietal side and prevent adhesions on the visceral side.

Special Procedures

Component Separation According to Ramirez

- Mobilization technique of the fascia to close large gaps of the median lines.
- Useful in combination with mesh reinforcement for large defects.

Surgical Procedure

Component Separation According to Ramirez

- Lateral: Longitudinal splitting of the external aponeurosis (approx. 1–2 cm lateral to the rectus sheath) = separation of the internal oblique muscle and external oblique muscle.
- Medial: Longitudinal splitting of the rectus sheath on both sides from the median line.
- Medialization of the rectus sheath blades = closure of the defect on the median line.

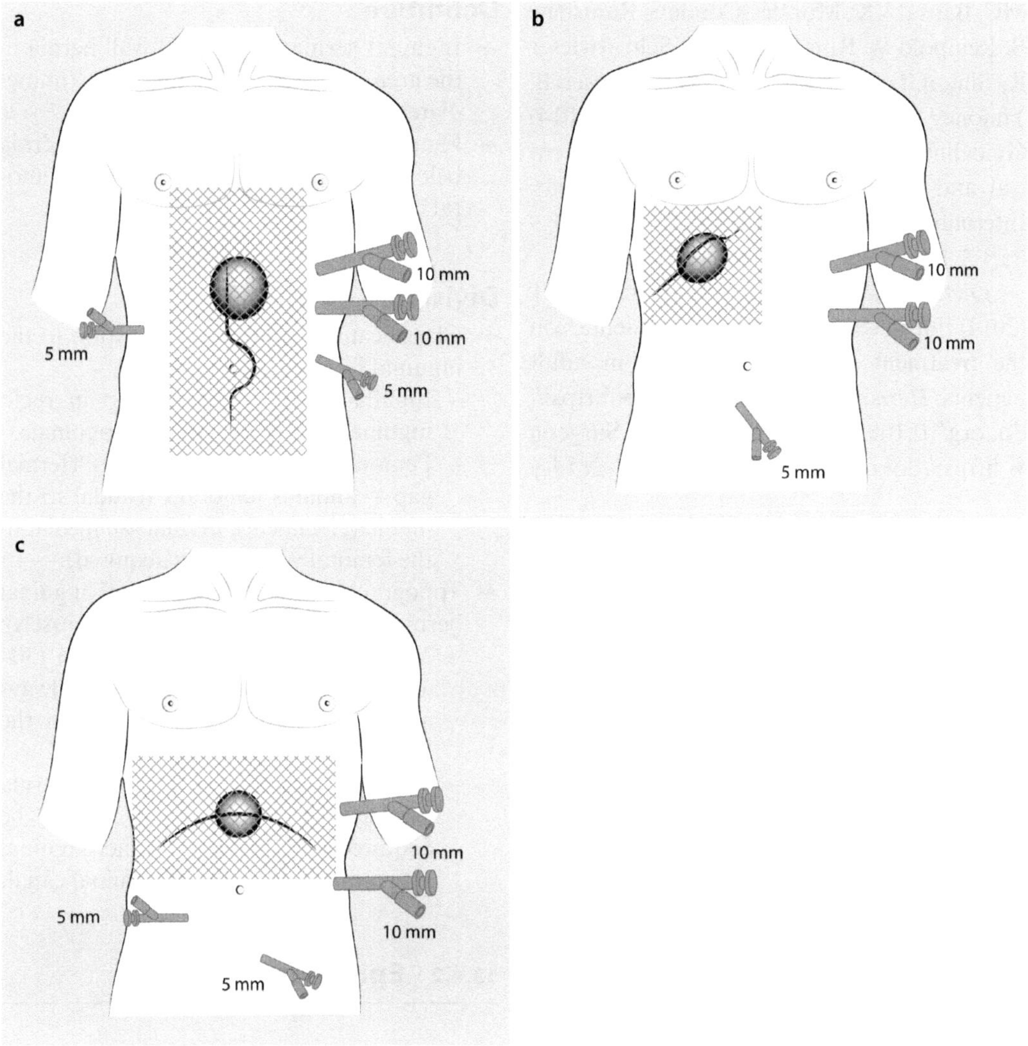

Fig. 13.2 Examples of mesh coverage. Trolar and Mesh placement in the case of: (**a**) Midline Incision Hernia; (**b**) Subcostal Incision Hernia; (**c**) Transversal Incision Hernia

13.3.7 Guidelines

Bittner R, Bingener-Casey J, Dietz U, Fabian M, Ferzli GS, Fortelny RH, Köckerling F, Kukleta J, Leblanc K, Lomanto D, Misra MC, Bansal VK, Morales-Conde S, Ramshaw B, Reinpold W, Rim S, Rohr M, Schrittwieser R, Simon T, Smietanski M, Stechemesser B, Timoney M, Chowbey P, IEHS (2014) Guidelines for laparoscopic treatment of ventral and incisional abdominal wall hernias. International Endohernia Society (IEHS) – Part 1. Surg Endosc 28: 2–29.

Bittner R, Bingener-Casey J, Dietz U, Fabian M, Ferzli GS, Fortelny RH, Köckerling F, Kukleta J, Leblanc K, Lomanto D, Misra MC, Bansal VK, Morales-Conde S, Ramshaw B, Reinpold W, Rim S, Rohr M, Schrittwieser R, Simon T, Smietanski M, Stechemesser B, Timoney M, Chowbey P, IEHS (2014) Guidelines for laparoscopic treatment of ventral and incisional abdominal wall hernias. International Endohernia Society (IEHS) – Part 2. Surg Endosc 28: 353–379.

Bittner R, Bingener-Casey J, Dietz U, Fabian M, Ferzli GS, Fortelny RH, Köckerling F, Kukleta J, Leblanc K, Lomanto D, Misra

MC, Bansal VK, Morales-Conde S, Ramshaw B, Reinpold W, Rim S, Rohr M, Schrittwieser R, Simon T, Smietanski M, Stechemesser B, Timoney M, Chowbey P, IEHS (2014) Guidelines for laparoscopic treatment of ventral and incisional abdominal wall hernias. International Endohernia Society (IEHS) – Part 3. Surg Endosc 28: 380–404.

Dietz UA, Wiegering A, Germer CT (2014) European Hernia Society guidelines on the treatment of inguinal hernia in adult patients; *Hernia* (2009) 13: 343–403; ▶ https://doi.org/10.1007/s10029-009-0529-7 Surgeon ▶ https://doi.org/10.1007/s00104-014-2814-y

13.4 Inguinal and Femoral Hernia

13.4.1 Anatomy, Definition and Classification

Anatomy

- Inguinal canal (= inguinal canal):
  - Course from the inner, lateral (= Anulus inguinalis profundus) to the outer, medial (= Anulus inguinalis superficialis) inguinal ring.
  - Contents: In the male spermatic cord + vessels supplying the testis; in the female Lig. rotundum.
  - Anatomical border: anterior wall = aponeurosis of the obliquus externus muscle; posterior wall = fascia transversalis and peritoneum; upper border = inferior border of the obliquus internus muscle and the transversus muscle; inferior border = inguinal ligament.
- Femoral canal (= thigh canal):
  - Anulus femoralis: entrance into the femoral canal; limited by V. femoralis, Lig. inguinale, Lig. lacunare and Pecten os pubis.
  - Canalis femoralis: 3–4 cm long canal in the medial section of the lacuna vasorum (femoral vessels).

Definition

- Inguinal hernia: abdominal wall hernia in the area of the trigonum inguinale (immediately above the lig. inguinale).
- Femoral hernia: abdominal wall hernia below the lig. Inguinale through the femoral canal.

Division

- Classification of hernias in relation to the inguinal ligament:
  - Inguinal hernia: hernial gap in regio inguinale, cranial of the lig. Inguinale.
  - Femoral hernia (= thigh hernia): Hernial gap = annulus femoralis (caudal to the inguinal ligament), hernial sac medial to the femoral vein (always acquired).
- Topographical classification of inguinal hernia (in relation to the epigastric vessels):
  - Medial (= direct) inguinal hernia (30–40% of all inguinal hernias, always acquired): Hernial gap directly in the area of the medial inguinal fossa.
  - Lateral (= indirect) inguinal hernia (mostly congenital, can also be acquired): Hernial gap = inner inguinal ring, course through the inguinal canal.

13.4.2 Epidemiology

Inguinal Hernia

- Incidence = 25% of all men and 2% of all women during their lifetime.
- Peak of manifestation: childhood and adolescence + older adulthood (>40 years).
- Bilateral findings = 15–30%.
- 220,000 interventions in Germany.
- Men: Women = 8: 1.
- In children almost always indirect; in adults 70% indirect.

Femoral Hernia

- Incidence = 5–7% of all hernias (significantly less frequent than inguinal hernia).
- Mostly women of advanced age (75%).
- Association with simultaneous inguinal hernia: Up to 9% in women; up to 50% in men.

13.4.3 Pathophysiology

- Risk factors:
  - Increased intra-abdominal pressure (e.g. obesity, chronic cough, COPD, prostatic hyperplasia or constipation).
  - Connective tissue disorders (e.g. Ehlers-Danlos syndrome, Marfan syndrome or osteogenesis imperfecta).
  - Change in collagen composition.
  - Smoking.

13.4.4 Clinical Presentation

Asymptomatic Small Inguinal Hernia

- Incidental finding in the course of a clinical or sonographic examination.
- Initially no indication for surgery = "watchful waiting".

Symptomatic Inguinal Hernia

- Visible/palpable protrusion (= size progression).
- Under stress (abdominal press, lifting weights, etc.) Pain in the groin region.
- Possibly swelling in the groin.

Complications

- Intestinal incarveration: severe, persistent pain + a palpable, turgid swelling of the groin region.
- Irreducibility: increase in symptoms → vomiting + ileus symptoms → intestinal perforation + peritonitis.

Caution

Intestinal incarceration, ileus or perforation = indication for immediate emergency surgery.

- Entrapment of parts of the omentum majus: often pressure-painful swelling.

Femoral Hernia

- Typical hernial growth below the inguinal ligament.
- Mostly unspecific feeling of pressure.
- Signs of incarceration.
- Differential diagnoses: lymphadenopathy, subsidence abscess, lymph node, lipoma.
  - Exclusion by sonography.

13.4.5 Diagnostic Procedures

Palpation of the Inguinal Canal

- Lying down + standing patient under abdominal pressure (cough) = assessment of potential hernia/hernial gap.
- Clarification of reproducibility.

Sonography

- In combination with palpation = reliable statement on hernia size, position, content, reducibility and incarceration.

CT/MRI Examination

- Only in exceptional cases (e.g. previous operations/obesity).

13.4.6 Therapeutic Principles

Evidence-Based Strategy (◘ Fig. 13.3)

EHS (European Hernia Society) Recommendation

- All male adults aged 30 years and older with symptomatic inguinal hernia → Surgical procedure with mesh implantation.
- Open Lichtenstein surgery/minimally invasive surgical procedures (TAPP and TEP) = best evidence-based methods for the treatment of a primary unilateral inguinal hernia.
- Suture procedure without mesh implantation (Shouldice procedure): Only in individual cases (e.g. young patient with a small hernia gap and sufficient fascial conditions or young patient with a desire to have children).

Principles

- Surgery = therapy of choice.

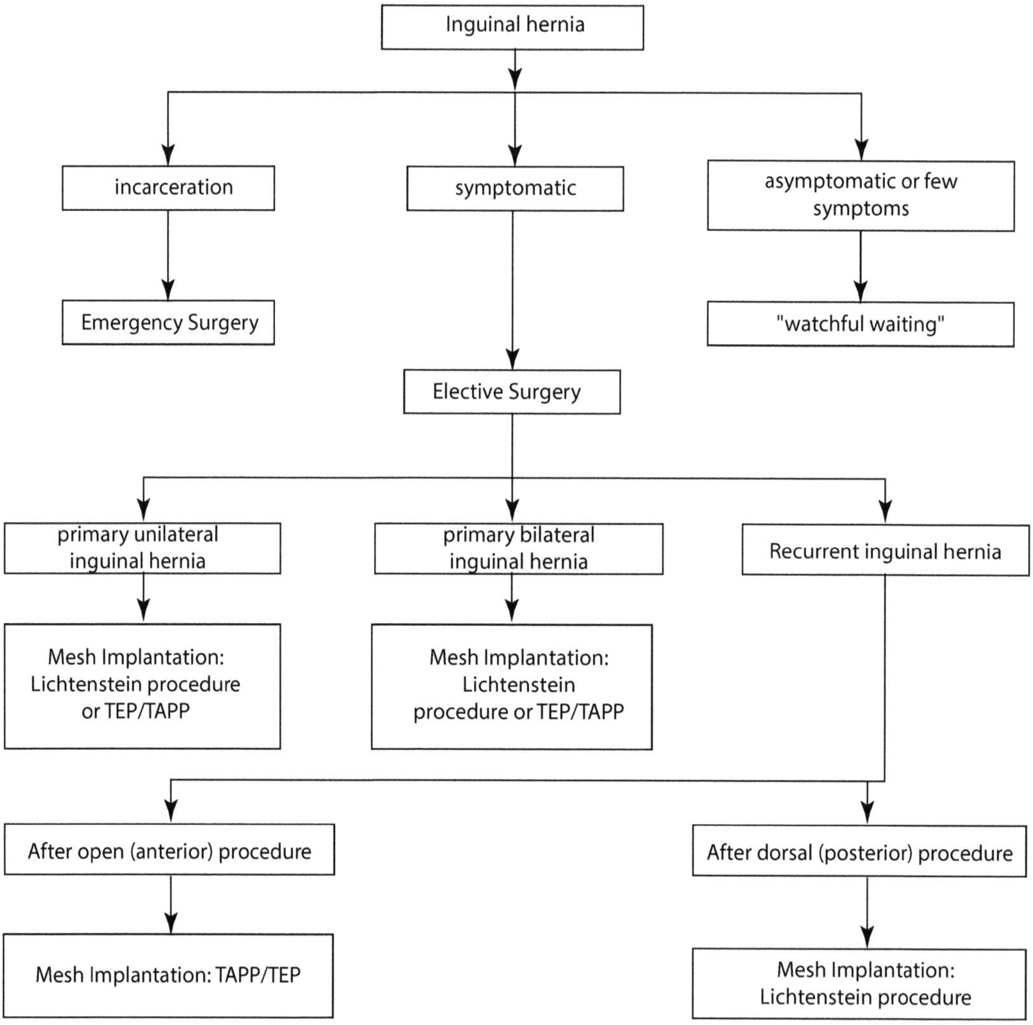

Fig. 13.3 Flowchart for the treatment of inguinal hernia (*IH*) in men aged 30 years and older; *TEP* total extraperitoneal plasty, *TAPP* transabdominal preperitoneal plasty. (European Hernia Society Guidelines 2009)

- Aim of the surgical procedures = reinforcement of the posterior wall of the inguinal canal by means of a mesh implant.
- Laparoscopic procedures (TAPP/TEP):
  - Lower rate of wound infection/hematoma formation.
  - Shorter convalescence time but longer OP time.

In women (high rate of femoral hernias) = laparoscopic repair procedures are more likely, since the possibility of clarifying the treatment of the femoral hernia is better.

- Open procedures:
  - Surgery under local anesthesia possible.
  - Intraoperative decision option pro vs. contra mesh (in case of strong fascia conditions and small hernia gap = suture procedure without mesh application, e.g. Shouldice possible).

Emergency Surgery

- Incarceration + signs of mechanical ileus = emergency surgery.
- Acute hernia incarceration (<6 h) = one reduction attempt + inpatient monitoring.
- Suspected bowel necrosis/acute abdomen = emergency surgery.

Complications

- Essential in preoperative education.
- Inguinal hernia recurrence (1–10%).
- Chronic groin pain:
  - Definition: Groin pain that has been present for 3 months or more.
  - Incidence: open procedure 18%; laparoscopic procedure 6%; however, after approx. 2.5 years the incidence is the same for both surgical procedures.
- Injury to the spermatic cord = potential infertility/testicular necrosis.
- Intraoperative conversion to open surgical technique, even median laparotomy in case of emergency.
- Injuries to the bowel, urinary bladder or iliac vessels.
- Wound infection (1–2%).
- Seroma formation.
- Bleeding (0.5%).
- Injury or compression of the femoral artery, femoral vein and femoral nerve (1%), thromboembolism (1%).
- Lethality <1%.

Caution
In case of incarceration with bowel resection: lethality up to 20%.

Intraoperative EHS Classification (2007)

- Assessment of:
  - Frequency of hernia (primary and recurrent).
  - Localization (medial, lateral, femoral, combined).
  - Size of hernial gap (1 = 1.5 cm corresponding to ≤1 finger, 2 = 1.5–3 cm corresponding to 1–2 fingers, 3 ≥ 3 cm corresponding to 3 fingers and more).
- Target:
  - Standardization of the hernia description.
  - Enabling large international comparative studies.

Surgical Technology

Inguinal Hernia

Operative Procedure

Shouldice Herniotomy

- Opening of the inguinal canal, attachment of the spermatic cord with appendages, separation of the hernia sac.
- Important = protection of the ilioinguinal nerve, iliohypogastric nerve and the rami genitales as well as femorales of the genitofemoral nerve.
- 2-row doubling of the fascia transversalis (continuous Prolene suture) starting at the tuberculum pubicum.
- Narrowing of the inner inguinal ring.
- Continuous suture of the transversus abdominis and obliquus internus muscles to the inguinal ligament (2-row).
- Continuous closure of the external aponeurosis, skin suture.

Surgical Procedure

Herniotomy According to Lichtenstein

- Opening of the inguinal canal, attachment of the spermatic cord with appendages, separation of the hernia sac.
- Important = protection of the ilioinguinal nerve, iliohypogastric nerve and the rami genitales as well as femorales of the genitofemoral nerve.
- Treatment of the hernia, resection of the preperitoneal lipoma if necessary; repair of the posterior wall with non-absorbable mesh (8 × 12 cm); continuous mesh fixation at the inguinal ligament.
- In the male, slit in the lateral part and new formation of the inner inguinal

ring around the spermatic cord and testicular vessels and subsequent closure of the slit.
- Externus aponeurosis closure.

Surgical Procedure
TAPP (= Transabdominal Preperitoneal Plasty)
- Only intubation anesthesia because of capnoperitoneum.
- Periumbilical camera trocar plus two working trocars, creation of the capnoperitoneum.
- Incision of the peritoneum + dissection of the preperitoneal inguinal region with visualization of the hernial gap, inguinal ligament and inguinal canal structures.
- Dissection of the hernia back into the peritoneal space.
- Placement of a non-absorbable mesh implant (mesh size at least 10 × 15 cm); fixation only if necessary by means of tissue adhesive, absorbable stapler – more important is sufficient overlapping of the mesh in relation to the fracture edge.
- Closure of the peritoneum (continuous suture).

Surgical Procedure
TEP (= Total Extraperitoneal Plasty)
- Preparation in the preperitoneal space by mechanical + CO_2 insufflation.
- Intubation anesthesia only.
- Subumbilical access to the preperitoneal space; CO_2 insufflation.
- Two additional working trocars in the midline and suprasymphysary: preparation of the preperitoneal inguinal region with visualization of the hernial gap, inguinal ligament and inguinal canal structures.
- Placement of a non-absorbable mesh implant (mesh size 10 × 15 cm); fixation with tissue adhesive/no fixation.
- Relief CO_2, fascial closure of the subumbilical incision, skin suture.

Surgical Procedure
Recurrence of Inguinal Hernia
- Supply principle depends on the previous operation.
- After open hernia repair = laparoscopic procedure recommended.
- After laparoscopic hernia repair = open procedure recommended.

Surgical Procedure
Femoral Hernia
- Optimal treatment possible with TAPP – Open surgery: visualization of the femoral portal via inguinal access/crural access.
- Closure of the hernial gap:
- Continuous suture of the pectineal ligament to the inguinal ligament (according to Moschkowitz/Fabricius).
- Single button sutures between M. obliquus internus and M. transversus abdominis and Lig. pectineale and Fascia transversalis (after Lotheissen/McVay).
- Closure of the hernial gap by mesh (Gilbert prosthesis via inguinal; plug from crural).

Aftercare

- Rule of thumb: do not lift more than 10–15 kg for 4–6 weeks.
- Immediately postoperative: pain-adapted stress possible.
- Refrain from heavy lifting/sporting activities for approx. 2–3 weeks, followed by pain-adapted loading.

13.4.7 Guidelines

European Hernia Society guidelines on the treatment of inguinal hernia in adult patients; *Hernia* (2009) 13: 343–403; ► https://doi.org/10.1007/s10029-009-0529-7

Simons MP, Aufenacker T, Bay-Nielsen M, Bouillot JL, Campanelli G, Conze J, de Lange D, Fortelny R, Heikkinen T, Kingsnorth A, Kukleta J, Morales-Conde S, Nordin P, Schumpelick V, Smedberg S, Smietanski M, Weber G, Miserez M (2009) European Hernia Society guidelines on the treatment of inguinal hernia in adult patients. Hernia 13: 343–403.

Bittner R, Arregui ME, Bisgaard T, Dudai M, Ferzli GS, Fitzgibbons RJ, Fortelny RH, Klinge U, Kockerling F, Kuhry E, Kukleta J, Lomanto D, Misra MC, Montgomery A, Morales-Conde S, Reinpold W, Rosenberg J, Sauerland S, Schug-Pass C, Singh K, Timoney M, Weyhe D, Chombey P (2011) Guidelines for laparoscopic (TAPP) and endoscopic (TEP) treatment of inguinal hernia [International Endohernia Society (IEHS)]. Surg Endosc 25: 2773–2843.

13.5 Umbilical and Epigastric Hernia

13.5.1 Umbilical Hernia

Definition

- Hernia.
- Incidence = approx. 5.
- Women > Men.
- Risk factors: Ascites, obesity, pregnancy…

Division

- Infantile umbilical hernias:
  - Hernia gap at the annulus umbilicalis.
  - Spontaneous closure in the first years of life (98%) = no indication for surgery before the age of 2 years.
- In adulthood:
  - Mostly paraumbilical hernia next to the umbilical pillar.
  - No spontaneous regression tendency at all.
  - Risk factors: Obesity, liver cirrhosis or ascites; in combination with rectus diastasis.

13.5.2 Epigastric Hernia

Definition

- Fascia defect in the linea alba between xyphoid and umbilicus.
- Incidence = approx. 5.
- Men > Women.
- Overview: Clinical presentation, diagnosis and indication for surgery is similar for umbilical and epigastric hernia.

13.5.3 Clinical presentation

- Unspecific abdominal pain.
- Pain when stretching or tensing the abdominal wall muscles.
- protrusion of the abdominal wall.
- Depending on the findings, up to intestinal obstruction, with ileus or strangulation.

13.5.4 Diagnosis

- Palpation.
- Sonography: fascial gap, hernia contents.

13.5.5 Therapy

- Small asymptomatic findings = "watchful waiting".
- Symptomatic findings (e.g. increase in size, incarcerations or also non-specific abdominal pain) = surgical therapy:
  - Small fascial defects (<1 cm): continuous sutureplasty (non-absorbable, transverse), joint to joint.
  - Fascia defects >1 cm and/or a BMI of >30: Additional mesh implant (alloplastic material).

13.5.6 Guideline

Guidelines for treatment of umbilical and epigastric hernias from the European Hernia Society and Americas Hernia Society N. A. Henriksen, A. Montgomery, R. Kaufmann, F. Berrevoet, B. East, J. Fischer,W. Hope, D. Klassen, R. Lorenz, Y.Renard, M. A. Garcia Urena and M. P. Simons5onbehalf of the European and Americas Hernia Societies (EHS and AHS).

Surgical Procedure
Umbilical Hernia

- Semicircular left lateral umbilical incision (extendable to cranial and caudal).
- Sharp detachment of the navel (**caution:** skin injury and blood circulation).
- Preparation of the hernia sac up to linea alba and hernia gap.
- Repositioning the hernia sac.
- Transverse hernia closure: Direct non-absorbable or slow-absorbable suture for small gaps less than 1 cm; mesh implantation in preperitoneal position (preperitoneal umbilical mesh plasty = PUMP) with an overlap of 3 cm for gaps of 1–4 cm.
- Refixation of the umbilicus and skin closure.

Surgical Procedure
Epigastric Hernia

- Transverse skin incision.
- Then procedure analogous to the umbilical hernia.

13.5.7 Differential Diagnosis: Rectus Diastasis

Definition

- Divergence of the rectus musculature in the area of the linea alba.
- **No** fascial defect: bulge-like protrusion.

Etiology and Pathogenesis

- Congenital rectus diastasis.
- Acquired rectus diastasis.

Clinical Presentation

- Protrusion in the area of the diastasis when tightening the abdominal muscles (or straightening).
- Mostly only an aesthetic problem.

Therapy

- In the absence of a fascial defect, no risk of incarceration = primary conservative therapy.
- Only rarely (e.g. for cosmetic reasons) correction indicated = procedure as for incisional hernia = mesh implant in retromuscular position (sublay).
- High recurrence rate without mesh reinforcement.

13.6 Parastomal Hernia

13.6.1 Definition

- Protrusion of any kind near a stoma.

13.6.2 Epidemiology

- Incidence depending on stomatal type:
  - Terminal colostomy: 4–48%.
  - Terminal ileostomy: 2–28%.
  - Loop colostomy: 0–31%.
  - Loop ileostomy: 0–6%.
  - High recurrence rate after treatment.

13.6.3 Risk Factors and Prevention

Risk Factors

- General risk factors (similar to the pathogenesis of incisional hernias, ► Sect. 13.3.3): Obesity, wound infections, advanced age, immunosuppression, COPD.

- Special risk factor = opening too large for stoma passage (fascial passage should be as narrow as possible).

Prevention

- Expulsion of the stoma through rectus muscle.
- abdominal wall gap (fascia gap) as small as possible.
- Tunneling technique under peritoneum (valve mechanism) (before abdominal wall passage).
- Prophylactic mesh implantation: Significant reduction in the rate of parastomal hernias = recommended for open/laparoscopic creation of permanent terminal small and large bowel stomas (Level 1 recommendation, Bittner et al. 2014).

13.6.4 Clinical Presentation

- Often symptomatic
- Especially supply problems with plate and bag.
- Voiding disorder, pain.
- Incarceration, ileus.

13.6.5 Relevant Complications

- Hernia incarceration.
- Ileus.
- Progressive voiding obstruction.
- Chronic pain and subileus conditions.

13.6.6 Therapy

- Mains supply = standard.

Open Procedures

- Local suture procedures with only fascia constriction (= recurrence rate 50 to 76%) = not recommended.
- Stomal Relocation:
  - Usually by means of relaparotomy.
  - Relocation alone without prophylactic mesh implantation = disappointing recurrence rates (30–45% parastomal hernias at the newly created stoma site) (analogous to initial placement).
  - Treatment of the defect at the initial stoma site in the sense of a scar hernia (in 33% here recurrent scar hernia).
  - A further disadvantage of relocation is scar fractures in the relaparotomy area in 10–20% of cases.
- Repair by means of mesh implantation (◘ Fig. 13.4):
  - Reduction of the fracture.
  - Fascia constriction and reinforcement using textile mesh implant;
  - Reticular tunneling and lateralization of the intestine (Sugarbaker technique).

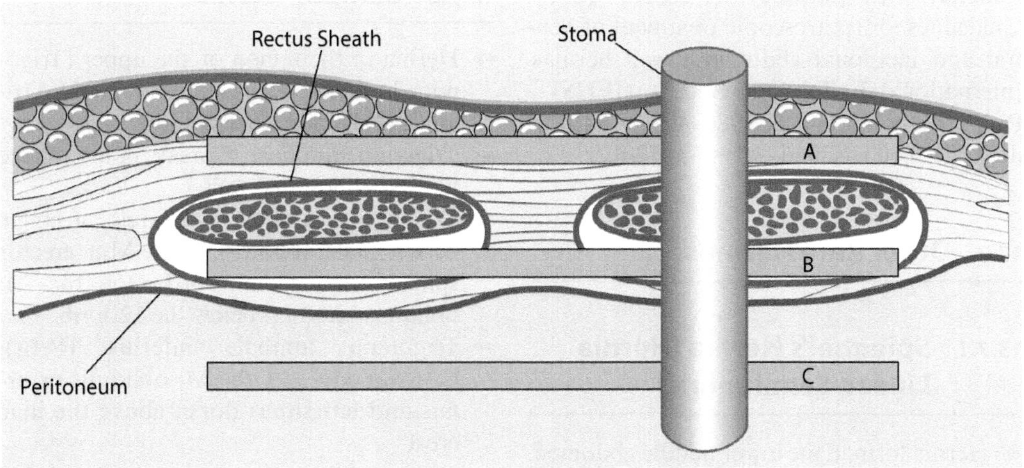

◘ **Fig. 13.4** Mesh position in parastomal hernia repair. **a** Onlay, **b** Sublay, **c** Intraperitoneal mesh position

- Classification of the technique according to mesh positioning: epifascial (onlay), retromuscular (sublay) intraperitoneal mesh reinforcement (■ Fig. 13.4).

Minimally Invasive Procedures

- Laparoscopic hernia reduction + intraperitoneal mesh reinforcement.
- Techniques:
  - IPST mesh (intraperitoneal stoma mesh): Mesh with a central tunnel (from 2–3.5 cm diameter) is placed around the terminal stoma and fixed to the abdominal wall.
  - Sugarbaker technique: reduction of the hernia + lateralization of the executing intestinal loop with a covering mesh.
  - Sandwich technique: reduction of the hernia + positioning of a keyhole-shaped mesh around the terminal intestinal loop + additional lateralization of this loop with another mesh in the sense of the Sugarbaker technique.

13.6.7 Guidelines

Bittner R, Bingener-Casey J, Dietz U, Fabian M, Ferzli GS, Fortelny RH, Köckerling F, Kukleta J, Leblanc K, Lomanto D, Misra MC, Bansal VK, Morales-Conde S, Ramshaw B, Reinpold W, Rim S, Rohr M, Schrittwieser R, Simon T, Smietanski M, Stechemesser B, Timoney M, Chowbey P, IEHS (2014) Guidelines for laparoscopic treatment of ventral and incisional abdominal wall hernias. International Endohernia Society (IEHS) – Part 3. Surg Endosc 28: 380–404. ► https://doi.org/10.1007/s00464-01m3-3172-4

13

13.7 Other Rare Hernias

13.7.1 Spieghel's Hernia (Hernia Lineae Semilunaris)

- Hernia form in the lower middle abdomen.
- Hernial gap: between the aponeurosis of the internal oblique muscle and the outer edge of the rectus sheath (linea semilunaris).

13.7.2 Hernia Obturatoria

- Hernia of the pelvic floor (■ Fig. 13.5).
- Hernial gap in the obturator foramen, along the vasa obturatoria/N. obturatorius.
- Especially for older women.
- Clinical presentation: Typically pain in the lower abdomen + radiation to the inner thighs.
- **Caution:** Not visible externally.

13.7.3 Hernia Ischiadica

- Hernial gap = foramen ischiadicum in the region of the gluteus maximus muscle (■ Fig. 13.5).

13.7.4 Hernia Perinealis

- Hernia through ischiorectal fossa (■ Fig. 13.5).
- Course: to the perineum or into the labia majora.

13.7.5 Lumbar Hernia

- Hernia in the region of the upper (Trigonum lumbale superius)/lower lumbar triangle (Trigonum lumbale inferius).
- Trigonum lumbale = weak point of the lumbar abdominal wall.
- Trigonum lumbale superius: triangle between lateral border of the Mm. erector spinae and medial border of the M. obliquus internus, below the 12th rib.
- Trigonum lumbale inferius (Petit): between edges of the M. obliquus externus and latissimus dorsi, above the iliac crest.

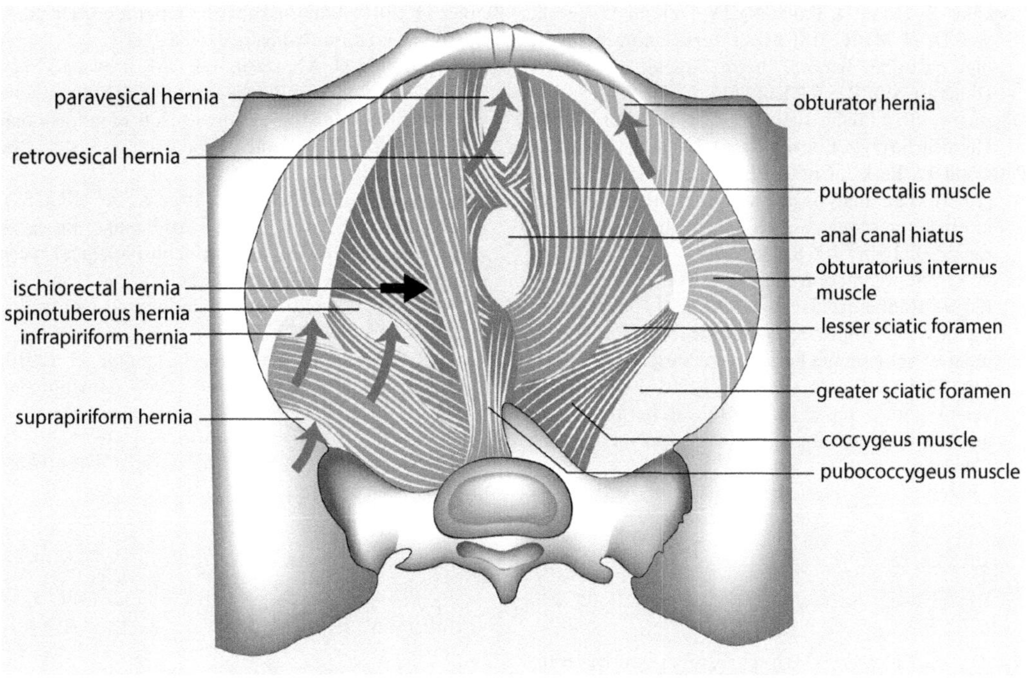

Fig. 13.5 Rare hernias of the pelvic floor

References

European Hernia Society guidelines (2009) on the treatment of inguinal hernia in adult patients. Hernia 13:343–403. https://doi.org/10.1007/s10029-009-0529-7

Schumpelick V (ed) (2011) Gastroenterologische Chirurgie, 3rd edn. Springer, Berlin/Heidelberg

Further Reading

Bakker WJ, Aufenacker TJ, Boschman JS, Burgmans JPJ (2020) Lightweight mesh is recommended in open inguinal (Lichtenstein) hernia repair: a systematic review and meta-analysis. Surgery 167: 581–589

Bernardi K, Olavarria OA, Holihan JL, Kao LS, Ko TC, Roth JS, Tsuda S, Vaziri K, Liang MK (2019) Primary fascial closure during laparoscopic ventral hernia repair improves patient quality of life: a multicenter, blinded randomized controlled trial. Ann Surg 271:434–439

Blonk L, Civil YA, Kaufmann R, Ket JCF, van der Velde S (2019) A systematic review on surgical treatment of primary epigastric hernias. Hernia 23:847–857

Bökkerink WJV, Koning GG, Malagic D, van Hout L, van Laarhoven CJHM, Vriens PWHE (2019) Long-term results from a randomized comparison of open transinguinal preperitoneal hernia repair and the Lichtenstein method (TULIP trial). Br J Surg 106:856–861

Bullen NL, Massey LH, Antoniou SA, Smart NJ, Fortelny RH (2019) Open versus laparoscopic mesh repair of primary unilateral uncomplicated inguinal hernia: a systematic review with meta-analysis and trial sequential analysis. Hernia 23:461–472

Caro-Tarrago A, Olona C, Millán M, Olona M, Espina B, Jorba R (2019) Long-term results of a prospective randomized trial of midline laparotomy closure with onlay mesh. Hernia 23:335–340

Gavriilidis P, Davies RJ, Wheeler J, de' Angelis N, Di Saverio S (2019) Total extraperitoneal endoscopic hernioplasty (TEP) versus Lichtenstein hernioplasty: a systematic review by updated traditional and cumulative meta-analysis of randomised-controlled trials. Hernia 23:1093–1103

Gutlic N, Gutlic A, Petersson U, Rogmark P, Montgomery A (2019) Randomized clinical trial comparing total extraperitoneal with Lichtenstein inguinal hernia repair (TEPLICH trial). Br J Surg 106:845–855

van den Hil LCL, van Steensel S, Schreinemacher MHF, Bouvy ND (2019) Prophylactic mesh placement to avoid incisional hernias after stoma reversal: a systematic review and meta-analysis. Hernia 23: 733–741

Kohler A, Lavanchy JL, Lenoir U, Kurmann A, Candinas D, Beldi G (2019) Effectiveness of prophylactic intraperitoneal mesh implantation for prevention of incisional hernia in patients undergoing open abdominal surgery: a randomized clinical trial. JAMA Surg 154:109–115

Lockhart K, Dunn D, Teo S, Ng JY, Dhillon M, Teo E, van Driel ML (2018) Mesh versus non-mesh for inguinal and femoral hernia repair. Cochrane Database Syst Rev 9:CD011517

Obermaier R, Pfeffer F, Hopt UT (eds) (2009) Hernienchirurgie. Elsevier Urban & Fischer, München

Patterson TJ, Beck J, Currie PJ, Spence RAJ, Spence G (2019) Meta-analysis of patient-reported outcomes after laparoscopic versus open inguinal hernia repair. Br J Surg 106:824–836

Sheen AJ, Montgomery A, Simon T, Ilves I, Paajanen H (2019) Randomized clinical trial of open suture repair versus totally extraperitoneal repair for treatment of sportsman's hernia. Br J Surg 106:837–844

Shrestha D, Shrestha A, Shrestha B (2019) Open mesh versus suture repair of umbilical hernia: meta-analysis of randomized controlled trials. Int J Surg 62:62–66

Berger D (2010) Laparoskopische reparation der parastomalen Hernie. Chirurg 81:988–992

Jones HG, Rees M, Aboumarzouk OM, Brown J, Cragg J, Billings P, Carter B, Chandran P (2018) Prosthetic mesh placement for the prevention of parastomal herniation. Cochrane Database Syst Rev 7:CD008905

Reinforcement of Closure of Stoma Site (ROCSS), Collaborative and West Midlands Research Collaborative (2020) Prophylactic biological mesh reinforcement versus standard closure of stoma site (ROCSS): a multicentre, randomised controlled trial. Lancet 395:417–426

Rosch R, Conze J, Junge K, Neumann U (2010) Konventionelle Reparation der parastomalen Hernie. Chirurg 81:982–987

Gastrointestinal Stromal Tumors and Sarcomas

Daniel Oertli, Holger Bannasch, Athanasios Tampakis, Christoph Kettelhack, and Tobias Keck

Contents

F. Billmann, T. Keck (eds.), *Essentials of Visceral Surgery*,
https://doi.org/10.1007/978-3-662-66735-4_14

14.1 Gastrointestinal Stromal Tumours (GIST)

D. Oertli and T. Keck

Key Points

- GIST = Most common soft tissue tumors in the gastrointestinal tract.
- Overexpression of the KIT tyrosine kinase receptor (CD 117):
  - Diagnostic marker.
  - Simultaneous target for systemic therapy.
- Smaller tumors consistently benign; with larger diameter = malignant potential (occasionally liver metastases).
- Radical surgical excision indicated (goal = R0 resection) = avoidance of local recurrences.
- Adjuvant/neoadjuvant antibody therapy: with imatinib ("first line")/with sunitinib ("second line").

14.1.1 Definition

- GIST (gastrointestinal stromal tumors) = soft tissue tumors of the GI tract.
- Malignant potential dependent on:
  - Differentiation (G = Grading).
  - Tumor size.
  - Metastasis.

14.1.2 Epidemiology and Tumour Localisation

Epidemiology

- Annual incidence = 1/100,000 in general population.
- Women: Men = 1: 1.
- Peak incidence = 5th–7th decade of life.

Localization

- Stomach: 60–70%.
- Small intestine: 20–30.
- Colorectum: <5%.
- Other localization: esophagus, omentum, mesentery <5%.

- Most GIST = sporadic.
- Solitary in 95% of cases.

Tumor Biology

- Locally displacing growth.
- Tumor originates from the tunica muscularis.
- Usually no lymphatic metastasis.
- Hematogenous or peritoneal metastasis possible, 20% of tumors are metastatic at diagnosis.

Risk Factors

- Neurofibromatosis.
- In the context of the Carney triad: extraadrenal paraganglioma, pulmonary chondroma, GIST.
- Familial accumulation possible.

14.1.3 Clinical Presentation

Manifestation

- 70% symptomatic.
- 20% Incidental finding during endoscopy or surgery.
- 10% autopsy finding.

Symptoms

- Often incidental finding.
- Gastrointestinal bleeding 52%; if localized in the stomach: bleeding in 70% of cases.
- Abdominal pain 32%.

Prognosis at Diagnosis

- 5-year survival of the total collective (SEER database) = 45%.
  - Primary tumor = 53% (5-year survival = 64%).

- Locoregional recurrence = 19%.
- Stage IV (metastatic) = 23% (5-year survival = 13%).

14.1.4 Pathology

Conventional Histology

- Homogeneous proliferation of mesenchymal cells.
- gastrointestinal tract: cells with characteristic features of interstitial Cajal cells (pacemaker cells for peristalsis located in muscle wall with characteristic features of both smooth muscle and autonomic nerve cells).
- Histological subtypes:
  - Spindle cell type (70%).
  - Epithelioid cell type (20%).
  - Mixed type (spindle + epithelioid cells = 10%).

Immune Phenotype

- KIT tyrosinase receptor (CD 117) overexpression: 95% of cases.
  - CD 117 = product of the c-KIT gene (= protooncogene).
  - Diagnostic marker in immunohistochemistry.
  - Most other mesenchymal tumors (except Ewing's sarcoma) = CD 117-negative.
- Other positive markers:
  - CD 34: 70%.
  - "Smooth muscle actin" (SMA): 25%.
  - S-100 <10%.
  - Desmin <5%.

Mutation Detection

- Mutation in KIT receptor / in platelet-derived growth factor receptor α (PDGFRA): Functionally corresponding to protooncogene.
- Mutated protooncogene permanently active: cell proliferation and tumor formation.

14

14.1.5 Diagnosis

Diagnostic Imaging

- Primary diagnosis by esophagogastroduodenoscopy (EGD), in case of tumor localization in the small intestine push/double balloon endoscopy (advancing the endoscope into the small intestine with the help of balloons) or capsule endoscopy necessary.
- In the case of unclear tumour extension or to exclude metastases, additional CT-scan.
- For tumor search in the small intestine: dynamic magnetic resonance examination with oral contrast medium (MRI-Sellink) useful.
- Standard diagnosis CT, MRI and FDG PET if necessary for therapy assessment.

Tissue Biopsy

- Indications:
  - If endoscopically accessible (± endoluminal sonography).
  - If tumor is unresectable or metastatic.
  - If neoadjuvant pretreatment is planned.
- Contraindication/no indication: If tumour appears to be primarily completely resectable.

Caution

Tumor seeding on biopsy and/or postinterventional bleeding from tumor.

14.1.6 Therapy

Surgical Therapy

Indication

- Surgery = standard therapy for resectable GIST.

General Principles

- Minimum distance to the tumour: of 1–2 cm sufficent under certain circumstances.

- Partial resection of the stomach possible (e.g. wedge resection): Gastrectomy necessary in rare cases.
- Segment resections of the small and large intestine.
- Local R0 resection of the rectum permitted.
- No systematic lymphadenectomy (because predominantly hematogenous metastasis).

Caution

A complete microscopic resection (R0 resection) should **always** be aimed for!

GIST of the Stomach

- Tumour diameter 0.3–6.5 cm = mostly "low risk".
- Small tumors: well localizable + resectable by laparoscopy +/intraoperative gastroscopy.

Caution

If tumor rupture (spontaneous, traumatic, iatrogenic, intraoperative) and tumor cell seeding:

- Adjuvant therapy (see below).
- Without imatinib high local recurrence risk.

Adjuvant Treatment

Antibodies (Ab) Against the Tyrosine Kinase Receptor

- Imatinib (e.g. Gleevec) = selective thyrosine kinase inhibitor on c-KIT and PDGFRA.
- Central role of the c-KIT mutation status (see below "Molecular genetic analysis").
- Dosage = 400–800 mg daily.
- Median time to maximum response: 197 days.
- Results
  - Complete remission = 5%.
  - Partial remission = 47%.
  - Disease stabilisation = 32%.

Molecular Genetic Analysis as a Guide for Ab Treatment

- c-KIT exon 11: mutation higher response rate than c-KIT exon 9 mutation.
- c-KIT mutation: Higher response rate than wild type.
- As a consequence 2 strategies possible:
  - Pro: High dosage (800 mg daily) in wild type and in exon 9 mutation.
  - Contra: 400 mg in all patients, increase to 800 mg if progression.
- Side effects: Anemia, neutropenia, fatigue, edema, rash, nausea, diarrhea.

Second-Line Therapy

- In case of resistance to imatinib (Gleevec):
  - 5% primary resistance.
  - 14% Secondary resistance.
- Sunitinib: Different clinical benefit depending on genotype: KIT exon 9: 63%; wild type 56%; KIT exon 11: 36%; PDGFRA 25%.

Neoadjuvant Treatment

Goals

- Achieving resectability in primary irrectable GIST.
  - Tumor regression (size): Can function-preserving surgery be facilitated? Can a multivisceral resection be avoided?
  - Minimization of tumor fragility.
- Based on imatinib (Gleevec).

Indications/Target Organs

- Locally advanced tumor.
- Target Organs:
  - Rectum.
  - Esophagus.
  - Pancreas.

Multimodal Therapy

- Indication depends on the risk of recurrence; this can be assessed, for example, with the score according to Fletcher et al. (2002a, b) (Table 14.1) or Miettinen and Lasota (2001).

Results of Neoadjuvant Therapy

- Maximum tumor response after 6–12 months: Surgery.
- Despite R0 resection: local recurrence (up to 76% of patients).

Table 14.1 Risk stratification according to Fletcher in GIST

Risk	Tumor size	Microscopy: number of mitoses
Very low	<2 cm	<5/50 HPF
Low	2–5 cm	<5/50 HPF
Interme-diary	<5 cm 5–10 cm	6–10/50 HPF <5/50 HPF
High	>5 cm >10 cm Any size	>5/50 HPF Each number >10/50 HPF

HPF high power field

- In this case salvage surgery: 15 months median survival.
- Prognostic factors (poor prognosis):
  - Tumor size.
  - Tumor localization (duodenum, rectum).
  - Incomplete resection.
  - High proliferation rate (Ki-67 index).
  - Mutation status (deletion in KIT exon 11).

Assessment of the Therapeutic Success in Imaging

Caution
Cross-sectional imaging needed to evaluate therapeutic success.

- Absence of increase in size of tumor and metastases = response.
- Especially if tissue density changes under Ab therapy.

Computer Tomography (CT scan)

- Therapy success = no increase in size (not necessarily shrinkage of the lesion).
- Decrease in measured density (in Hounsfield units) >15% = remission.

Positron Emission Tomography (PET)

- Decrease in SUV ("standardized uptake value") by more than 40% from baseline or SUV <3.4 = response to neoadjuvant therapy.

14.1.7 Guidelines

ESMO (2018) Clinical Practice Guidelines for diagnosis, treatment and follow-up. Ann Oncol 29 (Suppl 4): iv 68–78.

14.2 Soft Tissue Tumours of the Extremities

H. Bannasch

14.2.1 General: Classification

Key Points

- Benign soft tissue tumors 90% vs. Soft tissue sarcomas 10%.
- In 60% of cases = Extremities affected.
- Diagnosis: Ultrasound, MRI, PET.
- Prognosis: Depending on tumor size + grading.

Epidemiology

General Information

- Benign soft tissue tumors.
  - Large majority of all soft tissue tumours (at least 100 times more frequent than soft tissue sarcomas).
  - Incidence = approx. 300/100,000.
- Soft tissue sarcomas (STS)
  - Rare and heterogeneous group of malignant tumors.
  - Mesenchymal origin.
  - STS = only 1% of all adult malignancies.

- Incidence in adults = approx. 2–3/100,000.
- Incidence increase of STS in the last decades (possibly only apparent increase due to better data collection).
- No differences in the geographical frequency distribution.
- In children: Proportion of STS in all malignancies significantly higher (5–8%) despite lower incidence.

STS Body-Distribution Pattern

- 60% Extremities.
  - Lower extremity more often than upper extremity.
  - In each case, higher incidence for the proximal limb sections.
- 20–35% retro- and intraperitoneal sarcomas including GIST (▶ Sect. 14.1).
- 15–20% trunk, head and neck region.

Caution

Soft tissue sarcomas in adults vs. children: significant differences with regard to distribution pattern in the body, histological frequency distribution of the subtypes and tumor biology!

Rare Hereditary Risk Factors

- Li-Fraumeni Syndrome.
  - Very rare autosomal dominant disease with germline mutation of the tumor suppressor gene p53.
  - Very high risk for numerous malignancies.
- Neurofibromatosis type 1 (von Recklinghausen's disease).
  - Incidence approx. 35/100,000.
  - Autosomal dominant inherited multiorgan disease.
  - Mainly involvement of the skin and nervous system (phacomatosis).
  - including benign neurofibromas.
  - Lifetime risk of about 5–10% for malignant transformation of a (plexiform) neurofibroma into a malignant peripheral nerve sheath tumor (MPNST).

Acquired Risk Factors

- Postradiogenic sarcomas (latency of up to 20 years).
- Steward-Treves syndrome (angiosarcoma originating from chronic lymphedema).
- Viral infections in immunocompromised patients causally responsible for STS development:
  - HHV8 for Kaposi's sarcoma.
  - EBV for leiomyosarcoma.

Caution

Etiology of soft tissue sarcomas mostly unclear; rare hereditary and acquired risk factors known.

14.2.2 Clinical Presentation

- Leading symptom = mostly painless swelling of the extremities.
- Duration of symptoms often not ascertainable.
- Frequent anamnestic association with minor trauma (patient's need for causality).
- Rarely specific symptoms with peripheral functional deficits – vascular-nervous (blood flow, motor function, sensory function) deficits often only in advanced local stages.
- B-symptomatics only present in exceptional cases.

Caution

Increased delay in diagnosis:

- Due to the rarity of soft tissue sarcomas (often the possibility of a malignant tumour is not considered).
- Diagnosis in many cases in the context of an inadequate excision without prior diagnosis.

Anamnesis

- Despite oligosymptomatic: careful history and examination obligatory.
- Documentation of extent and duration of swelling/discomfort.
- Querying risk factors (see above).

Investigation

- Inspection of the extremities.
  - Differences in side circumference, swellings.
  - Sensory and motor function deficits.
- Palpation of the lymph node stations (rarely affected).

Caution
Swelling of the extremities resistant to therapy for longer than 4 weeks → further investigation needed.

14.2.3 Diagnosis

- Goals
  - Determination of the histology of the tumor.
  - Determination of tumor size + tumor location with reference to surrounding anatomical structures.
  - Staging: detection of distant metastases (mostly haematogenous).
  - Staging of children with soft tissue sarcomas: more complex + extensive than in adults.

Local Diagnosis

Ultrasound (Unclear Swelling of the Extremity)

- Helpful for initial descriptive purposes.
- Can be repeated without complications.
- Disadvantages: Investigator dependence and relative nonspecificity.

Native X-Ray Imaging in 2 Planes

- possible calcifications in case of extraosseous bone tumours.

Magnetic Resonance Imaging (MRI): Gold Standard

- Local presentation of a soft tissue tumor of the extremity.
- MRI is clearly superior to computed tomography (CT).
- Always with and without contrast medium.
- Provides valuable information about the size, location and contents of the tumour (necrosis, myxoid areas, haemorrhages, etc.).
- Assessment of the technical operability and evaluation of a necessary "down-sizing".

Fluorodeoxyglucose (FDG)-PET

- Not generally recommended.

Diagnosis of Local and General Spread

Pathophysiology

- Adult STS: Preferential metastasis = hematogenous-pulmonary.

Diagnosis

- MRI: for local extension.
- CT chest/(abdomen): Staging.
- Lymph node diagnosis: No evidence.
- Sentinel lymph node biopsy: No evidence.
- FDG-PET: Only useful in individual cases.
- Tumor markers: No evidence.

Biopsy

Caution
Suspicion of malignant soft tissue tumor: histological diagnosis is indicated and early referral to a specialized center indicated.

General

- Differentiation malignant vs. benign with imaging techniques: not possible with certainty.
- Multiple tumor characteristic features correlatable with ex post diagnosis of STS:
  - Tumour diameter > 5 cm.
  - Size increase.
  - Painfulness.
  - Deep localization.

Indication for Biopsy

- Any tumor = malignant until proven otherwise.
- Slow tumor growth = no definite evidence of benign disease.
- Only every 100th–200th soft tissue tumour = malignant.
- Conclusion: Therefore very generous indication for biopsy.

14

Excisional Biopsy

- Only if the tumour is definitely epifascial.
- Only for small (<5 cm) tumors.
- Only for tumors without high suspicion of malignancy!
- In case of malignancy:
  - Oncologic resection in these cases usually technically unproblematic.
  - No influence on prognosis.

Caution

Send every specimen for histopathologic examination!

Open Incisional Biopsy

- Open incisional biopsy = procedure of choice.
- In case of suspected malignancy always at the center.
- Ideally by the surgeon scheduled for oncologic resection.
- Principle: Obtaining sufficient material including the so-called pseudocapsule for:
  - Conventional + immunohistochemical examinations.
  - Molecular genetic examinations: Fluorescence in situ hybridization (FISH), polymerase chain reaction (PCR).
  - If necessary, pathology reference center (indicate generously).

Caution

Possible mistakes:

- Incision, which complicates a later ideal reconstruction (access path and drainage outlets have to be resected during the second operation).
- Insufficient haemostasis = haematoma formation + risk of cell spreading.
- Unfavorable drainage outlets far away from the surgical area: need for larger excision during second operation.

Punch Biopsy

- Possible in centres with sufficient expertise under sonographic control.
- Diagnostic certainty: punch biopsy > fine needle aspiration; punch biopsy = open incision biopsy.
- Molecular pathology also feasible with little tissue.

14.2.4 Classification

Histological Classification

- Overview: Internationally valid classification for soft tissue tumors:
  - WHO classification of tumours of the soft tissues and bone (Fletcher et al. 2002a, b).
- Diagnostic tools PCR and FISH: detection of numerous specific chromosomal translocations = supplementation of the classical pathomorphological diagnosis.
- Unchanged classification according to detectable line of differentiation.
- First classification principle = descent from probable tissue of origin (lipomatous, fibroblastic etc.)
- Second classification principle = within the entities with regard to their dignity: benign – intermediate (locally aggressive) – intermediate (rarely metastatic) – malignant.

Most Common Entities

- Leiomyosarcomas (15–25%).
- Liposarcomas (10–15%).
- Pleomorphic sarcoma (formerly called myxoid fibrous histiocytoma, MFH, 15–25%).

Staging and Grading

Staging

- TNM classification of the American Joint Committee on Cancer (AJCC) and the Union Internationale contre le Cancer (UICC; see below).
- Criteria (update 2017).

  - 4 tumor sizes (T1: ≤5 cm; T2: >5 ≤ 10 cm; T3: >10 ≤ 15 cm; T4: >15 cm).
  - Tumor site (formerly a = superficial, b = deep): omitted!
  - Lymph node metastasis.
  - Distant metastasis.

Grading

- 3-level scoring system of the FNCLCC (French Federation of Cancer Centers Sarcoma Group):
- G1 = Low-grade tumours.
- G2 and G3 = High-grade tumours.

UICC Stages According to the TNM Classification

- TNM classification of adult soft tissue sarcomas (AJCC/UICC, eighth amendment 2017).

IA	T1	N0	M0	G1
IB	T2, T3	N0	M0	G1, GX
II	T1	N0	M0	G2, G3
IIIA	T2	N0	M0	G2, G3
IIIB	T3, T4	N0	M0	G2, G3
IIIC	Each T	N1	M0	Each

14

14.2.5 Prognosis

Main Prognostic Determinants for Non-Metastatic Tumours

- Tumor size.
- Grading.

5-Year Survival for Patients with STS of the Extremities

- Allover approx. 70–75%.
- Depending on tumor size: <5 cm: 85%, 5–15 cm: 68%, >15 cm: 52%.
- Depending on the grading: G1: 80–90%, G2: 65–77%, G3: 42–50%.
- Depending on the UICC/AJCC stage: stage I: 85–96%, stage II: 72–78%, stage III: 50% and stage IV: 10%.

14.2.6 Therapeutic Principles

Sarcoma Centre: Tumour Board—Interdisciplinary, Multimodal Therapy

Key Points

- Oncosurgical resective surgery = central element of therapy.
- Reconstructive surgery afterwards.
- Radiotherapy = additional local therapy.
- Combination of pre- and postoperative chemotherapy with regional hyperthermia (± radiotherapy) for locally advanced tumor.
- Primary treatment at a certified STS centre = improved oncological outcome.
- Specialized certified sarcoma tumor board (general surgery, orthopedics, plastic surgery, radiotherapy, oncology, radiology, pathology).
  - Pre- and postoperative presentation.
  - Diagnosis and complete staging.
  - Multimodal therapy concepts (also for metachronous recurrences or metastases).

Surgery

Oncosurgical Resective Surgery

Wide Excision

- Goal = local tumor control to prevent local recurrence.
- Outcome: strongly dependent on initial metastasis.

Surgical Procedure

Wide Sarcoma Excision

- Resection of the tumor with sufficient safety margin (a few mm).
- Remove biopsy access and drainage of previous operations as well.
- Orientation based on preoperative MRI and intraoperative palpation.
- Consider relation of tumor to anatomical boundary structures (fasciae, intermuscular septa, epineurium, adventitia, periosteum) (achieve R0).
- Correct thread marking of the preparation at critical sites and correlating clip marking in the tumor bed.
- Photographic documentation.
- No general recommendation for frozen section.

No STS resection of the limb possible without knowledge of reconstructive options. Combination of the above techniques + radiotherapy allows limb preservation in 90–95% of cases.

Caution

- Enucleation at the edge of the pseudocapsule (marginal excision) is not an oncologic resection in sano!
- measurement of sufficient safety margin of a wide excision in sano is not clearly defined.
- Substantial = resection of the tumor with a sufficient margin of healthy tissue (= seeing the tumor itself).

Compartment Resection

- Radical removal of a complete compartment.
- largely abandoned (exaggerated radicality).
- Significant loss of function.

Limb Amputation

- Individual cases ("life before limb").
- Reconstructive techniques (e.g. Borggreve reversal plastic or stump lengthening using fillet flaps).
- Future inovations to be expected (bionic prosthetics).

Reconstructive Surgery

- Definition
  - Reconstructive-restorative measure = everything that goes beyond primary suture.
- Goal
  - Undisturbed wound healing.
  - Important for general rehabilitation and undelayed initiation of adjuvant therapies.

Surface Restoration

- Indication
  - Restoration of surface continuity = reconstruction of form and surface as accurately as possible under functional-aesthetic aspects.
- Technique/Strategy
  - Split-thickness skin grafting.
  - Flap plasty.
  - Random SkinFlaps.
  - Displacement-swivel-plasty for smaller defects.
  - Axial flap plasty for larger defects.
  - Microsurgical flap plasty with negligible lifting defect morbidity = indispensable component of modern extremity reconstruction.
  - Modern perforator flap plasties.

Functional Restoration

- Principle:
  - Functional reconstructions = simultaneous to surface reconstruction.
  - Nerve interposition (usually suralis cable graft interposition): For sensitive reconstruction.
  - Vascular replacement (proximal to elbow and knee by vascular surgeons).
- Motor Reconstructions:
  - Tendon interposition (palmaris longus or plantaris longus muscles).
  - Free functional muscle transfers rarely indicated (e.g. free gracilis transfer as motor long finger flexor replacement).

Caution

- Resection and reconstruction often possible in a single stage.

- MRI-guided surgical planning on the extremities = essential because of possible defects that are difficult to close.

Tumor Recurrence Surgery

- Surgical treatment of local recurrence = same principles as treatment of primary tumor.
- Renewed staging + renewed interdisciplinary discussion obligatory.

Tumor Metastases Surgery

- Lung = most frequent target organ of STS metastases.
- Resection of lung metastases = established procedure.
- Complete surgical resection of lung metastases = positive prognostic factor.

Radiotherapy

Principle

- Without surgery no cure.
- Palliative radiotherapy only in inoperable patients.
- Additive or adjuvant radiotherapy = in addition to surgery.
- In R1 situation, reoperation to be preferred if technically possible.

14

Application

- Total dose 60–66 Gy with conventional fractionation.
- Radiation field = tumor site + safety margin + all scars + drainage exit sites.
- Improved local control for G2 and G3 STS proven.
- Influence on overall survival = controversial.
- Rradiation therapy not indicated in R0-resected G1-STS.
- Do not irradiate complex reconstructions

Neoadjuvant Radiotherapy

- Equivalent to adjuvant radiotherapy in terms of local control.
- Smaller field size and lower dose (50 Gy).
- Fewer long-term consequences (fibrosis, edema) for soft tissue.
- For irresectable tumors: Consider multimodal combinations (radiochemotherapy or limb perfusion).

Caution

With neoadjuvant radiotherapy, the rate of early postoperative (sometimes severe) wound healing disorders of the lower extremity is significantly increased!

Intraoperative Radiotherapy

- Limited availability.
- Targeted application of a single dose of 12–20 Gy into tumor bed.
- Always in combination with neoadjuvant or adjuvant radiotherapy.
- Reduces percutaneous residual dose.

Chemotherapy

- STS generally little chemosensitivity.
- Exception: small, blue, round cell sarcomas such as extraosseous Ewing sarcoma, rhabdomyosarcomas, primitive neuroectodermal tumors (PNET) and desmoplastic, small and round cell tumors with a clear recommendation for neoadjuvant chemotherapy.
- "Molecular targeted therapy" very limited (Imatinib for dermatofibrosarcoma protuberans, Sorafenib for angiosarcoma).
- Limited benefit of chemotherapy: No general recommendation.

Hyperthermia/Isolated Limb Perfusion

- Combination of pre + postoperative chemotherapy with regional hyperthermia (± radiotherapy).
  - In locally advanced soft tissue sarcomas: improvement of local tumor control and progression-free survival.
- Isolated limb perfusion (ILP) with TNF-α and melphalan.

Tumor Follow-up

- Department of General Surgery, University Hospital Basel, BaselIndividualized, risk-adapted follow-up care for at least 10 years.

Local Tumor Follow-up

- Regular clinical examination.
- MRI.

Systemic Tumor Follow-up

- Regular oncological follow-up.
- every 6 months Chest Imaging.
- FDG-PET in individual cases.

14.2.7 Guidelines

AWMF soft tissue sarcoma guideline registry number 025–007; 3/2017; ► https://www.awmf.org/leitlinien/detail/ll/025-007.html.

Kandel R, Coakley N, Werier J, Engel J, Ghert M, Verma S; Sarcoma Disease Site Group of Cancer Care Ontario's Program in Evidence-Based Care (2013) Surgical margins and handling of soft-tissue sarcoma in extremities: a clinical practice guideline. Curr Oncol 20: e247-e254.

Schütte J, Hartmann JT, Reichardt P, Issels RD, Tunn PU, Budach V (2011) Soft tissue sarcomas, DGHO guideline. ► https://www.dgho-onkopedia.de/de/onkopedia/leitlinien/weichteilsarkome.

14.3 Retroperitoneal Sarcomas

A. Tampakis and C. Kettelhack

14.3.1 Epidemiology and Prognosis

Epidemiology

- 0.2–0.3% of all malignancies in adults.
- Annual incidence = 0.3/100,000 population (estimated).
- 15% of all soft tissue sarcomas.
- 1/3 of malignant retroperitoneal tumors.
- Associated genetic diseases:.
  - Li-Fraumeni Syndrome
  - Familial adenomatous polyposis.
  - Gardner Syndrome.
  - Carney-Stratakis Syndrome.

Prognosis and Prognostic Factors

- 5-year survival rate = 64.6%.
- Prognostic factor for overall survival, 5-year survival, and survival after relapse = histologic subtype: atypical lipomatous tumor (ALT, well-differentiated liposarcoma) vs. non-ALT liposarcoma vs. other subtypes.
- Median time to locoregional recurrence (23% at 5 years) = 41 months.
- Prognostic factors for local recurrence = size, histologic grade, and completeness of surgical resection.

Tumor size + malignancy grade = most important prognostic factors for overall survival.

14.3.2 Pathology

- Histology of retroperitoneal sarcomas (RPS): well-differentiated liposarcomas, malignant fibrous histiocytomas, dedifferentiated liposarcomas, leiomyosarcomas, malignant peripheral nerve sheath tumors, solitary fibrous tumors, and other sarcomas (◘ Table 14.2).

◘ **Table 14.2** Pathology of retroperitoneal sarcomas. (According to Nathan et al. 2009)

Histology	Number (*n*)	Share (%)
Liposarcoma	682	50
Leiomyosarcoma	358	26
Malignant fibrous histiocytoma	146	11
Fibrosarcoma	24	2
Rhabdomyosarcoma	21	2
MPNST	15	1
Hemangiopericytoma	13	<1
Hemangiosarcoma	10	<1
Malignant mesenchymoma	5	<1
Sarcoma NOS	91	7
Total	1365	100

MPNST malignant peripheral nerve sheath tumors, *NOS* not otherwised specified

14.3.3 Classification

AJCC/UICC

- TNM and staging.
- Malignancy grade: High significance in sarcomas.
- Pathology of retroperitoneal sarcomas (AJCC Soft Tissue Sarcoma Staging System; Feig and Ching 2012).

TNM Classification

- Primary tumor (T).
  - Tx Primary tumor cannot be assessed.
  - T0 No evidence of primary tumor.
  - T1 tumor ≤5 cm in the largest diameter.
    - T1a Above and no invasion of the fascia.
    - T1b Invasion of the fascia or below the fascia.
  - T2 Tumor >5 cm in largest diameter.
    - T2a Above and no invasion of the fascia.
    - T2b Invasion of the fascia or below the fascia.
- Regional lymph nodes (N).
  - Nx Regional lymph nodes cannot be assessed.
  - N0 No regional lymph node metastases.
  - N1 Regional lymph node metastases.
- Distant metastases (M).
  - Mx distant metastases cannot be assessed.
  - M0 No distant metastases
  - M1 distant metastases.
- Histopathological grading (G).
  - Gx: Grading cannot be assessed.
  - G1: Grade 1.
  - G2: Grade 2.
  - G3: Grade 3.

UICC Stages According to the TNM Classification

Stage IA	T1a, T1b	N0	M0	G1, Gx
Stage IB	T2a, T2b	N0	M0	G1, Gx
Stage IIA	T1a, T1b	N0	M0	G2, G3
Stage IIB	T2a, T2b	N0	M0	G2
Stage III	T2a, T2b	N0	M0	G3
	Each T	N1	M0	Each G
Stage IV	Each T	Each N	M1	Each G

14.3.4 Molecular Genetics

- Mesenchymal origin.
- Dysregulation of gene expression by aberrant chimeric transcription factors.
- Genetic-etiological 2 main categories:
  - Tumor-specific translocation.
  - Complex karyotypes (= characteristic feature of severe genetic + chromosomal instability).

14.3.5 Clinical Presentation

Early Symptoms

- Mostly missing.
- Due to large expansion potential of the retroperitoneum and the abdominal cavity (= progressive growth of retroperitoneal sarcomas unnoticed until advanced stages).
- At diagnosis: Retroperitoneal sarcomas >20 cm = 50%.

Clinical Symptoms (If Present)

- Mostly due to compression/invasion of neighbouring structures.
- abdominal distension.
- Changes in bowel movements.
- Abdominal pain.
- Weight loss/anemia (occasionally).

Caution

- In case of fever + night sweats: think of lymphoma as differential diagnosis.
- Testicular examination (clinical examination + ultrasound if necessary) in men = important, since retroperitoneal metastases from a primary gonadal tumor often present similarly.

Guidelines (main guidelines)
- NCCN(The *National Comprehensive Cancer Network*) Guidelines from 2014.
- European Consensus Guidelines of ESMO (European Society for Medical Oncology) 2014.

14.3.6 Diagnosis

Medical History and Clinical Examination
- Exclusion of lymphoma signs (see above).
- Clinical Examination:
  - Draining lymph node groups.
  - Testis: Exclusion of metastatic/advanced testicular tumor…
- Laboratory test: LDH + AFP + βHCG to exclude lymphoma/germ cell tumour.

Radiology

Multiphase Spiral CT scan
- Abdomen/Retroperitoneum/Pelvis: Most important diagnostic procedure.
- Thorax: for the detection of lung metastases/staging.

MRI
- Essential for vascular assessment, delineation of compartments, fasciae, nerves.

PET/PET-CT
- No required as standard examination.
- Potential use for response assessment in preoperative therapy.
- Possible use to exclude distant metastases.

Renal Scintigraphy
- Examination of the split renal function.
- Preparation for possible nephrectomy for en bloc multivisceral resections.

Biopsy
- Ideally preoperative image-guided punch biopsy.
- If large tumor heterogeneity on CT: Multiple biopsies.

No evidence for worsening of prognosis by percutaneous punch biopsy: In retroperitoneal sarcomas no influence of biopsy on local recurrence, disease-free survival, overall survival.

NCCN Guidelines
- In case of clearly resectable tumor: Surgery also justifiable without prior biopsy to confirm the diagnosis.

Caution
Surgical resection without prior biopsy: Only after interdisciplinary discussion in the sarcoma tumor board.

- Biopsy necessary before starting preoperative radio- or chemotherapy.
- Open incisional biopsy by laparoscopy or laparotomy not indicated.

14.3.7 Therapy

Surgical Therapy
- Surgical tumor resection with tumor-free resection margins = only curative therapy option.
- Incomplete resection = direct effect on outcome:
  - Increased risk of recurrence (mortality usually associated with local recurrence).
  - Increased risk of distant metastasis.
  - Worse overall survival.

Macroscopic complete resection possible in 40–60% of cases: Due to narrow anatomical relationship + locally advanced tumor extension.

En Bloc Organ Resection
- Traditionally only in case of direct infiltration through the tumor

Principle En Bloc Resection
- Tumors + adjacent organs (e.g. kidney, colon, psoas muscle, small intestine, pancreas tail, diaphragm).

- Critical structures: resection only in case of direct infiltration (duodenum/pancreas head, liver, stomach, large abdominal vessels and nerves, bones).
- Results: Significantly fewer locoregional tumor recurrences, no effect on survival rates.

Palliative resections to improve quality of life possible (e.g. for symptoms such as ileus, bleeding).

Morbidity and Mortality

- Morbidity 22–26% and perioperative mortality 1.7–3%.
- Most common complications:
  - Anastomotic insufficiencies.
  - Paralytic ileus.
  - Retroperitoneal fluid collections.
  - Bleeding.

Independent Predictive Factors Associated with a Lower Locoregional Tumor Recurrence Rate

- Complete tumor resection without intraoperative tumor rupture.
- Low-grade tumor.
- Histologically confirmed negative resection margins.
- Number of cases treated annually per institution; so-called hospital volume.
- Radical surgical strategy.

14

For completely resected RPS: 5-year local recurrence-free survival (LRFS) = 55%; 5-year distant metastasis-free survival = 66–79%.

Radiotherapy

Preoperative Radiotherapy (PrR)

Main Objectives of the PrR

- Increase in resectability.
- Local control.
- Lack of level 1 evidence for PrR
- Incidence of PrR use for RPS: 3% in 2005; 10% in 2011.

Theoretical Advantages of PrR (Nussbaum et al. 2014)

- Irradiation field aligned more precisely.
- Thickness of the tumor pseudocapsule increases after irradiation = better imageable margin layer between healthy tissue and tumor.
- Reduction of tumor size = higher probability of R0 resection.
- Morbidity and mortality after RPS resection + previous PrR: Not significantly increased.

- Mean dose of PrR in studies: from 45 to 50.4 Gy
- PrR tolerated with selective dose increase in the tumor area ("boost")

Intraoperative Radiotherapy (IORT)

Principle

- Displacement/Protection of sensitive normal tissue.
- Use of individualized shields.
- Limited penetration depth of electrons: Use of a biologically effective single large dose of radiation by IORT.

Limits of the IORT

- Limited availability of technology.
- Lack of data.

- ESMO guidelines: Efficacy of intraoperative irradiation not sufficiently proven so far, therefore not recommended outside studies
- NCCN Guidelines: IORT with or without external beam radiotherapy effective in local control and survival in patients with primary and recurrent RPS

Postoperative Radiotherapy (PostR)

- Indications
  - Narrow (Rx) or positive (R1) resection limits.
  - Especially recommended for high-grade tumors.

- General efficacy in retroperitoneal tumors = not sufficiently documented.
- Not indicated in the presence of metastases.

- ESMO Guidelines (2014): Adjuvant radiotherapy of limited value + significant short- and long-term toxicity: therefore use only in very selective cases.
- If PostR planned: Recommendation to use omentum or other placeholders to move the bowel out of the tumor bed = reduction of the risk of radiation-induced bowel toxicity.

Chemotherapy

Preoperative Chemotherapy

- No recommendation for neoadjuvant therapy.

Phase 3 multicenter randomized trial (Gaspar et al. 2015): Neoadjuvant chemotherapy (etoposide + ifosfamide + doxorubicin with/without regional hyperthermia) = better local tumor control in patients at high risk of tumor recurrence (grading 2 and 3, tumor diameter > 5 cm).

Adjuvant Chemotherapy

- No indication for adjuvant chemotherapy in retroperitoneal sarcomas.

14.3.8 Management of Recurrences

Incidence

- Recurrence = in 2/3 of patients.
  - Local in tumor bed.
  - Metastases: Lung, liver.
  - Sarcomatosis: Diffuse recurrence in the peritoneal cavity.
- In up to 40% of patients: Recurrence later than 5 years after initial surgery.

Treatment of the Recurrence

- If resectable: goal should be R0 resection.
- Isolated liver metastases: Resection/RFTA (radiofrequency thermoablation)/chemoembolization possible (if stable for months).

Resectability of local recurrence = decreasing with each recurrence: 57% of patients at first recurrence, 20% at second recurrence, 10% at third recurrence.

- Most important outcome predictor in local recurrence = resectability of recurrent tumors: median survival = 60 months in operated patients vs. 20 months in non-operated patients.

14.3.9 Follow up

Evidence

- Recommendations for follow-up = not sufficiently evidence-based.
- No evidence of improvement in recurrence-free or overall survival with intensive follow-up.
- Risk of recurrence and metastasis: highest in the first 2 years after primary surgery.

Strategy

- In high-risk patients:
  - CT (MRI) scan of the abdomen (and thorax) recommended at 3- to 4-month intervals for 2 years.
  - 6 months in the third year, then annually.
- After chemotherapy:
  - Laboratory examination every 3 months for the first 2 years, every 6 months in the third and fourth year and annually from the fifth year onwards.

14.3.10 Guidelines

AWMF soft tissue sarcoma guideline registry number 025–007; 3/2017; ► https://www.awmf.org/leitlinien/detail/ll/025-007.html

ESMO (2014) European Consensus Guidelines. ► https://www.nccn.org

NCCN (2014) Guidelines. ► http://oncologypro.esmo.org/Guidelines-Practice/ESMO-Consensus-Conferences

References

Feig BW, Ching CD (2012) The MD Anderson surgical oncology handbook, 5th edn. Lippincott, Williams and Wilkins, Philadelphia/Baltimore/New York/London

Fletcher CD, Berman JJ, Corless C et al (2002a) Diagnosis of gastrointestinal stromal tumors: a consensus approach. Hum Pathol 33:459–465

Miettinen M, Lasota J (2001) Gastrointestinal stromal tumors – definition, clinical, histological, immunohistochemical, and moleculargenetic features and differential diagnosis. Virchows Arch 438:1–12

Fletcher CDM, Unni KK, Mertens F (2002b) Pathology and genetics of tumours of soft tissue and bone. In: WHO classification of tumours, international agency for research on cancer. IARC Press, Lyon

Gaspar N, Hawkins DS, Dirksen U et al (2015) Ewing sarcoma: current management and future approaches through collaboration. J Clin Oncol 33(27):3036–3046

Nathan H, Raut CP, Thornton K, Herman JM et al (2009) Predictors of survival after resection of retroperitoneal sarcoma: a population-based analysis and critical appraisal of the AJCC staging system. Ann Surg 250:970–976

Nussbaum DP, Speicher PJ, Gulack BC et al (2014) The effect of neoadjuvant radiation therapy on perioperative outcomes among patients undergoing resection of retroperitoneal sarcomas. Surg Oncol 23:155–160

Perioperative Medicine

Maren Rudat and Sebastian Stehr

Contents

F. Billmann, T. Keck (eds.), *Essentials of Visceral Surgery*,
https://doi.org/10.1007/978-3-662-66735-4_15

15.1 Preoperative Phase

Key Points

- Risk stratification (patient-related, surgery-related risk factors, medication, laboratory chemistry).
- Determination of perioperative anticoagulation and medication management.

15.1.1 Risk Stratification

- Patient-related surgical risk depending on the patient's state of health and the invasiveness of the operation.

Identification of Patient-Related Risks

- Careful anamnesis, thorough examination.
- Presentation in the anaesthesia department (ideally max. 6 weeks before surgery).
- Initiate further diagnosis.
- General condition of the patient according to ASA classification:
  - Description of preoperative health status, 1 (healthy patient) to 6 (brain-dead patient at organ removal ◘ Table 15.1).

◘ **Table 15.1** ASA (American Society of Anesthesiologists) classification

Class	Criteria
ASA 1	Normal, healthy patient
ASA 2	Patient with mild general illness
ASA 3	Patient with severe general illness
ASA 4	Patient with a severe general illness that is a constant threat to life
ASA 5	Moribund patient unlikely to survive without surgery
ASA 6	Brain-dead patient whose organs are removed for organ donation

Systemic Diseases with High Postoperative Risk

- Cardiovascular System:
  - Various scores: RCR (Revised Cardiac Risk) index according to Lee (Lee et al. 1999), NYHA (*New York Heart Association)* classification, MET (metabolic equivalent).
  - Risk factors for cardiovascular complications: Coronary artery disease (CAD), heart failure, fresh myocardial infarction, chronic venous insufficiency (CVI), insulin-dependent diabetes mellitus (IDDM), chronic renal failure, cardiac arrhythmia (CAr), fresh insult.
  - Diagnosis: 12-lead ECG, echocardiography, exercise ECG, coronary angiography, carotid Doppler, chest X-ray.
- Pulmonary disease:
  - Different scores for the prediction of postoperative ventilation risk and re-intubation.
  - Increased risk in chronic obstructive pulmonary disease (COPD), asthma, obesity, obstructive sleep apnoea syndrome (OSAS) and smokers.
  - Diagnosis: chest X-ray, blood gas analysis BGA, lung function test.
- Diabetes mellitus:
  - Perioperative normoglycemic setting: blood glucose (BG) = 140–180 mg/dl and close-meshed BG controls.

Perioperative Risk (◘ Table 15.2)

- Depending on invasiveness, duration and possible blood loss.
  - Mild: minor endoscopic and outpatient procedures, breast surgery.
  - Moderate: intraperitoneal, intrathoracic surgery, orthopedics.
  - High: Aortic surgery, vascular surgery.

Intubation Conditions

- To estimate a possible difficult airway.
- Mallampati score (relation of tongue size to pharynx).
- Head reclination.
- Mouth opening.
- 3-3-2 rule (mouth opening >3 fingers, os hyoideum chin distance ≥3 fingers, thyromental distance >2 fingers).
- Aspiration risk.

Table 15.2 Risk of perioperative myocardial infarction or death within 30 days after surgery

Low <1%	Mean 1–5%	High >5%
Chest Tooth Eye Gynecology Minor orthopedic surgery (knee) Urology	Visceral surgery Carotid Angioplasty Endovascular aneurysms Head and neck Major orthopedic surgery Transplant Major urological surgery	Aorta Major vascular surgery PAOD Esophagectomy Cystectomy Pneumonectomy

PAOD peripheral arterial occlusive disease

15.1.2 Laboratory and Blood Products

Blood Management

- Preoperative anemia prevalence: approx. 30%.
- Risk factor for perioperative morbidity and mortality.
- Preoperative improvement through "patient blood management" by increasing erythropoiesis (erythropoietin, iron substitution).
- Preoperative blood transfusion.
- Preparation of packed red blood cells (PRBCs) depending on the planned procedure.
- **Caution:** PRBCs administration: increased morbidity, mortality and risk of complications.

Laboratory Diagnosis

- Blood tests dependent on:
  - Age.
  - ASA classification (see above).
  - Operation.
  - Risk profile of the patient.
- Small blood count, electrolytes, coagulation, BG, creatinine, transaminases.
- No routine screening.

15.1.3 Additional Investigations

ECG

- Preoperative ECG not necessary in asymptomatic and anamnestically unremarkable patients.
- ECG recommended for
  - Patients with cardiac symptoms and/or
  - Abnormal cardiac history.

Chest X-Ray

- Indicated for new onset or acutely symptomatic respiratory symptoms.

Pulmonary Function Diagnosis

- Indicated for severity assessment in new-onset or acutely symptomatic pulmonary disease, lung surgery.

15.1.4 Perioperative Anticoagulation

Coronary Artery Disease and Stent Implantation

- Metal stents: dual platelet aggregation inhibition up to 3 months.
- DES (Drug Eluting Stent): Time interval up to 12 months.
- If possible, no elective operations during this period.
- Commonly used: Acetylsalicylic acid (ASA), dipyridamole, clopidogrel, prasugrel, ticagrelor.
- Perioperative discontinuation: Increased rate of cardiovascular events due to rebound phenomenon = continue ASA.
- Bleeding risk:
  - ASA only moderate bleeding risk, exceptions: NCH (neurosurgery), prostate resection…
  - Dual platelet aggregation = high risk of bleeding: discontinue 7–10 days prior to major procedures, procedures in closed body cavities, and spinal anesthesia close to the spinal cord.

Perioperative Thrombosis Prophylaxis

- Venous thromboembolism = still clinically relevant complication.
- The more morbid the patient, the higher the risk of thrombosis.
- Incidence can be reduced by 50% through prophylaxis.
- Parenteral: Unfractionated heparin (UFH), low-molecular-weight heparin (LMWH), Fondaparinux.

Caution
Heparin-induced thrombocytopenia type II (HIT II) in UFH and LMWH.

- Alternative anticoagulants:
  - Argatroban (Agarta): for HIT II.
  - Bivalirudin (Angiox): Alternative to UFH for coronary intervention.
  - Phenprocoumon.

New Oral Anticoagulants (NOACs/DOACs)

- Pradaxa (dagibatran etexilate) and Xarelto (rivaroxaban) for:
  - Knee and hip joint replacement.
  - Stroke prophylaxis in atrial fibrillation.
  - Therapy for venous thromboembolism.
- Eliquis (apixaban) approved for knee and hip replacements.

15.1.5 Medication Management

Continue

- Antianginal, antihypertensive and antiarrhythmic medication:
  - Beta-blockers: otherwise increase in mortality due to rebound phenomenon; preoperative new medication can be considered with sufficient distance to surgery and high-risk patients.
  - Calcium antagonists: Otherwise possible preoperative blood pressure increase.
  - Nitrates: risk of myocardial ischemia.
  - Antiarrhythmic drugs: risk of arrhythmias.
- Corticosteroids:
  - Continue substitution for longer than 5 days if substitution is already in place.
  - In addition, 50–200 mg hydrocortisone perioperatively over 48 h in patients with long-term medication above the Cushing's threshold, depending on the severity of the procedure.
- Statins:
  - Continue perioperatively.
  - New prescription after vascular surgery.
  - Reduce perioperative risk of infarction.
- Anticonvulsants: triggering seizures.
- Parkinson's drugs: enhancement of extrapyramidal symptoms.
- Thyroid hormones.
- Psychotropic drugs:
  - Tricyclic antidepressants.
  - Neuroleptics.
  - Selective serotonin reuptake inhibitors.
  - Third generation MAO (monoamine oxidase) inhibitors.

Caution
Perioperative drug interaction.

Convert

- Phenprocoumon: convert to heparin 3–5 days before surgery.
- MAO inhibitors: Switch to reversible and selective third generation MAO inhibitors 2 weeks prior to surgery.

Discontinue

- Diuretics
  - Otherwise risk of hypovolaemia with hypotension.
  - Immediate restart after surgery in stable patients.
- ACE (angiotensin converting enzyme) inhibitors and AT II (angiotensin II) blockers
  - Danger of perioperative hypotension in operations with high volume shifts, otherwise due not discontinue.
- Digitalis
  - Controversially discussed.
  - Long half-life, short-term discontinuation associated with little benefit.
  - Continue in patients with normofrequency absolute arrhythmia.

- OAD (oral antidiabetic drugs)
  - Risk of hypoglycaemia: Regular perioperative BG measurements.
  - Metformin: Risk of lactic acidosis, discontinue 48 h before surgery.

Endocarditis Prophylaxis

- Depends on operation and patient-related risk
  - Patients with valve replacements (mechanical and biological prostheses), patients with reconstructed valves using grafts for 6 months after surgery.
  - Patients after endocarditis.
  - Patients with congenital heart defects (cyanotic, postoperative).
  - Patients after heart transplant, with cardiac valvulopathy.
- For interventions in the gastrointestinal tract or urinary tract
  - Prophylaxis only in cases of an infection of these organs.
  - Amoxicillin: 2 g single dose 60 min before surgery.
  - In case of penicillin or ampicillin allergy: Clindamycin 600 mg.

15.1.6 Information from the Anaesthetist's Point of View

Legal Situation (Germany)

- Any medical interference with bodily integrity: criminal offence of bodily harm.
- Consent of the patient only legal after detailed explanation and documentation.
- If possible, 24 h before planned surgical intervention.

Prerequisite

- The patient has to understand and decide, voluntariness.
- Patients who have reached the age of majority and have the capacity to consent and make decisions.
- In the case of minors and persons incapable of giving consent: Parents, legal guardians.

Requirement

- Explanation of the relevant information.
- Procedure with risks typical of procedures and anaesthesia.
- Various therapy options with risk-reward consideration.
- Understanding the patient.
- 3 phases of enlightenment according to hick:
  - Comprehensive information.
  - Summary.
  - Decision of the patient.

Elements of Consent

- Decision for a course of action (alternatives).
- Placement of the treatment order.
- **Caution:** Documentation is obligatory (in writing).

Outpatient Interventions

- For minor surgery: Consent is possible directly prior to surgery (without premedication).

Living Will or Health Care Proxy

- For major procedures or anticipated intensive care stays, inquire about.

15.2 Intraoperative Phase

Key Points

- Essential intraoperative monitoring.
- Central importance of volume management, thermal homeostasis and hemodynamics.

15.2.1 Intraoperative Monitoring According to AAGBI and BDA Guidelines

- WHO checklist, team time-out before start of surgery.
- Essential Equipment:
  - Ventilation system with CO_2 –, O_2 – and ventilation pressure measurement.
  - Pulse oximetry.

  - NIBD (non-invasive blood pressure measurement).
  - ECG.
  - Relaxometry.
  - Temperature measurement.
  - Defibrillator and cardiopulmonary resuscitation equipment.
  - Infusion pumps.
- In addition, according to the severity of the intervention and the morbidity of the patient:
  - Invasive blood pressure measurement and haemodynamic monitoring.
  - Transesophageal Doppler.
  - Cerebral measurement of oxygen saturation.
  - Blood glucose meter.
  - BIS (Bispectral Index) Monitor.

15.2.2 Volume Management

- Avoid preoperative exsiccosis and malnutrition.
- Hemostasis and coagulation management.
- Surgical technique and careful haemostasis decisive.
- Implementation of an evidence-based perioperative transfusion regime.
- Measures to save foreign blood.
- Normothermia and avoidance of acidosis.
- if necessary, use of hemostatic drugs (tranexamic acid, Minirin).

15.2.3 Hemodynamics

Pathophysiology

- MAP (mean arterial pressure) <60 mmHg: decrease in cerebral and renal blood flow.
- Critical perfusion pressure of the coronaries dependent on cardiac output (CO).

Risk Factors for Hypotension

- Age.
- ASA classification.
- Duration of the operation.
- Combined regional and general anaesthesia.
- Premedication.
- Storage.
- Intraoperative hypotension associated with increased 1-year mortality.

Principles/Goals

- MAP >60 mmHg, in hypertensive patients >80 mmHg.
- Early initiation of volume and catecholamine therapy, if necessary with hemodynamic monitoring.

15.2.4 Heat Retention

- Perioperative hypothermia = risk factor for
  - Worsened outcome.
  - Wound healing disorder.
  - Extended length of stay in hospital.

15.2.5 Perioperative Antibiotic Therapy

Incidence of SSI ("Surgical Site Infection")

- Wound healing disorders in approx. 10% of all operations.
- 16% of all nosocomial infections.
- Up to 24.5% after gastrointestinal surgery.
- Lead to longer hospital stays.
- Additional costs.

Risk Factors

- Patient-Related:
  - Diabetes mellitus.
  - Obesity.
  - Clotting disorder.
  - Age.
  - Malnutrition.
  - Medication.
- Patient-independent:
  - Hygiene standards.
  - Operating time.
  - Inadequate perioperative antibiotic therapy.

Pathogen Spectrum

- According to the type and location of the intervention
  - Frequently mixed infections with enterobacteria, approx. 2/3 of all infections by: E. coli, Enterococcus spp., Bacteroides spp., Pseudomonas aeruginosa.
- Multi-resistant germs:
  - MRSA (methicillin-resistant Staphylococcus aureus).
  - MRSE (coagulase-negative staphylococci with methicillin/oxacillin resistance).
  - VRE (vancomycin-resistant enterococci).
  - ESBL (extended spectrum beta-lactamases).

Prevention

- Avoid preoperative medications: NSAIDs (non-steroidal anti-inflammatory drugs), chemotherapy, phenprocoumon.
- Optimize concomitant diseases.
- Perioperative antibiotic administration.
- Hygiene measures: Hand disinfection, area clothing, asepsis.
- Wound closure without impairment of local blood circulation.
- Drains as short as possible in situ.

Caution
No recommendation for irrigation of the abdominal cavity before wound closure.

Perioperative Antibiotic Prophylaxis (PAP)

- Requirement: bactericidal, i.v. application, tolerable
- Two goals:
  - Reduction of bacteria introduced into the surgical area.
  - Prevention of systemic germ introduction.
- Antibiotic of choice: aminopenicillins plus beta-lactam inhibitor or first or second generation cephalosporins.
- Second choice antibiotic: third or fourth generation cephalosporins in combination with metronidazole or carbapenem.
- Time of application: 1 h before to 2 h after skin incision.

Caution
Vancomycin or fluoroquinolones have a longer infusion duration (60 min).

- In case of bacteriological sample collection (e.g. blood culture), administration after sample collection.
- 1–2 doses only for 24 h after surgery, if necessary only single dose.
- For long operations second dose intraoperatively.

15.3 Postoperative Phase

Key Points

- Determination of a strategy for postoperative analgesia.
- Prevention/treatment of PONV, delirium, POCD.
- Principles of fast-track surgery.

15.3.1 Analgesia

Pathophysiology

- Prevention:
  - Delirium.
  - Chronification.
  - Cardiorespiratory problems.
  - Delayed mobilization.

Evidence-Based Analgesia

- Evidence-based analgesia positive for:
  - Earlier hospital discharge.
  - Reduce morbidity.

Pain Measurement

- Measurement of pain by:
  - VAS (visual analogue scale).
  - NRS (numerical rating scale).
  - If possible 2-hourly in the first 24 h.

Caution
Increase in pain or new onset of increased analgesic consumption: indication of complications.

Principles

- Individual adaptation to patient, comorbidity.
- Stepwise therapy according to WHO analgesic ladder.
- Administration of opioids as sparingly as possible.
- Use coanalgesics such as clonidine, spasmolytics.
- Prefer perioperative epidural anesthesia.

15.3.2 Postoperative Nausea and Vomiting (PONV)

Forecasting Systems

- For the assessment of postoperative nausea and vomiting.
- E.g. Apfel Score:
  - Female.
  - History of PONV/kinetosis.
  - Non-smoker.
  - Opiate administration.

Prophylaxis

- Regional anaesthesia, no volatile anaesthetics, avoid opiates.
  - Medications:
    - Corticosteroids (dexamethasone).
    - 5-HT_3 antagonists: administration at the end of surgery.
    - No butyrophenones or benzamines because of possible extrapyramidal motor effects.
- Adjuvants: Acupuncture/acupressure on the wrist, aromatherapy, ginger.

Therapy

- Quick action.
- 5-HT_3 antagonists as first-choice drugs.
- Dexamethasone only slow onset of action, only in combination.
- Alternative: haloperidol, dimenhydrinate, promethazine.

15.3.3 Delirium/Postoperative Cognitive Deficit (POCD)

Epidemiology

- Prevalence 15–50%, ventilated patients up to 80%.
- Longer hospital stay, increased mortality, and cognitive late effects on long-term follow-up.

Division

- Three types:
  - Hyperactive.
  - Hypoactive.
  - Mixed type.
- Three forms of postoperative cognitive deficit:
  - Emergence Delirium: at discharge.
  - Postoperative delirium.
  - Transient cognitive impairment.

Preoperative Evaluation of Risk Factors

- Age.
- Morbidity.
- Cognitive skills.
- Severity of the surgical procedure.
- Hypoxia.
- Infection.

Prevention

- Avoid preoperative food restriction and fluid deficit.
- Stress avoidance (isolation, lack of daylight, restraint).
- Communication aids (glasses, hearing aid).
- Early mobilization.
- Avoid prodelirant drugs (e.g. benzodiazepines, opiates, sedative hypnotics).

Early Screening

- CAM-ICU (Confusion Assessment Method/Intensive Care Unit), ICU:

- Acute onset or fluctuating course.
- Attention Deficit Disorder.
- Changes in awareness.
- Disorganized thinking.
- Nu-DESC (Nursing Delirium Screening Scale), PACU.

Therapy

- Most important tool: Recognition of delirium.
- Reduce risk factors.
- Strengthen reorientation.
- Drug therapy:
  - Haloperidol.
  - Atypical neuroleptics.
  - Dexmedetomidine.
- **Caution:** Haloperidol: QT time, extrapyramidal symptoms at more than 4.5 mg/day.

15.3.4 Recovery Room (PACU)

- Regular documentation of vital parameters.
- Surveillance:
  - State of alertness according to AVPU ("alert, voice, pain, unresponsive") scheme, protective reflexes present.
  - Circulatory situation: blood pressure, heart rate, ECG.
  - Airway: pulse oximetry, oxygen supply and if necessary airway protection e.g. by Wendl tube.
- Assessment of dressings and drains.
- Recognize and Treat:
  - PONV.
  - Shivering.
  - Restlessness.
  - Postoperative pain.
- Transfer if:
  - Patient awake, cooperative, preserved protective reflexes.
  - No more risk from anaesthesia and perioperative respiratory or circulatory problems.
  - Discharge criteria met.
  - Responsibility for discharge lies with anaesthetist.
  - Transfer to another ward/home.

15.3.5 Intensive Care Unit (ICU)/ Intermediate Care (IMC)

- In addition to the tasks of the PACU listed above:
  - Ward with monitoring and treatment of patients after extensive operations.
  - Monitoring and treatment of patients with high morbidity/mortality after minor surgery.
  - Circulatory the rapy.
  - Weaning.
  - Pre-operative stabilisation and preparation for surgery.
  - Organ-specific support.

15.4 Fast Track Surgery

Key Points

- Evidence-based multimodal interdisciplinary perioperative treatment concept.
- Goals = Shortening of treatment duration + Reduction of perioperative complications.

15.4.1 Definition

- Multimodal interdisciplinary perioperative treatment concept according to defined clinical treatment algorithms.
- Objectives
  - Shortening the duration of treatment.
  - Reduction of perioperative complications.

15.4.2 Preoperative Management

- Short preoperative food abstinence.
- Premedication with short-acting substances.

15.4.3 Intraoperative Management

- Atraumatic surgical technique.
- Anaesthetic guidance with short-acting substances.
- PONV prophylaxis.
- Peridural analgesia: Improves perioperative mortality and reduces tumor recurrence rate.
- Balanced volume therapy.
- **Caution:** Intestinal edema.
- Avoid hypothermia.
- Periopertiave antibiotic prophylaxis.

15.4.4 Postoperative Management

Analgesia

- Peridual anesthesia instead of systemic opiate administration.
- Analgesia according to WHO stage scheme.

Caution
Gastrointestinal bleeding is possible with NSAIDs.

Early Mobilization

Optimized Diet

- Epidemiology: mortality rate in ICU patients with gastrointestinal failure 43.7% vs. 5.3% without gastrointestinal failure.
- Pathophysiology:
  - Operation = motility disorder.
  - Motility disorder = passage disorder (bacterial density increased) + barrier function impaired.
  - Causes of motility disorder:
    - Drugs (opiates).
    - Immobilization.
    - Electrolyte derailments.
    - Shock.
    - Inflammation of the intestinal wall due to cytokine release also during surgical interventions.
    - Bowel wall edema.
    - Increased sympathetic tone with vasoconstriction in the splanchnic area.
- Fast track therapy.
  - Keep alimentation interruption as short as possible.
  - Start enteral nutrition early.
  - Laxatives (lactulose, macrogol).
  - Prokinetics (metoclopramide, erythromycin, neostigmine).
  - Opiate receptor antagonist (Relistor).

15.4.5 Guidelines

ESC/ESA (2014) Guidelines on non-cardiac surgery: cardiovascular assessment and management. Eur Heart J 35:2383–2243.

Reference

Lee TH et al (1999) Derivation and prospective validation of a simple index for prediction of cardiac risk of major noncardiac surgery. Circulation 100:1043–1049

Emergency Surgery

Benjamin Weixler, Raoul A. Droeser, Robert Mechera, Christian A. Nebiker, Debora Nowakowski, Heidi Misteli, and Henry Hoffmann

Contents

F. Billmann, T. Keck (eds.), *Essentials of Visceral Surgery*,
https://doi.org/10.1007/978-3-662-66735-4_16

16.1 Polytrauma: Abdominal Trauma

B. Weixler and R. A. Droeser

Key Points

- Abdominal trauma (in Europe): ≥80% blunt, ≤20% penetrating; mainly due to traffic and occupational accidents.
- Stabilization according to ATLS (Advanced Trauma Life Support) criteria: Airways, **Breathing**, Circulation, Disability, Exposure (ABCDE).
- FAST (Focused Assessment with Sonography in Trauma) examination: for all patients.
- Contrast-enhanced computed tomography (CT): only for patients hemodynamically stable.
- Circulatory unstable patients with positive FAST: immediate laparotomy.
- Circulatory stable patients without evidence of hollow organ perforation: non-operative approach.

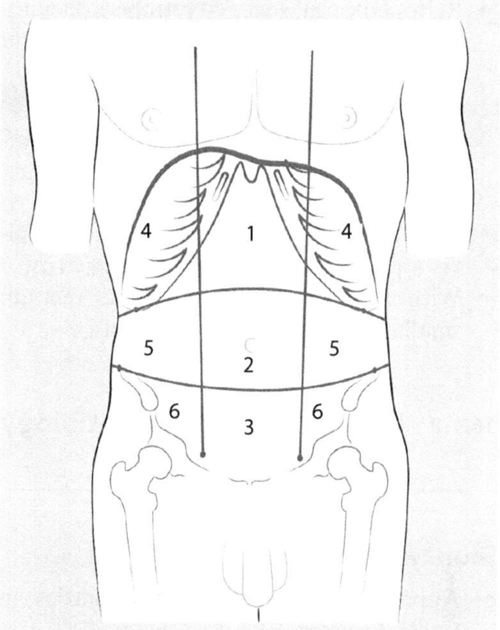

Fig. 16.1 Regional division of the abdominal wall

16.1.1 Anatomy of the Abdomen

External Divisions

Anterior Abdominal Wall

- From costal margin to symphysis.
- On both sides from midline to anterior axillary line.

Lateral Abdominal Wall (= Flank)

- Between anterior and posterior axillary line.
- 6. intercostal space to iliac crest.

Abdominal wall = anterior +2 lateral abdominal walls.

Quadrant/Sector Breakdown

- Regional structure of the abdominal wall (Fig. 16.1).
- Sector breakdown:
  - Epigastric region.
  - Umbilical region.
  - Pubic region.
  - Left and right hypochondrium.
  - Left and right lateral abdominal region (= Regio hypogastrica = Flank).
  - Left and right inguinal region (= groin).

Internal Divisions

Abdominal Cavity

- Definition: Abdominal cavity = peritoneal cavity + preperitoneal and retroperitoneal cavity.
  - Peritoneal cavity.
  - With liver, pancreas, spleen, small and large intestine, uterus (in pregnant women), filled urinary bladder.
  - Intracostal abdomen: special subdivision of the abdominal cavity, in the rib cage, with diaphragm, liver, pancreas, spleen.

- Retroperitoneal space (= retroperitoneum).
  - With kidneys, ureters, pancreas, aorta and v. cava.
  - Continuity with preperitoneal space and infraperitoneal space.

Pelvis

- Definition: pelvic cavity = true pelvis = peritoneal + infraperitoneal cavity.
- With urinary bladder, urethra, rectum, small intestine, ovaries and uterus.

16.1.2 Injury Mechanisms (Aetiology and Pathophysiology)

Blunt Abdominal Trauma

- Approx. 80% of abdominal injuries in Central Europe.
- Mainly: traffic and work accidents.

Deceleration Trauma

- Shear forces with traction on organs and vascular trunks.
- Injuries: Spleen (40%), liver (35%), small intestine (10%).

Crush Injury

- Between abdominal wall and spine and posterior thoracic wall.
- Especially vulnerable = solid organs (liver, spleen, kidneys).

Compression Injury

16

- Due to impacts, external compression (e.g. seat belt).
- Abrupt increase in intra-abdominal pressure: rupture of a hollow organ.

Penetrating Abdominal Trauma

- Often criminal/suicidal intent.
- Mostly single cavity, rarely double cavity injuries.

Stab Wound

- Prognostically most favourable form of injury.

Gunshot Wound

- Different injury patterns.
- Impact/Prognosis dependent on:
  - Velocity of projectile.
  - Type of projectile.
  - Firing distance.

Impalement Injury (Due to Accidents)

- Degree of injury depending on shape and penetration depth.
- Combination injuries (impalement + blunt trauma) possible.

16.1.3 Management and Diagnosis

Primary Management

Treatment According to ABCDE Rules (ATLS): Simultaneous Identification + Stabilization of Life-Threatening Injuries

- Airway/cervical spine protections ("**A**irway, with cervical spine protections").
- Ventilation, ensure gas exchange ("**B**reathing").
- Hemodynamic stabilization ("**C**irculation").
- Neurological status ("**D**isability").
- Exposure, complete undressing ("**E**xposure").

Anamnesis

- Rapid investigation of accident mechanism and timing.
- Allergies, medications, etc.

Clinical Presentation

- Inspection (ecchymosis, "seat belt sign", eviscerations, foreign bodies).
- Palpation, percussion, auscultation.
- Rectal examination (prostate protrusion for urethral lesion, evidence for bleeding, sphincter tone for neurological status).

Caution
- Intra-abdominal blood loss and/or small bowel rupture may remain asymptomatic for a prolonged period; development of peritonism takes several hours!
- Overlooking blunt abdominal trauma in unconscious patients.

Laboratory Tests
- Haemoglobin + haematocrit, electrolytes, creatinine and urea levels, blood coagulation, blood gas analysis, glucose, serum amylase, alcohol level, urinalysis, drug screening in urine and pregnancy test if necessary.
- Blood grouping + irregular antibody search; in case of circulatory instability, crossmatch red cell concentrates.

Diagnostic Imaging

X-ray
- Conventional images = low significance in abdominal trauma.

Ultrasound Examination
- FAST examination (Focused Assessment with Sonography for Trauma).
- Detection of free fluid and possible organ rupture (liver, spleen, kidney).
- Poor sensitivity compared to CT (82%).

Computer Tomography
- Whole-body spiral CT "Trauma spiral CT" in polytrauma; abdominal and pelvis CT scan in isolated abdominal trauma.
- No oral contrast agent necessary.
- Sensitivity for intra-abdominal injuries 98%, specificity 99%.

Caution
- Repeated clinical examination of the abdomen in addition to ultrasound + CT in the presence of a significant trauma mechanism.
- CT only if patient is hemodynamically stable.
- Diaphragmatic ruptures, intestinal perforations and pancreatic injuries often not visible at the beginning; in case of suspicion: repeat CT after 36–48 h.

16.1.4 Therapeutic Procedure

Conservative Therapy

Key Points
- Conservative therapy only in stable patients without relevant coagulation disorder.
- Conservative therapy never in case of hollow organ injury!

Blunt Abdominal Trauma
- Continuous (intensive medical) monitoring; also possible in the case of major injuries to parenchymatous organs.
- For liver and spleen injuries:
  - Regular clinical, laboratory and ultrasound control.
  - Conservative approach successful in over 80% of cases.
- Selective arteriography: for liver/spleen/vascular injury.
- Rarely also other interventional measures (drainage, stent placement, etc.)

Penetrating Abdominal Trauma
- Exploration of the wound:
  - Deep fascia intact: Conservative management possible.
  - Deep fascia injured: Diagnostic laparoscopy with evidence/exclusion of penetration of the parietal peritoneum, laparoscopic bowel revision if necessary (only reliable with sufficient overview).

Surgical Therapy

Circulatory Instability
- Patients with positive FAST: emergency laparotomy.
- If FAST not conclusive: If possible, stabilize patient so that CT can be performed…

Circulatory Stability

- Negative FAST and/or CT: Think of other sources of bleeding/shocks.

Major Visceral Trauma/Complex Surgery

- High mortality: due to intraoperative metabolic disturbances.
- Avoid lethal triad at all costs:
  - Coagulopathy.
  - Hypothermia.
  - Metabolic acidosis.
- Strategy:
  - Damage-control laparotomy: find source of bleeding quickly + stop bleeding; stop leakage of bowel contents, close bowel with GIA (blind closure), remove perforated sections.
  - Stabilization in the intensive care unit with the goal of euvolemia + coagulation recovery + warming up of the patient.
  - Planned second-look relaparotomy after 24–48 h for definitive treatment of the abdominal injuries, stoma creation if necessary.

Surgical Procedure

Damage Control Concept (Damage Control Laparotomy)

- Access always via median laparotomy.
- Abdominal packing: Packs inserted in all 4 quadrants, systematic exploration of all 4 quadrants.
- Emergency subdiaphragmatic clamping of the aorta, if necessary.
- Identification of the source of bleeding.
- In case of bleeding from liver parenchyma: possibly Pringle manoeuvre (temporary clamping of the hepatoduodenal ligament), debridement of avital parts of the parenchyma, possibly perihepatic packing (especially in case of coagulation disorder).
- For bleeding from the spleen: splenectomy.
- Bleeding from aorta and iliac vessels: sutures for small lesions, intra-arterial shunt for larger injuries.
- Injury to the vena cava: direct suturing, packing retrohepatic vena cava.
- After hemostasis: look for hollow organ perforations: Direct suture for small perforations; resect larger ones using linear stapler; no anastomosis, no enterostomy! Stomas are only created on the occasion of the second-look laparotomy.
- Leave the abdomen open (= avoid compartment syndrome; ► Sect. 16.3).
- Possibly postoperative angiography for interventional embolisation.

16

16.1.5 Guidelines

Como JJ, Bokhari F, Chiu WC, Duane TM, Holevar MR, Tandoh MA, Ivatury RR, Scalea TM (2010) Practice management guidelines for selective nonoperative management of penetrating abdominal trauma. J Trauma 68:721–733.

AWMF Guideline Polytrauma/Serious Injury Treatment, Register Number 012–019; ► https://www.awmf.org/leitlinien/detail/ll/012-019.html.

► https://www.wses.org.uk/guidelines.

Benz D, Balogh ZJ (2017) Damage control surgery: current state and future directions. Curr Opin Crit Care 23(6):491–497. ► https://doi.org/10.1097/MCC.0000000000000465.

16.2 Ileus/Obstruction

R. Mechera and C. A. Nebiker

16.2.1 Definition—Classification

Definition

- Intestinal ileus = intestinal obstruction = (small/large) bowel obstruction.
- Interruption of the flow of gastrointestinal contents from oral to aboral direction.
- Distinction:
  - Functional ileus = paralysis.
  - Mechanical ileus = mechanical obstruction.

Classification

- By course: Acute vs. subacute vs. chronic.
- By completeness: Complete vs. incomplete.
- According to localization: high vs. deep small bowel ileus vs. large bowel ileus.

16.2.2 Epidemiology

- Common clinical picture.
- Approx. 300,000 laparotomies in USA/year due to small bowel obstruction = approx. 850,000 hospitalization days = 1.3 billion USD per year.

16.2.3 Pathophysiology

"Circulus Vitiosus" of Ileus

- Numerous feedbacks.
- Based on intestinal distention.

Intestinal Distention

- Increase in wall tension → consecutive microcirculatory disturbance: intestinal wall edema + hypoxia of the intestinal wall.
- Consequences of bowel wall edema and bowel wall hypoxia:
  - Transmigratory peritonitis: hypoxia → impaired mucosal barrier and additional stasis → bacterial overgrowth + transmigration.
  - Increase in fluid sequestration into the intestinal lumen, intestinal wall and abdominal cavity.
  - Activation of biogenic amines, kinins and release of interleukins → formation of prostaglandin E with protein degradation, leukocyte increase and fever.
  - Ileus disease = hypovolemic, septic-toxic shock up to multi-organ failure (as final stage).

Normal postoperative normalization of intestinal transit

- Small intestine: 5–24 h.
- Stomach: 1–2 days.
- Colon: 2–3 days (from oral to aboral).

16.2.4 Diagnosis

Key Points

- Previous surgery as a clue of possible adhesions.
- Clinical presentation: palpation + auscultation.
- Abdominal CT scan: increasingly imaging of choice.
- Electrolyte and fluid balance: In the time interval between diagnosis and surgery.

Medical History and Symptoms

- Previous surgery as a clue of possible adhesions (bands).
- Previous changes in bowel habit (more often than complete ileus/obstruction) as the first symptom.
- Pencil thin stool.
- Weight loss.
- Family history.
- Fever.
- Night sweats.
- Loss of appetite, nausea, vomiting.
- Stool and wind retention.
- Acute onset pain: spasmodic/nonspecific.
- Increase in abdominal girth (meteorism).

Clinical Examination: Status Survey

- Fluid status and vital signs.
- Inspection: Surgical scars, hernias.
- Palpation:
  - Abdominal point tenderness.
  - Blumberg's sign/rebound tenderness.
  - Abdominal guarding ("défense musculaire").
  - Resistances.
- Percussion: Meteorism
- Auscultation:
  - Hyperperistalsis in mechanical ileus (high-pitched, metallic bowel sounds).
  - Intestinal sounds sparse or absent (so-called dead silence) in paralytic ileus.
- Digital rectal examination obligatory:
  - Stenoses.
  - Rectal Tumor.
  - Impacted stool.
  - Blood on the glove, if any.

Lab

- Signs of dehydration (hematocrit, creatinine, urea, electrolytes, acid-base balance)
- Infection parameters (CRP, leucocytes).
- Lactate and LDH: sign of vascular ileus (**caution:** normal in 40%).
- Additional parameters to exclude other causes and differential diagnoses: amylase, lipase.

Quantity/Quality of Gastrointestinal Contents Discharged

- Quantity/quality of gastrointestinal contents drained (gastric tube).

Imaging

Ultrasound

- Dilated fluid-filled intestinal loops.
- Intestinal peristalsis.
- Stenoses/strictures.
- Incarcerated hernias.
- Small bowel intussusception.
- intestinal wall thickening.
- Extraluminal free fluid with ineffective peristalsis (in severe ileus) ("to-and-fro" or "whirling" appearance of intra-luminal contents).
- Detection of obstruction: sensitivity 83%, specificity 100%, localization: 70%, etiology: 23%.

Conventional Abdominal Radiograph

- Supine and standing or left lateral position (abdominal overview).
- Obstruction sign:
  - Gas-fluid levels if the study is erect: interface between air/liquid in the intestine.
  - Free air, aerobilia (in 50% with gallstone ileus), shadowing concretions, foreign body.
  - Obstruction localization: eventually possible using gas-fluid level arrangement.
  - Hyperinflation/distention of the caecum in colonic ileus.
- Detection of obstruction: sensitivity 77%, specificity 50%, localization 60%, etiology: 7%.

16

Contrast-Enhanced (Gastrographin) Conventional X-Ray

- 100 mL gastrographin p.o./gastric tube, abdominal X-ray after 4–6 h.
- Statement possible about the level and extent of ileus.
- ileus resolved if contrast medium in colon in 24 h (sensitivity 97%, specificity 96%).
- Important in "high" proximal small bowel ileus, as no gas-fluid level formation in the normal abdominal radiograph.
- In addition, therapeutic laxative effect.

Caution

Contrast agent can convert a subileus into a complete ileus.

Computer Tomography (CT scan)

- Increasingly imaging modality of choice.
- Pathognomonic ileus signs = local wall thickening due to wall edema and caliber jump (dilated small bowel loops >2.5 cm up from outer wall to outer wall proximal to obstruction and normal caliber or collapsed loops distally) ± evidence of free abdominal fluid.
- Detection of obstruction: Sensitivity 93%, Specificity 100%, Localization: 93%, Etiology: 87%.

16.2.5 Mechanical Ileus (Mechanical Obstruction)

- Important measure: Balancing the electrolyte and fluid balance: In the time interval between diagnosis and surgery.

Etiology and Pathogenesis

Etiology (Table 16.1)

Pathogenesis

- Classification according to the type of obstruction:
  - Luminal obstruction (from inside).
  - Compression (from outside).
  - Strangulation (single band, adhesion, volvulus, abdominal wall hernias).

Table 16.1 Causes of mechanical obstruction

Mechanical small bowel obstruction	
External cause	Adhesions, Single band Internal and external hernias Tumors (pancreas, bile duct, etc.) Volvulus Intraabdominal abscess Intraabdominal hematoma Pancreatic pseudocyst Superior mesenteric artery compression syndrome Intra-abdominal drains Peritoneal carcinomatosis
Intraluminal causes	Neoplasms Gallstones Foreign bodies Bezoar
Intramural causes	Neoplasms Strictures (Crohn's disease, etc.) Hematomas Intussusception Actinic enteritis Regional enteritis
Mechanical large bowel (colon) obstruction	
Common causes	Malignancies Volvulus Diverticulitis Pseudo-obstruction (Ogilvie syndrome) Hernia Anastomotic stricture
Rare causes	Intussusception Stool impaction Strictures Foreign bodies External pressure

- Classification according to localization:
  - Small bowel obstruction (80% of all intestinal peristalsis disorders; high vs. low); bands, malignancies, hernias, adhesions (= 90% of the etiologies).
  - Large bowel (colonic) obstruction (10–15% of all intestinal peristalsis disorders): Stenosing cancer, diverticulitis, volvulus, etc.

Specific Symptoms

High Small Bowel Ileus

- Colicky pain.
- Severe biliary or clear vomiting.
- But: meteorism may be absent.

Low Small Bowel Ileus

- Colicky pain.
- Meteorism.
- Fecal vomiting (Miserere).

Large Bowel Obstruction

- Meteorism.
- Less pain.

Complications

- Ischemia.
  - In case of strangulation with vascular involvement.
  - Especially in the case of mobile small intestine (e.g. in the context of a single band obstruction, in the case of incarcerated hernia, etc.).
- Paralysis

16.2.6 Paralytic Ileus/Functional Obstruction

Etiology and Pathogenesis

Etiology (Table 16.2)

Pathogenesis

- Impairment of the muscular function of the intestinal wall (motility disorder).
- Reaction to various organ diseases, consequences of inflammation, injuries, circulatory or metabolic disorders.
- Reflective:
  - After major abdominal surgery.
  - For intra-abdominal pathology.
  - Response to acute extra-abdominal diseases.
- Special form: Intestinal pseudoobstruction (Ogilvie syndrome) = peristalsis disorder of the colon due to various causes with distension of the caecum.

Table 16.2 Causes of paralytic ileus

Primary forms		
	Myopathic chronic familial pseudoobstruction	
	Neuropathic chronic pseudoobstruction	
Secondary forms		
Intra-abdominal pathologies	Inflammatory	Peritonitis, abscess, colitis
	Mechanical	Operation, Foreign Body
	Chemical	Gastric juice (perforated gastric ulcer), bile, blood
	Autoimmune	Serositis, vasculitis
	Intestinal ischemia	Arterial, venous
Retroperitoneal pathologies		Pancreatitis Haematoma Trauma, e.g. vertebral body fracture Urolithiasis Pyelonephritis, etc.
Extraabdominal disease	Thoracic pathologies	Myocardial infarction Pneumonia Decompensated heart failure Rib fractures
	Metabolic changes	Electrolyte imbalance, e.g. hypokalemia Porphyria Hypothyroidism Hypoparathyroidism Uremia Lead poisoning
	Drugs	Opiates Anticholinergics Antihistamines Catecholamines Antidepressants
	Sepsis	
	Chemotherapy or radiotherapy	
	Trauma	Craniocerebral trauma Thoracic trauma Spinal cord injuries

Specific Symptoms

- Symptoms of the underlying pathology → Symptoms of obstruction → Symptoms of "ileus disease."

16.2.7 Therapy

Key Points

- Always general measures ± antibiotic therapy.
- Absolute indication for surgery:
  - Complete mechanical ileus.
  - High small bowel ileus.
  - Peritonitis with/without paralysis.
  - Strangulation Ileus.
  - Vascular ileus.
  - Gallstone ileus.

Conservative Therapy

General Measures

- Parenteral nutrition therapy (caloric intake).
- Monitoring and compensation of the fluid/electrolyte loss.
- Gastric tube (relief of gastrointestinal tract distension, electrolyte balance, reduction of aspiration risk).
- Regular clinical examination by experienced surgeon.

Antibiotic Therapy

- In the case of bacterial translocation.

Drug Stimulation in Paralytic Ileus

- Sympathicolysis (e.g. peridural catheter).
- Parasympatheticomimetic agents (e.g. neostigmine).
- Prokinetics (e.g. metoclopramide, cisapride).
- Erythromycin: stimulation of gastric peristalsis.
- Hyperosmolar substances.
- If Emergency surgery unlikely; hyperosmolar gastrographin:
  - Reduces bowel wall edema.
  - Promotes peristalsis.

Surgical Therapy

Goals

- Intestinal Decompression.
- Restoration of gastrointestinal patency and blood circulation.

Emergency Indications

- Complete mechanical ileus.
- High small intestine ileus.
- Peritonitis with/without paralysis.
- Strangulation ileus.
- Vascular ileus.
- Gallstone ileus.

Relative Indications

- Chronic recurrent ileus (abdominal adhesions).
- Subileus due to chronic inflammatory bowel disease.
- Peritoneal carcinomatosis.
- Ogilvie's syndrome.

Surgical Procedure

Surgery for Ileus

- Perioperative antibiotic therapy.
- Median laparotomy (extended, if necessary); eventually laparoscopy if single band expected.
- Access to the peritoneal cavity.
- Adhesiolysis: to localize obstruction + to treat obstruction.
- Possibly bowel segment resection (injury, stenosis, tumor, ischemia).
- **Careful** bowel decompression (**caution:** serosal lesions, endotoxin washout, postoperative atony).
- Assessment of blood flow/vitality of the intestine.
- Schedule second-look laparotomy if needed.

16.2.8 Specific Therapy for Certain Types of Ileus

Paralytic Ileus

Conservative Therapy

- Basic therapy as outlined (▶ Sect. 16.2.7 “Conservative therapy”).
- Drug stimulation.
- Elimination of triggering factors.

Surgical/Endoscopic Therapy

- Only in case of severe intestinal distension with consecutive risk of wall ischemia and rupture (especially in the cecal region).
- Endoscopic decompression, decompression tube.
- Surgical creation of a fistula/stoma.

Vascular Ileus

- Revascularization.
  - Embolectomy.
  - Thrombectomy.
  - Aortomesenteric bypass.
- Resection of avital bowel segments.

Strangulation Ileus

- Mechanical ileus with impaired blood circulation.
- Adhesiolysis, single band resection (possibly laparoscopic), hernia repair.
- Resection of avital bowel segments.

Postoperative Ileus

- Wait and see.
- Supportive therapy.

Caution: make the difference between postoperative ileus and ileus due to surgical complications:

- E.g. anastomotic insufficiency, intra-abdominal abscess.
- In case of surgical complications: Revisional surgery/intervention = necessary.

Ogilvie’s Syndrome

- Indication for surgery: In case of hyperinflation of the caecum >10 cm
- Interventions:
  - Ileostomy creation.
  - Colon resection.
  - Possibly endoscopic decompression.

Large Bowel Obstruction Due to Colon Cancer

- Procedure dependent on:
  - Localization of the cancer.
  - General condition of the patient.
  - Local intraoperative findings.

Conservative Therapy

- Palliative.
- Colonoscopic stent insertion.

Bridge-to-Surgery

- Goal = staged surgery (tumor operation in a second step).
- Indications:
  - Compensated ileus (= no distension of the small intestine).
  - Obstruction in the left hemicolon/rectum + mild symptoms.
- Methods:
  - Colonoscopic stent insertion.
  - Creation of ileostomy or colostomy.
  - Colonoscopic decompression tube.

Primary Resection

- Indication = Decompensated ileus.
- On the Right side (caecum to mid-transverse): Single-stage resection with simple or extended hemicolectomy and aspiration of the contents of the small intestine.
- On the Left side:
  - Resection with primary anastomosis, possibly insertion of a defunctioning ileostoma.
  - Discontinuity resection (Hartmann’s procedure).

Gallstone Ileus

- Removal of stone via enterotomy, cholecystectomy.
- Resection of the cholecystoduodenal fistula controversial (high morbidity).

Volvulus

- Attempt at colonoscopic derotation/decompression.
- If necessary staged surgical colopexy.

16.3 Abdominal Compartment Syndrome

D. Nowakowski and H. Misteli

16.3.1 Definitions

Key Points

- Abdominal compartment syndrome (ACS) = multiorgandysfunction.
- Intra-abdominal hypertension = origin of dysfunction.
- Mostly in critically ill patients.
- Wide range of medical and surgical clinical pictures.

Intra-Abdominal Pressure (IAP)

- Abdomen = polycompartment model.
  - Bounded by rigid, bony (ribs, pelvis, spine) and flexible (abdominal wall, diaphragm) structures.
  - Closed space with physiological pressure = intra-abdominal pressure (IAP).
- IAP:
  - Normally in a “steady state”.
  - Changes depending on wall characteristics (external influencing factors)/filling state of the abdominal cavity (internal influencing factors).
- Measurement (gold standard):
  - Indirect measurement: bladder pressure (in mmHg) (▶ Sect. 16.3.4 Bladder pressure measurement).
  - Normal levels: 5–7 mmHg in a healthy person, up to 10 mmHg in an intensive care patient.

IAP:

- Good correlation between bladder pressure and IAP.
- Aterated level in: Adhesions, pelvic hematoma or fracture, pelvic girth, neurogenic bladder.

Abdominal Perfusion Pressure (APP)

- Calculation: APP = mean arterial pressure (MAP) minus IAP (APP = MAP – IAP).
- Provides conclusions about perfusion of the abdominal organs.
- APP >60 mmHg: correlation with better survival in ACS.

Intra-Abdominal Hypertension (IAH)

- IAP continuous or over a prolonged period ≥12 mmHg.
- Classification:
  - Grade I: IAP = 12–15 mmHg.
  - Grade II: IAP = 16–20 mmHg.
  - Grade III: IAP = 21–25 mmHg.
  - Grade IV: IAP > 25 mmHg.

Abdominal Compartment Syndrome (ACS)

- Prolonged elevation of IAP >20 mmHg + new onset of organ dysfunction/failure.
- Distinction: Acute vs. chronic ACS.
- Destructive course of the disease comparable to ACS of the extremities.

16.3.2 Aetiology

Classification of Abdominal Compartment Syndrome (ACS, ◘ Table 16.3)

- Primary ACS: Due to intra-abdominal injury/disease (abdominal trauma, hematoperitoneum, pancreatitis).
- Secondary ACS: Without initial abdominal focus (hemorrhagic shock, infusion therapy, mesenteric ischemia, and reperfusion).

Pathophysiology

- IAH = Restriction of organ function → ACS.
- At the cellular level: swelling, hypoxia, dysfunction.
- Cardiovascular IAH = diaphragmatic elevation induced:
  - Decreased cardiac output.

Table 16.3 Classification and causes of abdominal compartment syndrome (ACS)

Division	Etiology
Primary ACS (= acute)	Penetrating abdominal trauma Intraperitoneal bleeding Pancreatitis External compression: e.g. after polytrauma, traffic accident, explosion Pelvic fracture Ruptured abdominal aortic aneurysm Perforated gastric ulcer
Secondary ACS (no acute event, subacute fluid accumulation with IAH)	Large volume administration during resuscitation (>3 L) Large-scale combustion (especially third degree combustion) Penetrating/blunt abdominal trauma without visible injury Postoperative After packing and fascial closure Sepsis
Chronic ACS	Peritoneal dialysis Morbid obesity/ extreme adiposity Cirrhosis Meigs' syndrome Intraabdominal mass

IAH intra-abdominal hypertension

16

  - V. cava compression (reduced backflow, blood pooling to the pelvis and lower extremities).
  - Decreased compliance and contractility due to direct compression.
- Pulmonary IAH = decreased thoracic volume induced:
  - Atelectasis + oedema (reduced oxygen diffusion).
  - Increased ventilation pressures needed (parenchymal lesion).
  - Ventilation-perfusion mismatch (increased intrapulmonary shunt fraction, increased alveolar dead space volume).
- Renal IAH = venous compression induced:
  - Decreased venous outflow.
  - Arterial vasoconstriction (activation of the renin-angiotensin-aldosterone system).
  - Decrease in glomerular perfusion and diuresis.
- Gastrointestinal IAH = decreased mesenteric blood flow induced:
  - Decreased mucosal perfusion.
  - Compression of the mesenteric veins.
  - Wall Edema.
  - "Circulus vitiosus" with end result of intestinal ischemia, lactic acidosis and possible bacterial translocation, sepsis, multiple organ failure.
- Liver IAH = decreased portal return induced by compression:
  - Decreased degradation of lactate.
- Cerebrovascular IAH = increased intracranial pressure:
  - Critical cerebral perfusion → cerebral ischemia.

IAH:
- Increased risk of thrombosis due to blood pooling in the lower extremities.
- Visceral "Circulus vitiosus": End result = intestinal ischemia.

16.3.3 Clinical presentation

Key Points

- Key role: compliance of the abdominal wall + intra-abdominal volume.
- Mostly lack of communication with severely ill patients.

Risk Factors

- Key role: compliance of the abdominal wall + intra-abdominal volume.
- "Deadly triad": acidosis + hypothermia + coagulopathy.
- Massive fluid substitution with crystalloids (hemorrhage, sepsis, burns).

- Anthropomorphology:
  - Male (intra-abdominal fat distribution).
  - Higher age.
  - Obesity.
  - Small size.
- Comorbidities and/or increased intrabdominal volume:
  - Ascites.
  - Fluid-filled intestinal loops (ileus, mesenteric ischemia).
  - Hepato-/splenomegaly.
  - Pancreatitis.
- Increased tension of the abdominal wall/diaphragm.
  - Fascia closure after damage-control laparotomy.
  - Active muscle contraction (pain).
  - "Body Builder".
  - Anasarca.
  - Abdominal wall hematoma (especially rectus sheath hematoma).
  - COPD (chronic obstructive pulmonary disease), mechanical ventilation (PEEP, "positive end-expiratory pressure"), pneumonia.
  - Burns.

Symptoms

- Distended abdomen.
- Oliguria to anuria.
- Hypercapnia and hypoxia (increase in ventilation pressure).
- Circulatory insufficiency.
- Decreased organ perfusion to lactic acidosis.
- Decreased cerebral and limb perfusion.
- Hypotension, tachycardia, increased jugular venous pressure, peripheral oedema, diffuse abdominal pain.

If ACS is imminent = usually lack of communication in a seriously ill patient.

16.3.4 Diagnosis

Key Points

- Bladder pressure = gold standard.
- Mortality in abdominal compartment syndrome = 40–100%.

Bladder Pressure Measurement (Gold Standard)

- Measurement in mmHg, at the end of expiration, in supine position.
- Reference point = mean axillary line.
- Instillation of 25 ml saline solution into an empty bladder.
- Regular measurement in intensive care patients with risk factors for ACS (4 to 6 h).

Clinical Presentation

- Poor predictor (▶ Sect. 16.3.3).

Imaging

- Not helpful for diagnosis; mostly CT.
- Signs on imaging: Visible IAH.
  - Diaphragmatic Protrusion.
  - Vein compression (especially inferior vena cava).
  - Abdominal distension.
  - Renal compression.
  - Bilateral inguinal hernias.

Caution

- Clinical diagnosis (detection) should be made before the formation of ACS at the stage of IAH.
- Mortality of ACS = 40–100%.

16.3.5 Therapy

Key Points

- Supportive measures + surgical pressure relief.
- Temporary → definitive abdominal closure.

General Principles of Therapy

WSACS Guidelines

- WSACS = "World Society of the Abdominal Compartment Syndrome": Recommendation of a Therapy Algorithm, Update 2013 (▶ Sect. 16.3.6).

Supportive Measures

- To lower the IAP ± surgical abdominal decompression.

Goals

- Improvement of abdominal wall compliance.
- Reduction of intra-abdominal volume.

Conservative Measures

Improvement of Abdominal Wall Compliance

- Analgesia.
- Sedation.
- Relaxation + anxiolytic therapy, respiratory support.
- Neuromuscular blockade.

Decrease in Intra-Abdominal Volume

- Balanced fluid management, fluid restriction if possible.
- Gastric/colonic compression:
  - Gastric tube/rectal tube (intestinal tube).
  - Enemas.
  - Prokinetics (metoclopramide, erythromycin, neostigmine).
  - Endoscopy: decompression of hollow organs.
- Drains:
  - Percutaneous drainage for obvious intraperitoneal fluid accumulation (ascites, hematoperitoneum).
  - Interventional drainage of an intra/retroperitoneal collection (abscess, pseudocyst).

Surgical Measures

- Surgical decompression = definitive therapy.
- Relevant complications of surgical therapy.
- Mortality up to 50% (depending on the etiology of ACS).

Decompressive Laparotomy

- Standard procedure.
- Median laparotomy (opening the linea alba + abdomen).

New Alternatives

- Minimally invasive percutaneous endoscopic component separation technique.
- Subcutaneous linea alba fasciotomy (SLAF).

Temporary Abdominal Closure

- Initially: leaving open (the fascia) of the abdomen.
- Abdominal wound dressing with bridging of the fascial ends (= prevention of evisceration/heat loss).
  - Vicryl mesh.
  - "Bogota bag" (sterile plastic bag).
  - "Packing" with wet cloths.
  - Vacuum dressing (= gold standard).

Caution

- Operative measures for all strategies: risk = small bowel fistula.

Definitive Abdominal Closure

- Recommendations:
  - Early.
  - If possible in the same hospitalization (usually within 5–7 days).
- For long-term open abdomen:
  - Often "loss of domain" of the abdominal organs (= covering with granulation tissue).

16

- Needed closure with "mesh graft": transplantation or cutaneous displacement flap.
- Subsequent fascial closure: only aim for after 9–12 months after.

16.3.6 Guidelines

Kirkpatric AW, Roberts DJ, De Waele J, Jaeschke R, Malbrain ML, De Keulenaer B, Duschesne J, Bjorck M, Leppaniemi A, Ejike JC, Sugrue M, Cheatham M, Ivatury R, Ball CG, Reintam Blaser A, Regli A, Balogh ZJ, D'Amours S, Debergh D, Kaplan M, Kimball E, Olvera C; Peditric Guidelines Sub-Committee for the World Society of the Abdominal Compartment Syndrome (2013) Intra-abdominal hypertension and the abdominal compartment syndrome: Updated consensus definitions and clinical practice guidelines from the World Society of the Abdominal Compartment Syndrome. Intensive Care Med 39:1190–1206.

Sosa G, Gandham N, Landeras V, Pauline Calimag A, Lerma E (2019) Abdominal compartment syndrome. Dis Mon 65(1):5–19.

Rogers WK, Garcia L (2018) Intraabdominal hypertension, abdominal compartment syndrome, and the open abdomen. Chest 153(1):238–250. ► https://doi.org/10.1016/j.chest.2017.07.023

Leppäniemi A, Hienonen P, Mentula P, Kemppainen E (2011) Subcutaneous linea alba fasciotomy, does it really work? Am Surg 77(1):99–102.

16.4 Intestinal Ischemia

B. Weixler and H. Hoffmann

16.4.1 General

- Intestinal ischemia = mesenteric ischemia.
- Classification of intestinal ischemia:
  - Due to the speed of formation/evolution.
  - Due to the severity of intestinal circulatory disorders.
- Two types of intestinal ischemia:
  - Acute intestinal ischemia (= acute mesenteric ischemia).
  - Chronic intestinal ischemia (= chronic mesenteric ischemia).

16.4.2 Acute Intestinal Ischaemia

Key Points

- Causes of acute mesenteric ischemia (AMI): embolus (50%), arterial thrombosis (25%), nonocclusive (20%), venous thrombosis (5%).
- Causes of ischemic colitis: Nonocclusive (95%).
- Clinical presentation: extent of subjective abdominal pain often in contrast to indolent abdominal examination.
- Three-phase clinical course: Acute pain interval (0–6 h); pain-free interval with intestinal paralysis, so-called "rotten peace" (7–12 h); renewed pain interval with peritonitis and septic shock with intestinal necrosis (12–24 h).
- Diagnosis: abdominal CT angiography with contrast medium.
- **Caution:** Normal lactate does not exclude intestinal ischemia!
- Therapy: Rapid start with broad-spectrum antibiotics; always surgical embolectomy and/or arterial thrombectomy, resection of avital intestinal segments if necessary.

Epidemiology

- Prevalence: approx. 1% of all patients with acute abdomen.
- In >70-year-olds: Prevalence = 10%.
- 60–70% of all intestinal ischemias = acute mesenterial ischemia (AMI).

Etiology and Pathogenesis

- Mesenteric artery embolism (50%):
- Cardiac embolus (most common).
- Ruptured plaque of the proximal aorta.
- Mesenteric artery thrombosis (25%):
  - Atherosclerosis (most common cause).
  - Arteritis.
  - Dehydration.
- Nonocclusive Mesenterial Ischemia (NOMI; 20%): Hypoperfusion and/or vasoconstriction in the splanchnic area (in heart failure, sepsis, cardiac or abdominal surgery, use of vasopressors, ergotamines, cocaine).
- Mesenteric vein thrombosis (5%):
  - Genetic hypercoagulability (>75%).
  - Paraneoplastic.
  - Cirrhosis of the liver.
  - Pancreatitis.
  - Pregnancy.

Ischemic colitis = most common form of intestinal ischemia: 95% of ischemic colitis due to NOMI in the area of the vascular anastomoses of the colonic arteries (left flexure and rectosigmoidal junction).

Clinical Presentation

Non-Specific Clinical Presentation

- Sudden onset of periumbilical abdominal pain.
  - Often in discrepancy with the inconspicuous abdominal examination.
  - Often accompanied by nausea, vomiting, diarrhea.
- Localized pain over affected bowel segment.
- In ischemic colitis, hematochezia/bloody diarrhea (typically only after 24 h).

16

Caution

- The first clinical examination of the abdomen may be completely normal!
- Compared to acute mesenteric ischemia, the pain associated with colonic ischemia is often not as severe.

3-Phase Clinical Course (Rarely Detectable)

- Acute pain interval: colicky pain + vomiting, diarrhoea, shock (after 0–6 h).
- Pain-free interval: intestinal paralysis, acidosis, "rotten peace" (7–12 h).
- New pain interval: peritonitis + septic shock with intestinal necrosis (12–24 h).

Diagnosis

Anamnesis

- Previous thromboembolic events.
- Postprandial abdominal pain (= "abdominal angina").

Laboratory Tests

- Lab levels unreliable; suggest AMI, but can **never** rule it out!
- Marked leukocytosis (>15,000/µl in 75% of patients).
- Elevation of lactate, LDH, CK or amylase = indicators for extent of tissue damage.
- Lactate increase = late; a lactate that remains constant during the course must suggest other diagnoses (sensitivity 90–96%, specificity 60–87%).

Important: If AMI is suspected (with normal laboratory) = no delay due to further diagnosis.

Caution

Lactate levels:

- Only increased lactate = indicative.
- Normal lactate = no exclusion of mesenterial ischemia!
- Explanation for normal levels: complete circulatory arrest in the ischemic area = no drainage of accumulated lactate = no lactate in the peripheral circulation.

Diagnostic Imaging

- CT angiography of the abdomen with contrast medium:
  - Imaging of vessel occlusion (= Contrast Medium stop).
  - Exclusion of tissue necrosis (intramural gas in the GI tract-pneumatosis intestinalis, portal venous gas: gas in the V. portae-hepatis branches).
  - Exclusion of bowel perforation (abdominal free air).

Therapy

Caution
As a principle: If there are clinical signs of intestinal necrosis = generous indication for exploratory laparotomy!

Stabilization
- Always intensive medical monitoring/ treatment.
- Oxygen administration + circulation stabilization + fluid balancing.
- Broad-spectrum antibiotic therapy (after only a few hours of ischemia = disintegration of the mucosal barrier = bacterial translocation).

Acute Mesenteric Artery Embolism
- Emergency laparotomy (see "Operative procedure" below).
- Embolectomy.

Acute Mesenteric Artery Thrombosis
- Emergency laparotomy (see "Operative procedure" below).
- Surgical thrombectomy.
- Alternative option = angioplasty within 8 h after symptom onset in stable patients without peritonism.

Acute Mesenteric Vein Thrombosis
- Emergency laparotomy: if evidence of bowel necrosis.
- Conservative therapy: Only in the absence of intestinal necrosis:
  - Heparin bolus 80 U/kg BW, not exceeding 5000 U, then infusion at 18 U/kg BW/h.
  - ICU-Monitoring.

Ischemic Colitis and Nonocclusive Mesenteric Ischemia (NOMI)
- Intensive care monitoring in the absence of gangrene or perforation: surgery necessary in only about 20% of patients (gangrene/perforation):
  - Improvement in heart function.
  - Correction of hypovolemia and metabolic acidosis.
  - Stop vasopressors.
  - Anticoagulation = no evidence.
- Emergency laparotomy if signs of intestinal necrosis (see "Operative procedure" below).

Surgical Procedure
Acute Mesenteric Artery Embolism
- Access via median laparotomy.
- Exposure of the superior mesenteric artery (SMA) in the mesenteric root: At the inferior border of the pancreas (lesser sac – bursa omentalis)/through inframesocolic access (transverse colon).
- Vascular incision proximal to the embolus + embolectomy (Fogarty catheter size 3/4).
- Examination of intestinal vitality (peristalsis and colour); examination of blood flow using vascular Doppler probe.
- If embolectomy not satisfactory: mesenteric vascular bypass if necessary.
- Resection of necrotic bowel + creation of primary anastomosis, ileostomy if necessary.
- In case of inconclusive exploration/ findings: laparostoma (leaving the abdomen open; e.g. insertion of an abdominal vacuum dressing + second-look laparotomy within 24–48 h).

Surgical Procedure
Acute Mesenteric Artery Thrombosis
- Access via median laparotomy.
- Exposure of the superior mesenteric artery (SMA) in the mesenteric root: at the inferior border of the pancreas (lesser sac – bursa omentalis)/through inframesocolic access (transverse colon).
- Identification of the affected arteries and intestinal segments (inspection, Doppler).
- Thrombectomy + arterial reconstruction; aortomesenteric bypass if necessary.

- Checking the vitality of the intestine/if necessary, segment resections with primary anastomosis.
- In case of inconclusive exploration/findings: Stapler closure of the bowel ends + laparostoma, second-look laparotomy within 24–48 h.

16.4.3 Chronic Mesenteric Ischaemia (CMI)

- Chronic mesenteric ischemia = chronic intestinal ischemia.

Etiology and Pathogenesis

Etiology

- Atherosclerosis of the mesenteric vessels (>95% of CMI).

Median Arcuate Ligament Syndrome (= MALS = Dunbar Syndrome)

- Controversially discussed clinical entity.
- Chronic intestinal ischemia = possible clinical presentation.
- Pathogenesis: Compression of the coeliac trunk by the median arcuate ligament (diaphragm).
- Rare: Diagnosis of exclusion, sometimes posture or respiration dependant pain.

16

Pathogenesis (= Atherosclerosis)

- Lack of increase in blood flow while increased demand.
- Reduced inflow.

Clinical Presentation

- Postprandial pain (typical "abdominal angina").
  - 10 min-3 h after food intake.
  - Mostly epigastric or periumbilical.
- Food aversion.
- Weight loss.

Diagnosis

- Diagnostic imaging.
  - Angiography = gold standard.
  - CT angiography (sensitivity 96%, specificity 94%): Additional information (e.g., topographic relationships).
  - MRI angiography (often only 25% of the course of IMA can be visualized).
  - Duplex ultrasound (SMA can be visualized in 90%, coeliac trunk in 80%).

Therapy

- Elective surgical vascular reconstruction.
- Percutaneous transluminal angioplasty (PTA).
- "Acute-on-chronic mesenteric ischemia = treat as an emergency.

16.4.4 Guidelines

Hirsch AT, Haskal ZJ, Hertzer NR, Bakal CW, Creager MA, Halperin JL, Hiratzka LF, Murphy WR, Olin JW, Puschett JB, Rosenfield KA, Sacks D, Stanley JC, Taylor LM Jr., White CJ, White RA, Antman EM, Smith SC Jr., Adams CD, Anderson JL, Faxon DP, Fuster V, Gibbons RJ, Hunt SA, Jacobs AK, Nishimura R, Ornato JP, Page RL, Riegel B (2006) ACC/AHA 2005 Practice Guidelines for the management of patients with peripheral arterial disease (lower extremity, renal, mesenteric, and abdominal aortic): A collaborative report from the American Association for Vascular Surgery/Society for Vascular Surgery, Society for Cardiovascular Angiography and Interventions, Society for Vascular Medicine and Biology, Society of Interventional Radiology, and the ACC/AHA TAsk Force on Practice Guidelines (Writing Committee to Develop Guidelines for the Management of Patients with Peripheral Arterial Disease). Circulation 113:e463–654.

American Gastroenterological Association Medical Position Statement: guidelines on intestinal ischemia (2000) Gastroenterology 118:951–953.

Pecoraro F, Rancic Z, Lachat M, Mayer D, Amann-Vesti B, Pfammatter T, Bajardi G, Veith FJ (2013) Chronic mesenteric ischemia: critical review and guidelines for management. Ann Vasc Surg 27:113–122.

Bala M, Kashuk J, Moore EE, et al. (2017) Acute mesenteric ischemia: guidelines of the World Society of Emergency Surgery. World J Emerg Surg 12:38. Published 2017 Aug 7. ► https://doi.org/10.1186/s13017-017-0150-5

Correction to: Endocrine Organs

Franck Billmann, Courtney Elizabeth Gibson,
and Robert Udelsman

F. Billmann, T. Keck (eds.), *Essentials of Visceral Surgery*,
https://doi.org/10.1007/978-3-662-66735-4_6

There was a mistake in the author's middle name spelling "Courtney Elisabeth Gibson" in Chapter 6, which has been now corrected as "Courtney Elizabeth Gibson".

The updated original version of this chapter can be found at
https://doi.org/10.1007/978-3-662-66735-4_6

F. Billmann, T. Keck (eds.), *Essentials of Visceral Surgery*,
https://doi.org/10.1007/978-3-662-66735-4_17

GPSR Compliance

The European Union's (EU) General Product Safety Regulation (GPSR) is a set of rules that requires consumer products to be safe and our obligations to ensure this.

If you have any concerns about our products, you can contact us on ProductSafety@springernature.com

In case Publisher is established outside the EU, the EU authorized representative is:

Springer Nature Customer Service Center GmbH
Europaplatz 3
69115 Heidelberg, Germany

Batch number: 10731393

Printed by Printforce, the Netherlands